# "Right for *Your* Body"

"With all the studies and claims about nutritional
supplements, it's awfully hard to design a supplement
program for your specific needs. That's why I'm so
enthusiastic about the publication of the second edition of
Lieberman and Bruning's *The Real Vitamin & Mineral Book*.
In this unique book, the authors will guide you
step-by-step in deciding what's right for *your* body."

**Melvyn R. Werbach, MD**
Author, *Nutritional Influences on Illness*

# "Highly Recommended"

"Time to take charge of your own health? Want to
prevent both everyday illness and problems common
in your family? *The Real Vitamin and Mineral Book*
by Dr. Shari Lieberman and Nancy Bruning is an
excellent place to start. Highly recommended for
anyone whose path to good health includes
basic good diet, vitamins, and minerals."

**Jonathan V. Wright, MD**
Tahoma Clinic, Kent, Washington

# "Valuable Information"

"Dr. Lieberman and Ms. Bruning provide valuable
information on how to use nutrients wisely and safely
to maintain good health and treat illness."

**Alan R. Gaby, MD**
Past President of American Holistic Medical Association

# THE REAL
# VITAMIN &
# MINERAL
# BOOK

## SHARI LIEBERMAN, PhD
## AND NANCY BRUNING

**Avery Publishing Group**

Garden City Park, New York

The nutritional, medical, and health information presented in this book is based on the research, training, and personal experiences of the authors, and is true and complete to the best of the authors' knowledge. However, this book is intended only as an informative guide for those wishing to know more about vitamins, minerals, and other supplements. It is not intended to replace or countermand the advice given to you by your physician. Because each person and each situation is unique, the publisher urges the reader to check with a qualified health professional before using any procedure where there is any question as to its appropriateness.

The publisher does not advocate the use of any particular diet and supplement program, but believes that the information presented in this book should be available to the public. Because there is always some risk involved, the authors and publisher are not responsible for any adverse effects or consequences resulting from the use of any of the suggestions in this book. Please feel free to consult a physician or other qualified health professional. It is a sign of wisdom, not cowardice, to seek a second or third opinion.

Cover Design: William Gonzalez and Rudy Shur
In-House Editor: Joanne Abrams
Printer: Paragon Press, Honesdale, PA


Cataloging-in-Publication Data
Lieberman, Shari.
    The real vitamin and mineral book: using supplements for optimum health / Shari Lieberman, Nancy Bruning.—2nd ed.
        p. cm.
    Includes bibliographical references and index.
    ISBN 0-89529-769-8

    1. Vitamins—Popular works. 2. Minerals in the body—Popular works. I. Bruning, Nancy. II. Title.

    QP771.L543 1997612.3'99
    QBI96-40554

# CONTENTS

*Shari Lieberman dedicates this book to the memory*
*of her father and mother,*
*Mort and Sheila Lieberman.*

*Nancy Bruning dedicates this book to her mother,*
*Anne Marie Jacelon,*
*and to her friends, who continue to nourish her*
*in ways beyond comprehension.*

# ACKNOWLEDGMENTS

Dr. Shari Lieberman would like to thank Kirk Hamilton, for *CP Currents,* his superb monthly newsletter review of the scientific literature.

# FOREWORD

The reliable information concerning supplements given in *The Real Vitamin and Mineral Book* by Dr. Lieberman and Ms. Bruning is of paramount importance. Recently, the Pracon Study, commissioned by the Council for Responsible Nutrition, estimated that $8.7 billion could be saved on five major diseases if Americans consumed optimal levels of the antioxidants vitamin C, vitamin E, and beta-carotene. Diets optimal in vitamin C, vitamin E, and beta-carotene can lessen costs for breast, lung, and stomach cancer, and these same antioxidants could dramatically reduce the incidence and/or severity of cataracts in the older population. Although much benefit could be derived from diet alone, many individuals, for whatever reason, do not eat the five servings of fruits and vegetables suggested by the National Cancer Institute. A 1990 analysis by NHANES II found that less than 10 percent of Americans actually consume two servings of fruits and three of vegetables per day. Further analysis of data from this study revealed that 50 percent of Americans eat no vegetables, and 70 percent eat no fruits or vegetables rich in vitamin C.

The average American seeks means to attain a longer and healthier life. Many reasons exist to encourage the use of supplements to lengthen lifespan and reduce the severity of chronic diseases among the general population. To accomplish this, two broad concepts much be considered. The first concept is that genes play a significant role in the overall health and longevity of an individual. This is evident because people have a proclivity to develop maladies similar to those of their ancestors, e.g., early onset of cardiovascular disease. While much research has gone into discovering important genes involved in overall health and chronic diseases, suffice it to say that little can be done now to favorably alter genetic makeup. However, all is not lost when considering the second broad concept affecting long-term health. We can control our destiny to some extent, because environmental conditions, principally nutrition, also play a significant role in overall health. For example, the rapid increase in cardiovascular diseases found among Americans in the first half of the twentieth century was attributed to the "modern diet," which featured an increased intake of fats and sugars at the expense of complex carbohydrates and fibers. An inadequate intake of certain vitamins and minerals is also a feature of the modern diet. In turn, the more recent reversal of this same trend has been attributed to an awareness of the benefits of low fat consumption and the use of vitamin and mineral supplements. Accordingly, genes may have a significant role in determining whether we live a long, healthy life. But within the constraints that genes impose on us, good nutritional practices can markedly influence health, as well.

Some years ago, my research led me into the field of nutrition. Although I initially focused on a small area of nutrition, in time, I became aware that there was much more I needed to know. Following a conversation with Dr. Lieberman, she provided me with the first edition of *The Real Vitamin and Mineral Book*. I appreciated the brevity and clarity of each chapter on a specific topic. The book was highly informative and persuasive. Using what I learned, I started my own supplement plan after careful thought. As a long-time member of the Risk/Benefits Committee at Georgetown University Medical Center, I have examined human studies designed to evaluate therapeutic interventions. From reading the first edition of this book, I was impressed with the favorable risk/benefit ratios of many supplements. Although the evidence of therapeutic benefit may not be 100 percent conclusive in each case, there is often great potential to be gained from taking supplements with little risk involved.

Like the first edition, this edition of *The Real Vitamin and Mineral Book* is designed to provide maximal information in a concise fashion. After a brief but persuasive discussion supporting the use of supplementation, updated chapters follow on fat-soluble and water-soluble vitamins and minerals. The section concerning "other nutrients" has undergone extensive revisions to include chapters on DHEA, melatonin, and carnitine. No debate is necessary over the timeliness of these chapters. The appendix contains reference abstracts, allowing the reader to pursue in greater depth topics of interest. Accordingly, the setup of the book provides the reader with a guide to the nutritional supplements he or she really needs in their most effective dosages.

I believe that each individual should become acquainted with all aspects of supplements, good and bad. This book is an excellent starting point. With knowledge gained in reading this comprehensive guide and the good advice of a professional health care provider, one can make wise decisions concerning supplementation, keeping in mind that individual programs should be updated as new information becomes available.

Harry G. Preuss, MD, FACN
*Professor of Medicine and Pathology*
*Georgetown University Medical Center*
*Washington, DC*

# WHAT'S YOUR VITAMIN AND MINERAL IQ?

You've probably heard so many contradictory statements regarding vitamins and minerals that you may be feeling confused about the benefits that can actually be derived from each supplement. The following quiz was designed to test your vitamin and mineral IQ. However, if after completing it you find your knowledge on the subject to be less than you'd hoped, don't worry. The information in this book will give you all the facts you'll need to design your own supplementation program.

1. Vitamin E has been shown to:
   A. Improve your sex life
   B. Help prevent cancer
   C. Prevent baldness
   D. None of the above

2. Enriched white bread is just as nutritious as whole wheat bread.
   A. True
   B. False

3. Which drug(s) increases your need for certain vitamins and/or minerals?
   A. Antibiotics
   B. Aspirin
   C. Birth control pills
   D. All of the above

4. Who generally requires a higher intake of vitamins and minerals?
   A. Senior citizens
   B. Body builders
   C. Marathon runners
   D. All of the above

5. Which mineral(s) has been shown to protect against many forms of cancer?
   A.  Calcium
   B.  Magnesium
   C.  Selenium
   D.  None of the above

6. When is the best time to take supplements?
   A.  In the morning
   B.  In the evening
   C.  With meals
   D.  On an empty stomach

7. As long as you take supplements, you can eat whatever you want.
   A.  True
   B.  False

8. Vitamin C has been shown to _____ colds.
   A.  Cure
   B.  Prevent
   C.  Shorten the duration of
   D.  All of the above

9. Which nutrient(s) may be effective in preventing cardiovascular disease?
   A.  Calcium
   B.  Vitamin E
   C.  Niacin
   D.  All of the above

10. The more supplements you take, the better.
   A.  True
   B.  False

## ANSWERS

1. **B.** Many studies have shown that vitamin E helps protect us against the harmful effects of a variety of carcinogens and toxins, including carbon tetrachloride, mercury, lead, benzene, ozone, and nitrous oxide. It prevents the formation of potent carcinogens called nitrosamines from the nitrates found in air pollution, cigarette smoke, and some foods. Vitamin E also prevents vitamins A and C, two other vitamins that protect us from carcinogens, from losing their potency in the body. Although severe vitamin E deficiency did cause infertility in experimental animals, no studies have shown this nutrient to improve the sex life of humans. Vitamin E does not prevent baldness. (For more information, see Chapter 8.)

2. **B.** The flour used to make white bread has been depleted of *over twenty*

nutrients, including up to 40 percent of the vitamin C, 85 percent of the vitamin B6, and 72 percent of the zinc. The manufacturers then put back a handful of these nutrients (five, to be exact), and call the result "enriched"! Whole wheat bread is much higher in almost every vitamin and mineral, including trace minerals such as chromium, selenium, and manganese. It is also higher in protein and fiber. (For more information, see Chapter 2.)

3. **D.** It is widely recognized that many drugs interact with nutrients in the body, often causing nutrient depletion. Antibiotics have been shown to interfere with the B vitamins, vitamin C, and calcium. Antibiotics may also destroy useful bacteria in the colon, thus hindering vitamin K synthesis. Estrogen-containing medications, such as birth control pills, deplete the body of vitamin B6, folic acid, and vitamin C. Even aspirin, if used over a long period of time, may deplete the body's stores of vitamin C and folic acid. (For more information, see Chapter 2.)

4. **D.** Because of their exercise regimens, marathoners and body builders are under physical stress, which increases their need for many vitamins and minerals. In addition, people who exercise heavily tend to eat large amounts of carbohydrates, which increase the need for thiamin. Finally, sweating has been shown to increase the excretion of certain essential nutrients. Many studies have shown that because of reduced absorption and poor eating habits, the elderly are also at great risk for having low levels of nutrients, especially calcium; vitamins B6, B12, E, and D; folic acid; and zinc. (For more information, see Chapter 2.)

5. **C.** There is a higher incidence of cancer among people who live in geographical areas where the soil is lower in selenium. Studies have correlated many forms of cancer, but especially breast cancer, with a low selenium intake. There is some evidence that calcium may protect against colon cancer, but the data is too preliminary to draw any firm conclusions. (For more information, see Chapter 29.)

6. **C.** Vitamin and mineral supplements are best absorbed when taken with food. It is even better if doses are divided throughout the day. Although some people believe it is advantageous to take certain nutrients in the morning and others in the evening, at this point, there is no evidence to support this theory. (For more information, see Chapter 4.)

7. **B.** Supplements are just that—supplements. They should be taken *in addition* to an intelligent diet to make up for the nutrients lost in our food as a result of shipping, storage, processing, and other factors. Supplements are not meant to overcome a diet that is too high in fat and sugar and too low in fiber. They are designed to be part of a total health program that includes good fresh food, exercise, stress reduction, and avoidance of substances known to be harmful to the body. (For more information, see Chapter 5.)

8. **C.** Vitamin C has been shown to shorten the duration of colds and lessen the severity of the symptoms. Vitamin C is necessary for the optimum function of the immune system, but has never been conclusively proven to either prevent or cure the common cold. (For more information, see Chapter 20.)

9. **D.** Many studies correlate a higher calcium intake with lower blood pressure. Vitamin E may reduce cholesterol in the blood, and increase levels of HDL (high-density lipoproteins, the "good" type of cholesterol). It may also help prevent platelets from clogging the arteries. Niacin has been shown to be effective in reducing cholesterol and triglycerides in the blood. In fact, two studies recommend niacin as the treatment of choice for these conditions. (For more information, see Chapters 8, 13, and 21.)

10. **B.** For each individual, there is an optimum amount of each nutrient beyond which the benefits are small or nonexistent. There is no reason to take, for example, 150 milligrams of the B vitamins if 50 milligrams will do the job. Although even very high doses of vitamin and mineral supplements are generally not harmful, it makes no sense economically or healthwise to take more than you really need. (For more information, see Chapter 4.)

## Your Score

- 7–10 Correct: Excellent
- 4–6 Correct: Average
- 0–3 Correct: Poor

# THE PURPOSE
# OF THIS BOOK

My becoming a nutritionist—as well as my writing this book—occurred in a rather roundabout way. Initially, I wanted to be a medical doctor. I was interested in science, and I wanted to work with people, to help them. I thought that being a physician would allow me to do this.

However, as a premed student, I learned that traditional Western medicine takes quite a rigid and fragmented approach to health. It is primarily concerned with treating isolated symptoms and diseases, rather than promoting the health of the whole person. I realized that although conventional medicine has its place and can do a lot of good—even perform miracles—prevention is a far more potent tool in the larger scheme of things. In addition, it became clear to me that as long as an illness or condition is not life threatening, nutrition should be the first line of defense. Compared with modern Western medicine, the nutritional approach is a safe, nontoxic, effective alternative.

My interest in nutrition was originally piqued at the age of fourteen, when I came down with mononucleosis. An avid tennis player, I was crushed when my doctor told me that I would need three months of bed rest to recover. However, my father started me on a program of vitamin A and C supplements. Imagine my physician's surprise when I returned to my tennis two weeks later! As I continued to take supplements, I noticed that not only was I free of colds, but I felt absolutely great.

As I grew older, another compelling reason to explore the potential impact of nutrition took shape. I discovered that I had a hereditary predisposition to heart disease. It seemed everybody in my family was dying of heart disease at a relatively early age: Both my grandfathers had heart attacks, my mother's mother died of a stroke, my father's two brothers had heart problems, and my own father died of a heart attack at the age of fifty-nine. There I was, at the age of twenty-two, with a cholesterol count of 225 and HDLs of 46. Although conventional medicine considered these levels acceptable, my research of the medical literature showed that this was an overly complacent attitude. Some researchers were saying that cholesterol levels higher than 200 in people under forty years of age increased the risk of heart disease.

Although the research then was new and sketchy, an alarm went off somewhere inside me. Was I doomed to watch my cholesterol gradually climb up and up, while I stood idly by? Was my future to consist of toxic drug therapy in an attempt to control my cholesterol, which would otherwise zoom sky high? Fortunately, there was also some research showing that simple dietary changes, certain supplements, and regular aerobic exercise could make a difference. Although this research was also new and controversial, I decided to take action. My cholesterol is now below 200, and my HDLs above 95. As a result, I now have a much lower risk of heart disease. I am happy to report that I have had similar results with my patients, as have other practicioners.

My co-author, Nancy Bruning, also came to nutrition and the writing of this book because of a very personal concern and involvement. Because she had heard that I work with cancer patients who are undergoing chemotherapy, she interviewed me for her book, *Coping With Chemotherapy*. A former cancer chemotherapy patient herself, Nancy was primarily interested in researching therapies that could be used to complement conventional chemotherapy to make it more comfortable, less damaging, and perhaps more effective. Although she learned firsthand the important role that nutrition plays in such circumstances, she also realized that disease prevention is a superior tactic, and that nutrition can have a tremendous impact on overall health. Fifteen years postdiagnosis, and in excellent health, she specializes in writing about disease prevention and about the advantages of combining mainstream medicine with complementary approaches such as nutrition.

My research and clinical experience in working with a wide variety of people have shown me that in today's world, most people do not get all the nutrients they need from food. As a result, not only do they not enjoy optimum health, but they are setting the stage for poor health in the future. Although nutritional supplements may be our best protection against future health problems, supplementation is an individual matter. Up to now, it has been difficult, if not impossible, for the average person to determine what he or she should take. My purpose in writing this book is to provide you with the guidelines you need to create your own personal supplement program, and with the scientific documentation that will help you feel confident that supplements have great potential to improve your health.

According to a 1991 Gallup Poll, 35 percent of the American population is taking one or more supplements. According to the Council for Responsible Nutrition, other national surveys indicate that an even greater portion of the population—50 percent—uses supplements at least occasionally. But do people know what to take, or why they are taking it? As a clinician, as a teacher, as a researcher, and as a lecturer, I have found that people want to individualize and optimize their vitamin regimens to suit their own needs, in much the way they want to individualize and optimize their workouts and diets.

As a nutritionist, I see people in my office every week. They are generally referred to me by their physicians for a variety of problems and needs. Some are specific, such as acne, HIV/AIDS, psoriasis, menstrual problems, blood sugar problems, intestinal disorders, high blood pressure, high cholesterol, an inability to sleep, fatigue, depression, or nervousness. These people turn to nutrition as an adjunct or an alternative to the treatment offered by their physicians. But most people who come to me are not obviously sick—they are interested in nutrition as a means of improving their health and preventing illness. They want to live longer, healthier lives; to feel better, look better, have more energy, withstand stress better, and be able to avoid or minimize diseases that range from the common cold to cancer. They come to me because they are very confused about supplementation. In spite of all the books and articles they've read, they still don't know how to apply the available information to their own lives.

In all its subtleties, nutrition is a very complex subject—one that is challenging for even the qualified professional. Moreover, the field is growing and becoming full of self-styled experts who bombard you with contradictory advice and information almost daily. Many people deal with this confusion by going to a clinical nutritionist or to a physician whose practice is nutritionally oriented. But practitioners who are up-to-date and proficient in the field of nutrition and knowledgeable about nutritional supplementation are not available to everyone. This book was written so that you can make your own intelligently designed supplement program. It is also a useful tool for practitioners who were not trained in nutrition, and are interested in learning about the progressive approach to this subject. I am grateful to know that many professionals recommend this book to both their colleagues and their patients.

Today, people say they either "believe" in taking vitamins, or they don't, as if this were some kind of religion, based on blind faith. I want to reassure you that the progressive nutritional approach to health is not a religion. It is an emerging science that is taking its rightful place alongside other health sciences. This poses two basic problems that I hope to correct with this book.

The first problem is that because supplementation is a science, the language can get very technical. My education and professional experiences have taught me how to translate highly technical data into a language that the average person can understand.

The second problem is that because nutrition is no longer a new science, the scientific literature is filled with studies on diet and supplementation. In writing this book, I have searched the most up-to-date professional journals, including foreign research journals, as well as attending numerous scientific conference and speaking with experts in the field of nutrition. I have interpreted the information and synthesized it to provide you with the most comprehensive, unified, and scientifically sound picture of what vitamins, minerals, and other dietary supplements can—and cannot—do for you.

As you will see in this book, people are not getting the government-established Reference Daily Intakes (the RDIs, formerly called the Recommended Daily Allowances, or RDAs) from their diets. In addition, the RDIs are not high enough for many people. *The Real Vitamin and Mineral Book* focuses on optimizing your health, rather than meeting the RDIs to prevent deficiency diseases by providing merely adequate amounts of nutrients for "normal healthy people," as recommended by the United States Food and Nutrition Board. This book is written from the viewpoint that amounts in excess of the RDIs can be preventive, therapeutic, and safe. I have called these greater amounts the Optimum Daily Intakes (ODIs)—a dosage range within which nearly everyone can find his or her individual amount. Every recommendation in *The Real Vitamin and Mineral Book* is based on the latest reliable scientific data, including studies published in well-respected professional journals and at scientific conferences, as well as on my own and other clinicians' successes with patients. It is not based on hearsay or on highly questionable studies. When contradictory or inconclusive data exist, I make it clear that further studies are needed. For example, I would very much like to say that large doses of vitamin C cure cancer, but the evidence so far has not supported this statement. On the other hand, the evidence is strong enough to recommend taking vitamin C as a *preventive measure* against certain cancers.

Nutritionists, physicians, and researchers are in agreement that vitamins and minerals are essential for human health. Opinions differ only as far as specific uses and amounts are concerned. Clearly, some of the claims for "megavitamins" are not as well supported as others. As a result, people are taking the wrong supplements in the wrong amounts for the wrong reasons. Many of them are wasting their time and money, either on multivitamins, which can be hit-or-miss, or on dosages that are either unnecessarily high or too low to have an appreciable effect. Other people would like to take supplements, but are confused, and so have never begun a supplement regimen.

If you, like many of my patients, have looked through or read other nutrition books but found them too technical, not specific enough, or just plain overwhelming, this book is for you. *The Real Vitamin and Mineral Book* dispels the confusion caused by medical jargon and conflicting information, taking the guesswork out of taking supplements. Moreover, this book deals only with supplements that are generally available to the public. This does not mean that you are getting *less* information, just *less distracting* information. You get clarity, not clutter. The information is presented in a straightforward, usable form, providing—in simple, honest, realistic terms—exactly the foundation you need to create a workable supplement plan for yourself.

**Part One** of *The Real Vitamin and Mineral Book* explains the RDIs and the ODIs, and guides you in using the remainder of the book. These introductory chapters give you a basic grasp of the concepts, goals, and guidelines of vitamin and mineral supplementation.

**Part Two** consists of individual chapters on each vitamin, including the doses I recommend to my patients both for general optimum health and for specific problems.

**Part Three** consists of individual chapters on minerals.

**Part Four** consists of chapters on nutrients that are not vitamins or minerals, but may have specific health benefits.

**Part Five** provides handy reference tables and sample worksheets to help you apply what you have learned to the custom design of your individual supplement program. I have also included reference abstracts for each nutrient chapter—summaries of the most recent scientific studies for anyone who wishes to research the subject further.

With the help of this book, you will find it easy to create a personal supplement plan. To get an overall picture of what supplements can do for you, I recommend that you first read through Part Two, "The Vitamins"; Part Three, "The Minerals"; and Part Four, "Beyond Vitamins and Minerals." Then tear out or photocopy the worksheet on pages 238 and 239 and, pen in hand, go through the book again, chapter by chapter, filling in your individual Optimum Daily Intake for each nutrient.

*If you have any medical condition, please consult your physician before taking any vitamin or mineral supplements. If he or she is not versed in nutrition, bring this book to the office. The ODIs are not meant to be a substitute for any medications, therapies, or medical treatments. In most cases, they may be used in addition to the recommended medical treatment. However, once again, consult your physician first.*

# TROUBLESHOOTING FOR DISORDERS

As you will learn in the following chapters, vitamins, minerals, and other nutrients can not only help you maintain optimum health, but also allow you to control a variety of symptoms and disorders. The following table will quickly guide you to those nutrients that are particularly important in the prevention or alleviation of specific conditions. Once you've identified these nutrients, turn to the appropriate chapters to learn how you can make these vitamins and minerals part of a balanced supplement program.

| At-a-Glance Nutritional Therapy | |
|---|---|
| **Symptom or Disorder** | **Suggested Key Nutrients** |
| Acne | A, Beta-carotene |
| Aging-Related Disorders | Beta-carotene, C, DHEA, E, Glutathione, Melatonin, N-acetylcysteine |
| Allergies and Asthma | C, Essential fatty acids, Flavonoids, N-acetyl-cysteine |
| Anemia | $B_{12}$, Folic acid, Iron |
| Arthritis and Other Joint Problems | Essential fatty acids, Manganese, Pantothenic acid, Selenium |
| Cancer Prevention | A, Beta-carotene, C, E, Essential fatty acids, Flavonoids, Garlic, Manganese, Selenium |
| Cardiovascular Disease Prevention | C, Coenzyme $Q_{10}$, E, Essential fatty acids, Flavonoids, Garlic, N-acetylcysteine, Selenium |
| Carpal Tunnel Syndrome | $B_2$, $B_6$, Niacin |

| Symptom or Disorder | Suggested Key Nutrients |
|---|---|
| Cataracts | Beta-carotene, C, E |
| Cholesterol-Related Problems | $B_3$, C, Chromium, Coenzyme $Q_{10}$, E, Garlic, Niacin, Pantothenic acid |
| Circulatory Problems | $B_3$, E, Flavonoids |
| Colds and Flu | C |
| Depression | $B_1$, $B_2$, $B_3$, $B_6$, $B_{12}$, Folic acid, Pantothenic acid |
| Diabetes | Chromium, E |
| Eczema | A, Beta-Carotene |
| Fatigue, Chronic | Coenzyme $Q_{10}$, Iron, Magnesium malate |
| Fibrocystic Breast Disease | E, Essential fatty acids |
| Gastrointestinal Problems | A, Beta-Carotene |
| High Blood Pressure | Calcium, Coenzyme $Q_{10}$, D, Magnesium |
| HIV/AIDS | A, Beta-carotene, C, Coenzyme $Q_{10}$, Garlic, Glutathione, N-acetycysteine, Quercetin, Zinc |
| Hypoglycemia | Chromium |
| Immune Problems | A, Beta-carotene, C, E, Essential fatty acids, Garlic, Glutathione, N-acetylcysteine, Zinc |
| Infection | C, Flavonoids, Garlic, Zinc |
| Insomnia | Calcium, Melatonin |
| Menopause Symptoms | E |
| Menstrual Pain | Essential fatty acids |
| Muscle Cramps | Calcium, Magnesium |
| Osteoporosis | Boron, Calcium, Copper, D, Magnesium, Manganese, Zinc |
| Premenstrual Syndrome | $B_6$, E, Essential fatty acids |
| Prostate Conditions | Zinc |
| Respiratory Problems | A, Beta-carotene, N-acetylcysteine |
| Skin Problems | A, Beta-carotene, Essential fatty acids, Zinc |

| Symptom or Disorder | Suggested Key Nutrients |
| --- | --- |
| Stress and Anxiety | $B_1$, $B_2$, $B_3$, $B_6$, $B_{12}$, C, Folic acid, Pantothenic acid |
| Wound Healing | C, E, Zinc |

# Part One

## THE CASE FOR SUPPLEMENTATION

# Chapter 1

# WHAT ARE VITAMINS AND MINERALS?

Vitamins and minerals are nutrients that are essential to life. They are often called *micronutrients* because, in comparison with the four major nutrients—carbohydrates, proteins, fats, and water—they are needed in relatively small amounts.

Vitamins are organic compounds, meaning that they occur naturally in plants and animals. By and large, vitamins function as *coenzymes*. Enzymes are catalysts or activators in the chemical reactions that are continually taking place in our bodies. Vitamins are a fundamental part of the enzymes, much the way your muscles are a fundamental part of your arms and legs.

Most people are aware that our enzymes help us digest our food. But enzymes do more than digest food. They are at the very foundation of *all* our bodily functions. Enzymes are what make things happen, and happen faster. Without enzymes, you can't breathe, blink, or walk. Your body can't break down proteins into essential amino acids, electrons can't flow, and nerve transmissions can't occur. You can't pull your hand out of the fire (or put it there in the first place), smell a rose, see a sunset, or taste an apple. And without vitamins, the enzymes can't do their job. For example, consider a particular enzyme that is needed to transmit nerve impulses to your fingers. No matter how plentiful this enzyme is in your body, if you are deficient in $B_6$, this enzyme cannot be activated. As a result, you might feel some numbness in your fingers.

Minerals are inorganic elements, meaning that they are not produced by plants and animals. Like vitamins, many minerals function as coenzymes, enabling chemical reactions to occur throughout the body.

In addition to their role as coenzymes, some micronutrients have other functions. For example, vitamin E acts as an antioxidant; calcium, magnesium, and phosphorus form our bones; iron enables the transport of oxygen from the lungs to the body cells; and active vitamin D functions as a hormone.

After they have been absorbed, vitamins and minerals actually become part of the structure of the body—of the cells, enzymes, hormones, muscles, blood, and bone. As part of the "body pool," these substances remain in the body for varying amounts of time. Some are utilized immediately, and some are stored and utilized over a period of time.

The vitamins that stay in the body for a short period of time—two to four days—are called *water-soluble vitamins.* The B vitamins and vitamin C belong to this group. Utilization of water-soluble vitamins begins the minute they are absorbed through your digestive system. Thus, these nutrients must be replenished regularly. Since they are not stored, but are quickly excreted from the body, toxicities are virtually unknown.

*Fat-soluble vitamins,* on the other hand, stay in the body for a longer period of time. Vitamins A, D, E, and K belong to this group. Although these vitamins are usually stored in fat (lipid) tissue, some may also be stored in some organs, especially the liver. Therefore, you can have toxicity problems with some of the fat-soluble vitamins, but only when you take very large doses.

Minerals also belong to two groups: the *macro,* or bulk, minerals; and the *micro,* or trace, minerals. Macro minerals are needed in larger amounts than are micro minerals. The macro minerals include calcium, magnesium, and phosphorus. The micro minerals include zinc, iron, copper, manganese, chromium, selenium, iodine, potassium, and boron. Minerals are stored in various parts of the body—primarily in bone and muscle tissue. Therefore, it is also possible to overdose on minerals if you take extremely large amounts.

If you are concerned about toxicity, you must remember that there is no vitamin or mineral that is as toxic as are most of the drugs you can buy over the counter, including aspirin. To reach toxicity, you must go out of your way to abuse supplements by taking massive quantities, usually for a prolonged period of time. The dose ranges I suggest for nutritional supplements are completely safe and have been used in human clinical studies with no evidence of toxicity.

Other nutrients, such as flavonoids, essential fatty acids, garlic, coenzyme Q10, glutathione, N-acetylcysteine, and carnitine, have only recently begun to be studied, but may also prove to be essential for optimum health. The information we have for these substances is generally less extensive than that for vitamins and minerals. However, I discuss these nutrients in this book because ongoing studies have thus far yielded promising results and have shown that they are safe when taken in the recommended amounts. Unlike the better-documented vitamins and minerals, though, these nutrients either have not yet been proven to be needed by everyone, or may be obtained by most people in sufficient quantities from their diets. Because of this, and the fact that they tend to be costly, there are no ODIs for these nutrients, and I generally recommend that their use be limited to the treatment and prevention of specific disorders.

# Chapter 2

# THE RDIs—THE MINIMUM WAGES OF NUTRITION

C learly, vitamins are minerals are essential to good health, and even to life itself. But how do we know whether we are getting sufficient nutrients to ensure our well-being? For approximately fifty years, the Recommended Daily Allowances (RDAs) were our guidelines. They were the United States Food and Nutrition Board's estimates of the amounts of nutrients required by most people to prevent overt deficiency symptoms. Most statements such as "We can get everything we need from a well-balanced diet," and "Vitamin and mineral supplements are a waste of money," are based on a widespread acceptance of these guidelines. However, while the RDAs were a significant first step in understanding nutrition, we are beginning to realize that the RDAs—as well as their successors, the RDIs— have very important limitations.

After their creation, the RDAs were periodically evaluated and updated based on a continuing analysis of our rapidly expanding knowledge of nutrition. But in 1985, there was such widespread disagreement among the scientists involved that the National Research Council was unable to issue its scheduled new edition of the RDAs until 1989. This near inability of even the most conservative nutrition experts to agree illustrates some of the reservations about the RDAs that I and other nutritionists, physicians, and researchers expressed for some time.

The RDAs were fairly complex. For each nutrient, separate recommendations were made based on gender, age, and other factors. In an effort to provide simpler standards, the final version of the Nutrition Labeling and Education Act of 1993 replaced the RDAs with the RDIs (Reference Daily Intakes), which represent an *average* need. Since January 1997, the RDA nomenclature has no longer been used. The official term is now RDI. The term RDI is used throughout this book except in discussions of studies that based their doses on the RDAs. In those cases, the term RDA has been retained.

It should be noted that the RDI values are for children and adults of four or more years of age. The RDAs and RDIs are essentially the same values. In some cases, the RDIs are lower than the former RDAs; in some cases, they are higher. RDIs are still generally lower than the ODIs.

Just like the RDAs, the RDIs have three basic problems: (1) you cannot get all of the nutrients you need from today's food; (2) the RDIs reflect amounts that are adequate to prevent nutrient-deficiency diseases, and are not tailored for individual needs; and (3) the RDIs do not address or consider *optimum* health or the prevention of degenerative diseases such as cancer and heart disease. This chapter examines each of these problems in turn.

## PROBLEM 1: CAN YOU REALLY GET EVERYTHING YOU NEED FROM FOOD?

The RDIs are intended to be met solely through diet. However, it is virtually *impossible* to meet the RDIs by eating the food available to us today. As a clinician who sees real people, I know how impractical and misleading the typical well-balanced diet explained in nutrition handbooks can be. Such a diet does not take into consideration people's individual lifestyles, food preferences, and habits; nutrient bioavailability; the inaccuracy of the food value tables; or the loss of nutrients that occurs during storage, shipping, processing, and cooking.

### The Myth of the Well-Balanced Diet

Most people simply do not eat a well-balanced diet, which, according to the latest recommendations of the National Research Council, consists of approximately 30 percent fat, 20 percent protein, 35 percent complex carbohydrates (grains, breads, and starchy vegetables), and 15 percent simple carbohydrates (high-sugar foods such as sweets and fruits). Does a frazzled executive take the time to calculate her fat intake? Does an overworked teacher know how much complex carbohydrate he has eaten? Does a teenager or a senior citizen know how much protein is in a cheese Danish? Does even the most health-conscious marathon runner eat a perfect diet every day? Of course not.

In addition, there is the calorie problem. A diet that satisfies the RDIs is based on approximately 2,000 calories for women and 3,000 calories for men. This is about twice as much as is allowed on the average reducing diet, and it has been estimated that one-third of America is dieting at any one time. Even when we are not dieting, most of us cannot consume this many calories and still maintain a desirable weight. When we are dieting, the news is even worse. Researchers have found that of eleven published diet-book plans (the F-plan, Scarsdale, Pritikin, Richard Simmons, Atkins, Stillman, I Love New York, I Love America, Beverly Hills, Carbohydrate Craver's, and California diets), *none* provides a full 100 percent of the RDIs for thirteen vitamins and minerals. It seems that there's a new miracle diet every year, but they all say essentially the same thing—"eat less"—and that translates into fewer nutrients. This is especially significant when you realize that low levels of certain nutrients may actually sabotage weight-loss efforts. For example, preliminary reports suggest that *lipotropic* (fat-loving) nutrients, such as chromium, L-carnitine, and choline, may enhance fat loss, provided an individual is eating a low-fat diet and engaging in regular aerobic exercise. Someone who is dieting may not be getting enough of these nutrients through food, theoretically making it more difficult to burn body fat and lose weight. (Unfortunately, there still is no miracle supplement that magically melts away excess fat.)

The danger of large-scale deficiencies is not just theory. Many published reports in the United States, Great Britain, and Europe show that portions of even affluent societies may be highly deficient in certain nutrients. Women are especially at risk for deficiencies. For example, one American study found that women generally consume 60 percent as many calories as men, and therefore obtain about 60 percent as much of each nutrient as men do.

Although overt vitamin deficiency, evidenced by conditions such as scurvy, is rare in the United States, cancer and heart disease are not. And study after study has linked the growing incidence of such disorders with diets that are typically too high in fat, and too low in the vitamins, minerals, and other nutrients needed for good health.

I have found it especially interesting—and, frankly, amusing—that a survey of over 600 dieticians found that nearly 60 percent of them use nutritional supplements. Add to this the fact that a show of hands at a 1994 conference of the American College of Cardiology revealed that approximately two-thirds of the 700 physicians in attendance took daily doses of antioxidants. Apparently, a majority of the food experts who have traditionally espoused the view that a balanced diet provides all the nutrients you need—as well as a number of other health-care practitioners—now realize how unrealistic this view is, at least when it comes to safeguarding their own health.

## The Case of the Missing Nutrients

Evidence shows that the food tables that supposedly tell us the nutrient content of the foods we eat probably overstate nutritional value. As a result, the orange you just bought is probably not nearly as full of vitamin C as you may have been led to believe.

What's more, the nutrient content of foods, especially regarding minerals, fluctuates widely, depending on the growing conditions. Our soil is depleted of selenium in most parts of the country, and often has only marginal levels of zinc, magnesium, calcium, and other minerals. Without mineral-rich soils, it is impossible for fruits and vegetables to contain a rich supply of nutrients.

# The Caveman Diet

*Some researchers have argued that the best diet for us is one that resembles the diet of our remote ancestors. Our genetic constitution has changed very little since modern human beings appeared about 40,000 years ago. One of the factors that played a part in influencing our genetic makeup was the food that was available at that time. It stands to reason that one logical approach to estimating our needs would be to look at what our early ancestors actually ate. The fact that "cavemen" may have died at an early age is beside the point, as their existence was far more precarious than ours. The point is that these people did survive—at least until they were old enough to reproduce and pass on their genes.*

*In a study published in 1985 in "The New England Journal of Medicine," the authors found that Paleolithic nutrition differed significantly from our own. Among other findings, they concluded that from their diet of 35 percent animal foods and 65 percent plant foods, our early ancestors obtained 1,579 milligrams of calcium (the RDI is 1,000 milligrams), and nearly 400 milligrams of vitamin C per day (the RDI is 60 milligrams). They also probably obtained much higher amounts of the B vitamins than the current RDI recommends.*

*Among the "primitive" hunter-gatherer people of today, whose way of eating most closely resembles that of our ancestors, the so-called diseases of civilization—coronary heart disease, hypertension, diabetes, and some types of cancer—are virtually unknown, even in the elderly. It is generally agreed that our present diet—high in fat, and low in fiber, vitamins, and minerals— plays a role in the now epidemic spread of these diseases. We have already seen a change from the old dietary guidelines to a lower-fat, higher-fiber diet that is considered optimal and preventive. It is my hope that the RDIs for vitamins and minerals will one day be approached in this same way.*

Artificial fertilizers are widely used to increase crop yields, but, as is often the case, quantity does not necessarily equal quality. Of the twenty-six elements that have thus far been established as essential for human life, only sixteen are essential for plants. Plants contain elements they themselves don't require because they are part of the food chain: they philanthropically provide plant-eating animals, and thus meat-eating animals, with the nutrients those animals require. Artificial fertilizers that are based solely on plant needs overlook human requirements, and could be creating more problems than they solve.

Fruits and vegetables begin to lose nutrients from the moment they are picked. Most of the "fresh" fruits and vegetables we buy have actually been picked, then stored, then shipped, and then stored again—possibly for weeks or months. After we buy them, we store them some more. Then we may cook them, or at least cut or slice them. Or a food may be processed before we buy it. Each of these steps causes further nutrient loss.

For example, the vitamin C content of apples may fall by two-thirds after only two or three months. Potatoes may have 30 milligrams of vitamin C per 100 grams when they are freshly harvested in the fall; but by springtime, they have only 8 milligrams per 100 grams; and by summer, they have practically none. Green vegetables suffer even more—they lose almost all their vitamin C after a few days of being stored at room temperature. Everyone knows that orange juice is high in vitamin C. But few people realize that an orange loses 30 percent of its vitamin C soon after it is squeezed. Nonfortified commercial orange juice has almost no natural vitamin C left.

Most people aren't aware that a surprising amount of the total nutrient content in many foods exists in a form that is not bioavailable, meaning that our bodies can't absorb and use it. About 40 percent of the vitamin C that is left in fresh-squeezed orange juice is biologically inactive. According to the food value tables, one cup of green cabbage has 33 milligrams of vitamin C—over half the RDI. What the food table *doesn't* tell you is that it is present in a form that is very poorly absorbed.

Next, we must consider how the heat, light, water, and chemicals used to process foods further deplete their nutrients. Blanching, a process that vegetables undergo before they are canned or frozen, can destroy up to 60 percent of the vitamin C content, 40 percent of the riboflavin, and 30 percent of the thiamin. The sterilization process used to can foods further destroys vitamins. For example, 39 percent of the vitamin A may be destroyed, and 69 percent of the remaining thiamin. While freezing itself seems preferable to canning, vitamin C may be depleted by about 25 percent. After they are processed, foods are stored and continue to lose their nutrients.

Even the simple act of cutting fruits and vegetables encourages both vitamin and mineral losses. Cooking methods generally deplete about 50 percent of the less stable vitamins, especially vitamin C. By the time you put cooked peas on the table, only 44 percent (for fresh peas), 17 percent (for frozen peas), or as little as 6 percent (for canned peas) of the original vitamin C may be left.

Perhaps one of the greatest injustices inflicted upon foods occurs during the milling of grains. When wheat is processed into white flour, up to 40 percent of the vitamin C, and from 65 to 85 percent of various B vitamins, are depleted. In addition, many minerals are lost, including 59 percent of the magnesium and 72 percent of the zinc. Also lost are significant amounts of other vitamins, protein, and fiber. All in all, an appalling twenty-six essential nutrients are removed. The food industry then puts back a few cents' worth of iron, calcium, niacin, thiamin, and riboflavin—and calls its bread "enriched"!

As might be expected, our meats, which come from animals raised on some of the same nutrient-depleted foods that are available to us, are also lower in vitamins and minerals than indicated in food tables. The nutrient levels in our factory-farm livestock, which are fed artificial diets, also differ from those of animals that enjoy a more natural existence. And, of course, cooking robs meat of even more nutrients—up to half of its thiamin, $B_6$, and pantothenic acid.

## PROBLEM 2: ARE THE RDIs REALLY FOR EVERYONE?

The RDIs are "one size fits all." They are designed to satisfy the needs of a mythical "average healthy person," not individual needs. Unfortunately, this person does not exist in reality, just as the average American family, with its 2.2 children, never really existed. For instance, the RDIs do not take into account the twenty-five documented inborn errors of metabolism, some of which can increase an individual's vitamin requirements by a factor of 10 to 1,000. In Wilson's disease, for example, abnormal copper metabolism greatly increases the body's need for zinc, which is necessary to regulate copper absorption. Experiments have shown that it is highly probable that many individuals have more subtle difficulties with specific nutrients. While these problems may be harder to diagnose, they can diminish our quality of life and lead to future problems as serious as cancer and heart disease.

In addition to the individual biological blueprint with which each of us comes into the world, throughout life, we each continue to change and to undergo different experiences, such as environmental pollution, stress, disease, drug therapy, and aging. Each of these has the potential to increase our body's use of specific nutrients, interfere with nutrient metabolism, or otherwise affect our nutritional needs.

### Environmental Pollution

Today, there are an unprecedented number of chemicals all around us—in our food, our water, and the very air we breathe. The Environmental Protection Agency has estimated that 60,000 chemicals have been buried or dumped throughout the United States over the years, and are now penetrating our water supply. Automobiles and industry spew millions of pounds of pollutants into the atmosphere every year. Our food has become a chemical feast that is sprayed with pesticides, injected with hormones, fed with antibiotics, and adulterated with over 3,000 chemicals in the form of artificial colors, flavors, textures, and preservatives. Cigarette smokers not only pollute their own lungs, but also endanger the health of others through secondhand smoke. Living or working with smokers can be equivalent to smoking several cigarettes a day. Many of the chemicals now in our environment have been proven to pose hazards to human health. Others may be potentially hazardous.

Fortunately, it has been found that certain vitamins and minerals are protective against some of these toxic substances. For example, vitamins C and E have been shown to be protective against nitrosamine, a carcinogen your body forms from the nitrates and nitrites found in processed meats such as hot dogs, bacon, ham, and bologna. These same carcinogens form from pollutants in the air and in cigarette smoke.

In addition to being cancer-causing agents, toxic chemicals have become a prime suspect in male infertility. Sperm counts all over the world are half what they were in the late 1930s, and of low quality. But sperm counts of men who eat organically grown food are twice as high as average. And vitamin C and glutathione have been shown to increase the percentage of normal sperm, sperm motility, and sperm viability in infertile men with lowered sperm count. Whether the chemicals deplete nutrients or increase your requirements, I feel it's wise to superfortify your body so that you can withstand these chemical insults.

### Mental and Physical Stress

It has been well documented that when you are under any sort of stress, you deplete your store of certain vitamins and minerals more rapidly. Whether the stress is physical, such as strenuous exercise, or emotional, such as changing jobs, such a situation generally calls for higher intakes of vitamins and minerals. For example, female athletes appear to be at risk for iron deficiency. Athletic performance was enhanced in women who were anemic when they were supplemented with iron. Some male athletes may require iron as well, provided a diagnosis of iron deficiency anemia has been confirmed. There have been conflicting reports on the use of vitamins and minerals as "ergogenic aids"—substances that enhance exercise performance. However, some recent research focusing on the effect of oxidative stress on muscle soreness after exercise has shown that antioxidant supplementation both reduces oxidative stress and speeds muscle recovery.

### Disease and Disorders

There are many diseases that interfere with the ingestion, digestion, absorption, and requirement of nutrients. Diseases that affect the digestive system—such as celiac disease, Crohn's disease, irritable bowel syndrome, lactose intolerance, and bacterial, viral, and parasitic infections—are the most obvious. But infections in *any* part of the body can rapidly deplete stores of most vitamins and minerals. In addition, your appetite usually decreases during times of illness, which further depletes nutrient supplies. During the recuperation process following an illness, trauma, burns, or surgery, the body's stores of nutrients need to be replenished and the injured tissues repaired. Nutrients are also important for building up our immune systems, especially at critical times. Ironically, a downward spiral often occurs, in which illness depletes the body of nutrients, which lowers the resistance to infection, which in turn lowers the nutrient levels even more, and so on. The results of several studies have indicated that hospital patients as a group are some of the most malnourished people in the world. In one study, only 12 percent of the patients tested had normal levels of vitamins in their bodies. Yet most of them had been eating a "normal American diet."

As you will see in the upcoming chapters on individual vitamins and minerals, people with overt diagnosed medical conditions or diseases often have low levels of one or more vitamins or minerals in their bodies. This occurs even when these conditions are not usually associated with nutritional deficiencies. This may indicate either that nutrient deficiencies play a previously unacknowledged role in the development of a particular disease or condition, or that deficiencies are a direct or indirect result of the condition. Whatever the relationship between the illness and the deficiency, supplementation can often be an effective means of treatment and prevention. The therapeutic potential of supplementation has been particularly apparent in the accumulating reports on patients with HIV infection, AIDS, multiple sclerosis, rheumatoid arthritis, and chronic fatigue. For these patients, who have few treatment options, nutritional supplementation has often been not only beneficial, but also *safe*. Certainly, your present and past physical condition, as well as your family's health history, should always be considered when planning a nutritional regimen.

### Drugs

It is widely recognized that many drugs interact with nutrients in the body, often causing depletion. Tetracycline, a widely used antibiotic, interferes with the absorption of calcium, magnesium, potassium, zinc, and iron. Many other antibiotics are known to interfere with the B-complex vitamins. Hormones in medications such as oral contraceptives appear to reduce the levels of some of the water-soluble vitamins. Antacids, which coat the walls of the intestines to protect them from stomach acid, also prevent several nutrients—most notably, calcium—from being absorbed. Questran, a commonly prescribed drug used to lower cholesterol, limits the absorption of vitamins A, $B_{12}$, D, E, K, and folic acid. (For details on a number of drug-nutrient interactions, see pages 234 to 236.)

Alcohol is a another drug that can interfere with nutrient absorption. Alcoholics have multiple nutritional deficiencies both for this reason and because they use alcohol as a substitute for food.

## Aging

Studies have shown that your body changes throughout life. As you age, your organs generally tend to function less efficiently, your digestion may be affected, and absorption and utilization of nutrients are decreased. Moreover, as your level of physical activity diminishes and your metabolism slows, your overall food intake lessens, too, putting the elderly at particular risk for suboptimal nutrition.

Many studies of older people have shown that they are simply not getting enough nutrients from their diets. It may come as no surprise to learn that a survey of fourteen nursing homes found that not one of them provided meals that met the RDAs for all nutrients. But another study—this one of 270 healthy elderly people living in the area of Albuquerque, New Mexico—provided truly startling results. Although the subjects were Caucasian and highly educated, had higher-than-average incomes, and were considered to be "health conscious," it was found that up to 86 percent of the women and 85 percent of the men were getting less than the RDAs for vitamins $B_6$, $B_{12}$, E, and D; folic acid; calcium; and zinc.

As we age, we do require more nutrients—particularly calcium and magnesium. In addition, many diseases associated with aging, such as cancer, high blood pressure, heart disease, and diabetes, as well as the aging process itself, may raise our requirements for certain antioxidant nutrients. These effects are more fully discussed in Chapter 3 and in chapters on the individual antioxidant nutrients. For example, several recent studies—including work done at the Human Nutrition Research Center on Aging at Tufts University—have shown that supplementation with single nutrients, such as vitamin E, or with multivitamin and mineral supplements at levels above the RDA, result in improved immune response. Two Canadian studies showed lower rates of infectious disease and cataracts among elderly people who took antioxidant vitamins. In the United States, a large-scale ongoing study of 87,000 nurses, ages 45 to 67 years of age, has found that vitamin C supplementation which continues for over ten years reduces the risk of cataracts by 45 percent. Those subjects with the highest intake of vitamin A and beta-carotene had a 39-percent lower risk of cataracts. In another study, beta-carotene and related compounds also significantly reduced the risk of macular degeneration, a major cause of blindness in the elderly.

## PROBLEM 3: DO THE RDIs ENSURE OPTIMUM HEALTH?

The RDIs are designed to prevent only overt deficiency symptoms. Prolonged deficiency of a certain vitamin or mineral generally results in severe disease with easily observable signs. For example, vitamin A deficiency leads to night blindness and other eye problems; niacin deficiency causes pellagra, characterized by diarrhea, dermatitis, and dementia; and iron or $B_{12}$ deficiency results in anemia. There is no question that the estimated RDIs are sufficient to prevent severe deficiency disorders in most people. But are they high enough to maintain optimum health? And is looking at severe, overt deficiency symptoms an accurate way of determining what you need? Maybe there are subtle changes that occur in the cells before the deficiency manifests itself in overt symptoms such as skin sores, mental disturbances, or crippling bone loss. Chapter 3, which is devoted to this issue, explains how the alternative to the RDIs, the ODIs, may help to ensure *optimal* health, not just the absence of disease.

As it currently stands, the RDI is a limited concept, the meaning and usefulness of which are being questioned even by the experts who are responsible for establishing and maintaining it. In today's world, the RDIs are, with a few exceptions, the nutritional equivalent of the minimum wage. They are probably high enough to keep you alive—although even this is open to question. But they do not appear high enough to allow you to enjoy the *best* quality of life. And why should you not strive for the best?

# Chapter 3

# THE OPTIMUM DAILY INTAKES (ODIs)

Recent evidence indicates that most of the RDIs are far too low. Why? Because vitamins and minerals do more than just prevent the severe, overt symptoms that are traditionally associated with deficiencies. Remember: *Vitamins and minerals are used in every process of the body.* We now know, for example, that vitamin A does more than prevent night blindness, that thiamin prevents more than beriberi, and that vitamin C does much more than prevent scurvy. By optimizing our daily intake of nutrients, we don't simply prevent disease. We help ensure a state of optimal health.

## SUBCLINICAL DEFICIENCIES

State-of-the-art biochemistry shows that classic, overt deficiency symptoms, like those of beriberi, are merely the last event in a long chain of reactions in the body, the way an erupting volcano or earthquake is the last dramatic step in a series of underground processes. That we are not always aware of these processes does not mean that they do not exist, or that they will not eventually cause an explosion of ill health at some point in the future. When we do not get enough of a specific vitamin, the initial reactions occur on the molecular level. The first thing that happens is a depletion of the vitamin stores in the body. Then the enzymes, of which the vitamin is a part, become depleted. This, in turn, brings about changes on the cellular level: Some of the cells of the body, which depend upon these enzymes, can no longer carry out their normal functions. It is not until the depletion is prolonged and severe that the classic clinical signs of deficiency appear.

Such cellular changes are also known as *subclinical deficiencies* because they are not the kind of deficiencies that your doctor would necessarily discover through a routine physical exam and blood tests. But while they may not be obvious, easily definable, or immediately debilitating, these deficiencies *do* have an effect on the body's well-being. For example, volunteers who were depleted of vitamin $B_1$ showed no detectable body changes for the first five to ten days. After ten days, there was evidence of changes in the cells' metabolism. Classic anatomical signs of $B_1$ deficiency became obvious only after about two hundred days. However, during that time, the subjects experienced a gradual decline in their health with nonspecific symptoms of loss of weight, loss of appetite, general malaise, insomnia, and irritability.

The subtle, subclinical changes due to poor nutrition may be responsible for a broad range of diffuse, nonspecific conditions that can at first be merely annoying and reduce our overall health and quality of life. These conditions can include chronic fatigue, skin problems, recurrent or lingering infections and colds, digestive problems, sleep problems, headaches, hormonal problems, depression, and nervousness. Poor nutrient intake may also leave us more vulnerable to genetically predisposed diseases and conditions such as cardiovascular disease, diabetes, and cancer. The role that the other nutrients, such as fat and carbohydrates, play in these diseases is becoming more and more solidly documented. Why should we be surprised by the accumulating evidence that vitamins and minerals also play a part?

## NUTRITION—NATURE'S PROTECTOR

As already discussed, nutrients do far more than protect the body against deficiency diseases. By buttressing our immune system, they protect us from foreign invaders, and therefore help fight infection. By guarding us from the ravages of oxidative stress, they prevent or slow the progress of a variety of degenerative illnesses, including cancer. And by helping regulate the balance of fats in the body, they fight heart disease. A brief look at each of these functions will provide a clearer idea of the importance of optimum nutrient intake to good health.

### Nutrients and the Immune System

Our immune system is a complex system of blood cells and special proteins acting together to defend us from harm. Improving our immune defense system is the main thrust behind modern preventive medicine because it protects us in so many important ways. For example, the immune system has the ability to engulf and kill bacteria and viruses. It can also repair or destroy a damaged cell before it grows into a cancerous tumor. This system, though powerful, is extremely delicate, its parts exquisitely interdependent upon one another. If any one aspect is compromised, we may become more susceptible to infections; degenerative diseases such as cancer and diabetes; and, perhaps, cardiovascular disease and certain forms of arthritis.

In many studies, inadequate nutrition has been shown to weaken one or more of the components of our defense system. Insufficient protein, too little fiber, and too much fat have all been implicated in impaired immunity, as have vitamin and mineral deficiencies. On the other hand, excesses of the

RDIs of almost all vitamins and minerals have been shown to enhance immunity. Those that seem to exert the most profound effect are the antioxidants, vitamins C and E, beta-carotene, and selenium; minerals such as zinc; and specific B vitamins, such as vitamin B$_{12}$.

## Nutrients and the Control of Oxidative Stress

A *free radical* is an atom or group of atoms that has at least one unpaired electron. An electron is a negatively charged particle that usually occurs in pairs, forming a chemically stable arrangement. When an electron is unpaired, another atom or molecule can then easily bond with it, causing a chemical reaction. Because they join so readily with other compounds, free radicals can effect dramatic changes in the body, causing a great deal of damage—damage often referred to as *oxidative stress*. Oxidative stress, which can accumulate over time, has been associated with the signs of aging and with debilitating and life-threatening degenerative diseases, including arthritis, hardening of the arteries, and heart and kidney ailments. It has also been implicated in the development of cancer. In fact, there's accumulating evidence that damage from out-of-control free radicals may lead to over sixty degenerative diseases.

Free radicals are formed by exposure to toxic chemicals in our food, water, and air; by radiation; by excessive sunlight; and, in part, by normal bodily processes. When the body obtains nutrients through the diet, it uses both these nutrients and oxygen to create energy. In this process, oxygen molecules containing unpaired electrons are released. These oxygen free radicals can cause damage to the body when produced in extremely large amounts. A diet that is high in fat is particularly associated with increased free radical activity because oxidation more readily occurs in fat molecules than it does in protein and carbohydrate molecules.

Although the formation of free radicals is taking place all the time, our body has certain defense mechanisms that keep these processes under control. One of the body's defense mechanisms is to repair the cell damage caused by free radicals. Another such mechanism is interception of the free radicals *before* they do any harm. This is where antioxidants come in. *Antioxidants*—which include vitamins C and E, beta-carotene, and selenium—either help the body protect itself, or are themselves protective. For example, in one study, 400 milligrams of vitamin C a day reduced the lipid (fat) peroxide level—a measurement of oxidative stress—by 13 percent in one year. Supplements of both vitamins E and C reduced the level by 25 percent. This highlights the fact that antioxidants very often work synergistically with one another or with other nutrients in the body's defense. For example, vitamin E, which is known as a "scavenger" of free radicals formed by the oxidation of fats, works synergistically with selenium. It also protects vitamin C from oxidation, thus preserving the potency of another antioxidant.

Studies show that if our bodies become overwhelmed by free radicals, or if we are not getting enough of the protective vitamins and minerals from our diets, antioxidant supplements can help protect us against oxidative stress. One study published in 1993 focused on Linxian, China, which has one of the highest rates of esophageal stomach cancer and a persistently low intake of micronutrients. In this study, approximately 30,000 adults who were given supplements of beta-carotene, vitamin E, and selenium, showed a 42-percent reduction in esophageal cancer and a reduced risk of death from cancer. The China study confirmed the work of Dr. Gladys Block, a respected epidemiologist who has written comprehensive reviews of the available scientific literature on antioxidants in food and supplements. She found, for example, that of approximately 130 studies in which subjects either took supplemental vitamin C, beta-carotene, or vitamin E, *or* ate antioxidant-rich foods, 120 studies showed statistically significant reduced risks of many, many cancers, including cancers of the lung, larynx, esophagus, oral cavity, pancreas, stomach, cervix, rectum, colon, ovary, endometrium, breast, and bladder.

### Nutrients, Fats, and Heart Disease

Nutrition also plays an important role in the balance of fats in our body. Our blood contains a variety of fats (lipids) and fat-like substances. Although our body requires a certain amount of fat to function well, an excess of some types of fats has been implicated in cardiovascular disease. These "bad" fats include *serum cholesterol; low-density lipoproteins* (LDLs), often called "bad cholesterol"; and *triglycerides*. On the other hand, "good" fats—*high-density lipoproteins* (HDLs), often called "good cholesterol"—are actually associated with a lowered risk of heart disease. (For more information on cholesterol, LDLs, and HDLs, see the inset on page 32.)

The balance between good and bad fats is determined by several factors, including diet (nutrition), exercise, and heredity. Fortunately, we can manipulate two out of three of these factors to create a more desirable balance. For example, there is evidence that levels of both triglycerides—a type of fat that may increase the risk of heart disease—and cholesterol can be lowered by the consumption of certain supplements. These supplements, which include niacin, vitamins C and E, chromium, EPA (eicosapentaenoic acid), and coenzyme $Q_{10}$, may also lower LDL and raise HDL cholesterol. Moreover, antioxidants such as vitamin E, beta-carotene, garlic, and coenzyme $Q_{10}$ have been shown to protect LDLs from oxidizing and causing havoc in our arteries. Aerobic exercise and a very low-fat, high-fiber diet have also proven effective in this regard. Be aware that simply reducing the amount of cholesterol in your diet is a rather ineffective way of changing your blood cholesterol levels. The most effective plan for lowering blood cholesterol includes all of these measures. And unlike the drugs commonly used to lower cholesterol, this plan is *safe*.

Two large-scale ongoing Harvard-based studies have already demonstrated the power that nutrients can have in the prevention of heart disease. One, the Health Professionals Follow-Up Study, involves 40,000 male physicians; the other, the Nurses' Health Study, involves 87,000 female nurses. These studies have found that vitamin E supplementation reduces the rate of heart disease in both men and women by 40 percent; that high intakes of beta-carotene reduce the rate of stroke in women by 40 percent; and that beta-carotene supplementation reduces heart attack, stroke, and death rates by half in men with heart disease.

## THE CHANGING VIEW OF NUTRITIONAL SUPPLEMENTS

Traditionally, the medical community has been very skeptical of the use of vitamin supplements. However, this is starting to change, especially regarding antioxidant nutrients. That's because of the overwhelming evidence that antioxidants may help prevent, slow, and even reverse serious diseases and conditions such as atherosclerosis, cancer, and cataracts.

Two large-scale ongoing Harvard-based studies—the Health Professionals Follow-Up Study, and the Nurses' Health Study—stand out as the turning point for many health professionals. These studies, which were discussed above are demonstrating the beneficial effects of antioxidants in the prevention of coronary disease. Research such as this is gradually providing consistent enough evidence to convince many former skeptics that supplementation with reasonable amounts of vitamins and minerals provides us with the optimum protection we need. At a recent American College of Cardiology meeting, two-thirds of the audience of approximately seven hundred physicians acknowledged that they themselves took antioxidant supplements daily.

Dr. Anthony J. Verlangieri, director of the Atherosclerosis Research Laboratories and Professor of Pharmacology and Toxicology at the University of Mississippi School of Pharmacy, states, "Yes, absolutely, everyone should take supplementary vitamins." Based on twenty-five years of his research, he recommends that everyone take 200 international units of natural vitamin E, 4,000 milligrams of vitamin C, and either 2,500 international units of vitamin A or 15 to 25 milligrams of beta-carotene daily, in divided doses. He states, "It is a myth that we all get the vitamins we need in our daily diets." In addition, he points out that there are absolutely no toxicities associated with these levels of antioxidant supplementation. Many nutrition experts, such as those on a panel sponsored by the nonprofit aging research group called

# Understanding Cholesterol

*Currently, cholesterol has an unsavory reputation. Yet, cholesterol is actually necessary for the proper functioning of the body. Cholesterol is used by cells to build membranes, to produce hormones, and to manufacture bile acids. Problems often occur, however, when the amount of cholesterol in the body exceeds the amount needed for body functions. To understand how cholesterol levels can get out of control—or be kept in check—it is necessary to know a little about how this substance is produced and distributed in the body.*

*Most of the cholesterol in the body is produced by the liver, which makes all of the cholesterol we need for good health. Cholesterol then travels from that organ through the bloodstream by means of protein molecules called lipoproteins, which deliver cholesterol to cells throughout the body. After the cells take what they need, any excess cholesterol remains in the bloodstream until other lipoproteins pick it up for transport back to the liver. If excess cholesterol is not picked up promptly, it can form plaque, which sticks to artery walls and can eventually cause cardiovascular disease.*

*There are two basic types of lipoproteins: low-density lipoproteins (LDLs) and high-density lipoproteins (HDLs). LDLs are the molecules that transport cholesterol from the liver to the cells of the body. High levels of LDLs in the bloodstream can result in clogged arteries, causing high blood pressure, stroke, or heart disease. LDL is very susceptible to oxidative stress. This is why LDL is often referred to as "bad cholesterol."*

*HDLs, on the other hand, circulate in the bloodstream removing excess cholesterol from the blood and tissues. The HDLs then carry the cholesterol to the liver, where it is converted to bile acids and then eliminated through the intestines. High levels of HDLs are linked with a decreased risk of coronary heart disease. This is why HDL is often called "good cholesterol."*

*Clearly, the amount of cholesterol in your diet plays a part in determining your blood cholesterol level. However, dietary cholesterol is not the only deciding factor. Research indicates that saturated fats increase total blood cholesterol—especially the undesirable LDL portion. Polyunsaturated fats, on the other hand, have been shown to lower levels of both HDL and LDL. And monounsaturated fats have been shown to reduce total blood cholesterol without lowering levels of healthful HDL. In addition, a number of micronutrients—including niacin, vitamins C and E, and chromium—may also lower LDL and raise HDL, contributing to the maintenance of a healthful cholesterol level. Vitamin E, in particular, prevents LDL from oxidizing.*

Alliance for Aging Research, have also made specific recommendations regarding the amounts of vitamins that should be taken to prevent disease.

While it is not a rule that more is always better, some experiments have shown that amounts of nutrients in excess of the RDAs, whether from food or supplements, do have a more positive effect than lower amounts. Some doctors have claimed that any excess micronutrients are a "waste"—that they simply end up in the urine. Although excess vitamins and minerals are eliminated from the body, research indicates that even this may not be a waste. For example, studies in which animals or humans were given substantially higher doses of the RDA for vitamin C have suggested that any excess vitamin C that spills into the urine may have a protective effect against urinary and bladder cancer.

One factor that may be persuading some clinicians of the benefits of supplementation is that of cost. Several economists have estimated that by increasing our intake of vitamins and minerals, we would reduce health-care costs by 25 percent for cardiovascular disease, 16 to 30 percent for a variety of cancers, and 50 percent for cataracts. Another example of cost effectiveness relates to carpal tunnel syndrome. When vitamin $B_6$ is used to treat this problem, it costs about $5 for a three-month supply. Compare this amount with that of surgery, and the savings are clear.

## THE ODIs—A REDEFINITION OF HEALTH

We have gradually expanded our knowledge and our thinking to include the notion that health should no longer be negatively defined as the absence of disease. Our current concept of real health is not one of mere survival, but one of a positive state of total mental and physical well-being. We have drawn a distinction between maintaining *minimum* or *adequate* health—which is what the RDIs appear to do—and attaining and maintaining *optimum* health—which the RDIs do not ensure. We want to be as healthy as we can be in our daily lives. This includes taking advantage of the most current research on the prevention of disease and the integration of nutritional therapies with appropriate medical care during the early, most treatable stage of disease.

### Why Do We Need the ODIs?

In order to attain a state of optimum health and disease prevention, we must take into our bodies optimum—not minimum—amounts of vitamins and minerals. To distinguish them from the lesser amounts characteristic of the RDIs, I have called these amounts the *Optimum Daily Intakes,* or ODIs. The need for ODIs is based on six factors:

1. The RDIs are generally based on an amount that simply prevents overt deficiency diseases.

2. The RDIs do not take into account preventive or therapeutic levels of nutrients.

3. We cannot meet the RDIs even if we eat the "perfect" diet.

4. Because of many factors, including loss of nutrients through shipping, storage, and processing, the foods available to us do not contain the amounts of vitamins and minerals they should contain.

5. Owing to the constant bombardment of stress factors, from pollution to emotional stress, we require higher levels of vitamins and minerals than originally thought.

6. The vitamins and minerals in foods and supplements are never 100 percent absorbed.

In acknowledgment of the fact that people are individuals, and so require differing amounts of nutrients, each of the ODIs in this book is presented as a range of doses. Although a few ODIs are close to or the same as the RDIs, they are generally in excess of the RDIs, and are often many times that amount. However, they are not "megadoses"—a term that is not only limiting, but totally inaccurate. "Mega" has come to mean "ten times" in popular usage and in some scientific articles; however, the term literally means "million." In *The Real Vitamin and Mineral Book,* the ODI is often much more than ten times the RDI. However, it is never a million times the RDI.

**What Is the Basis for the ODIs?**

The ODIs are based on data from three sources: the most up-to-date research studies published in highly respected American and foreign professional journals, my own clinical experience, and the experiences of other well-known clinicians in the field. It should be noted that it is often difficult to draw firm conclusions when there is no uniform standard that allows us to compare study results fairly. Among various studies:

❑ Different amounts of supplements are used.

❑ Different forms of supplements are used—e.g., d-alpha (natural vitamin E) versus d,l-alpha tocopherol (synthetic vitamin E).

❑ Different study designs are used—e.g., supplements are given for varying amounts of time, and diet and daily habits may or may not be considered.

❑ Different study populations are used. That is, the study may test if something lowered the cholesterol levels in people who do not have elevated cholesterol; the study may test for a blood pressure-lowering effect on people who do not have hypertension; study subjects may be male or female; or studies may involve people in different age groups.

## Evaluating the Studies

It has been estimated that our knowledge of the biological sciences is doubling every five to ten years, and human nutrition is an especially fast-growing field. Many practitioners, including myself, are interested in new findings and new ideas. We prefer to look forward, rather than backward. This means that we are sometimes in the position of having to take sketchy, somewhat experimental data and apply it to real-life situations, perhaps before the data is completely understood. So in many instances, I have had to take the research studies a step further.

One example of this regards the stated uses of vitamin C. It has been shown that vitamin C blocks the formation of nitrosamine from the nitrates in food. Therefore, it stands to reason that the same would hold true for nitrosamines formed from air pollution in our lungs.

Another example of extrapolation regards animal studies. Wherever feasible, my recommendations have been based on human studies. However, sometimes animal studies are all that is available, in part because it would be unethical to use similar methods on humans. For instance, tumors are often induced in animals, after which supplements are given to assess their efficacy in suppressing tumor growth. The animals are usually killed after the experiment is completed to measure the effects of nutrition on various parts of the body.

According to the American Medical Association, the extrapolation from animal studies to humans is widely accepted in the medical profession. Many major breakthroughs in medicine, in fact, have occurred as a consequence of animal research. The efficacy and toxicity of almost all the drugs used in medical practice were originally based on animal research. Animal studies have also been generally accepted as sufficient proof that certain substances, such as cyclamates and red dye number 2, may be cancer-producing in humans. It is logical to conclude that in many cases, extrapolation of data from animal studies with respect to human nutrition is just as valid. For instance, as mentioned earlier, the ODIs reflect the fact that individual needs for nutrients vary. This is based not only on our knowledge of human beings, but also on our knowledge of animals. Nobel Prize winner Linus Pauling found that the vitamin requirements of individual animals within the same species vary by as much as 2,000 percent. He inferred that the same is probably true of humans.

A third example of extrapolation regards epidemiological studies—studies of the causes, distribution, and control of disease in populations. For instance, researchers may measure the level of a certain vitamin in the diet or blood of groups of people. They then see whether there is any correlation between vitamin levels and state of health. Many of the studies linking a higher level of vitamin A or beta-carotene with a lower risk of cancer are of this type.

Nutritionists and physicians have disputed many of the findings of the epidemiologists, and have demanded experimental "proof." They want to see the same kind of placebo-controlled double-blind studies that are required to evaluate drugs. In this type of study, subjects are divided into two groups, one of which gets the drug, while the other gets a placebo (a dummy or sugar pill). Both the subjects and investigators are "blind"; that is, neither one knows which group of subjects is getting the drug or the placebo until the study is over and the code is broken. The Food and Drug Administration requires that two such studies be multi-center trials and show efficacy before a new medication is approved.

There are a number of problems with requiring that nutrients be evaluated using this so-called "gold standard" of testing. First of all, these studies cost millions of dollars to conduct. Pharmaceutical companies, which may profit handsomely from a patentable drug, are better able to fund such studies than are nutritional supplement companies, because nutrients are rarely patentable. Second—and, actually, more important—this type of study is usually based on the "magic bullet" approach, in which a single specific drug is used to cure or relieve the symptoms of a disease. This approach makes less sense in nutrition. Nutrients are not single magic bullets. They do not work alone. They work synergistically, and their effects cannot be adequately appreciated when they are studied as isolated substances.

So although the medical community is accustomed to seeing double-blind placebo-controlled studies, many experts believe that these studies may not be applicable in the evaluation of nutrients. Researcher and educator Jeffrey Bland, Ph.D., doesn't believe that we'll ever have unequivocal proof that supplements work—nor that we need it in the same way we do for drugs. He argues, "You can't hold people on controlled diets with nutritional supplements for thirty years, with a placebo group, to find answers to these questions about something that at its worst does no harm."

In the Harvard School of Public Health's December 1985 issue of *Nutrition Reviews,* Dr. D.M. Hegsted addressed this issue, pointing out the inconsistency in the skeptics' reasoning. He notes, "There is a large body of science, as valid as any other science, which rests upon observation and deduction rather than experimentation—such as astronomy, geology, and archeology. Indeed, the crowning achievement of biology—the theory of evolution—is based upon observation and deduction."

Our bodies have the remarkable ability to adapt and protect us from the ever-increasing abuses of life. Some people can tolerate a good deal of these insults, while others are much more sensitive and need optimal nutritional protection. However, we have no way of knowing for sure who falls into which category. Taking the Optimal Daily Intakes recommended in this book means that you are joining the legions of nutritionally aware people who would rather be safe than sorry.

# Chapter 4

# HOW TO DESIGN YOUR OWN NUTRITIONAL SUPPLEMENT PROGRAM

To design a nutritional supplement program that is suited to your particular needs, I recommend that you first read through Part Two, "The Vitamins"; Part Three, "The Minerals"; and Part Four, "Beyond Vitamins and Minerals." This will give you an overall picture of what the various supplements can do. Then tear out or photocopy the Sample Worksheet on pages 238 to 239 in Part Five, and go through the book again, chapter by chapter, filling in your Optimum Daily Intake for each nutrient.

Remember: *You must never take just one nutritional supplement or just a select few.* Although each has its own biochemical function in the body, nutrients tend to work together synergistically. They help one another. You must take appropriate amounts of them all, and in proportion to one another, to get the most out of them. For example, vitamin C can regenerate vitamin E in our bodies and make it more effective. In addition, because supplements compete for absorption in the body, supplementation of a single nutrient may put you at risk for developing a deficiency of those nutrients which are not being supplemented.

**STEP 1: DETERMINE YOUR BASIC ODI**

Notice that in each nutrient chapter, I have provided a basic Optimum Daily Intake. This is a safe dose range for general optimum health, and will help prevent illnesses in most people. Using the basic ODI program given in the Sample Worksheet on pages 238 to 239 as a guide, your first step is to fill in your basic ODI for each nutrient. If you are in good health, with no particular health concerns, and are primarily interested in all-round disease prevention, I advise you to start at the lower end of this basic ODI range. If you continue to feel well, this is probably all you will need to take. If you are generally not feeling well, I recommend that you start at the low end and gradually increase the dose until you notice an improvement.

## STEP 2: INDIVIDUALIZE YOUR ODI

Some people are at higher risk for illness owing to personal or family health history, environmental pollution, or other forms of stress. That is why in each chapter I also provide specific examples of amounts that I have found useful for preventing specific conditions and concerns. These ODIs for specific uses generally go higher than the basic ODIs because, based on both research and my experience, certain circumstances require higher amounts. Although they are higher than the basic ODIs, they are still nontoxic, and will not result in any adverse effects. In some cases, these higher amounts have also been effective as the primary treatment for an already existing condition, or have proven valuable as an adjunct to appropriate medical treatment.

However, large doses of certain supplements may have undesirable effects in some individuals with medical conditions, or may reduce or enhance the effectiveness of any medication being taken. I cannot emphasize too strongly that if you have a suspected or diagnosed medical condition, for your own protection, you *must* check with your physician before taking any nutritional supplement. In general, pregnant women may safely take the low end of the basic ODI; but again, please check with your physician.

If you are at high risk for a particular disease, your next step is to decide how much more than the basic ODI you want to take of specific nutrients. For example, if cancer runs in your family, I recommend that you take higher amounts of vitamins A, B-complex, C, D, and E; the minerals zinc, chromium, and selenium; and the essential fatty acids GLA and EPA—all nutrients that have been shown to be protective against cancer. If you smoke, live or work with a smoker, or live in a polluted city environment, you also might want to take higher amounts of certain nutrients. The same holds true if you have a tendency towards high blood pressure or other forms of coronary disease, diabetes, premenstrual syndrome, fibrocystic breast disease, and so on. To serve as a guide, the worksheet includes programs for some of the most common specific concerns, such as emotional stress, immunity enhancement, cancer prevention, cardiovascular disease prevention, skin problems, and diabetes prevention.

In addition, you can use the examples on the following pages to get an idea of how supplement programs can be individualized for people in a variety of circumstances. When reading through the examples, keep in mind that, as mentioned earlier, I generally reserve supplements such as melatonin, DHEA, and coenzyme Q10 for the specific conditions listed in appropriate chapters, or for situations in which other supplements have failed to achieve the desired results.

I'll start with myself. I'm in my thirties, and I live and run my practice in New York City. I am under a lot of stress, both from my polluted environment and from business pressures. I play tennis, lift weights, and get regular aerobic exercise. My diet is optimal (low-fat, low-sugar, high-fiber), but there is a strong family propensity toward heart disease, high cholesterol, and high triglycerides. My supplement program looks like this:

| Supplement | Daily Dosage |
| --- | --- |
| Vitamin A | 5,000 IU |
| Beta-carotene | 100,000 IU |
| B complex | 50 mg |
| Vitamin $B_3$ (niacin) | 500 mg |
| Vitamin C | 4,000 mg |
| Vitamin D | 400 IU |
| Vitamin E | 400 IU |
| Bioflavonoids | 500 mg |
| Calcium | 1,000 mg |
| Coenzyme $Q_{10}$ | 100 mg |
| Copper | Obtained from food sources |
| EPA | 1,120 mg |
| Garlic | 1,000 mg |
| GTF chromium | 200 mcg |
| Iodine | 150 mcg |
| Iron | 25 mg |
| Magnesium | 500 mg |
| Manganese | 25 mg |
| Phosphorus | Obtained from food sources |
| Selenium | 250 mcg |
| Zinc | 50 mg |

My co-author, Nancy Bruning, is in her forties and is a professional, with her own business. She lives in San Francisco, and so is exposed to a fair amount of urban pollution. As a freelance writer, she is also subject to a fair amount of stress. Sixteen years ago, she was treated with surgery and chemotherapy for breast cancer, and now has no evidence of disease. She tends to have allergies and hormonal problems, with premenstrual syndrome being particularly problematic. Her program is:

| Supplement | Daily Dosage |
|---|---|
| Vitamin A | 10,000 IU |
| Beta-carotene | 75,000 IU |
| B complex | 50 mg |
| Vitamin B6 | 100 mg |
| Vitamin C | 4,000–5,000 mg |
| Vitamin D | 400 IU |
| Vitamin E | 800 IU |
| Calcium | 1,000 mg |
| Copper | Obtained from food sources |
| EPA | 1,500 mg |
| GLA | 140–240 mg |
| GTF chromium | 200 mcg |
| Iodine | 150 mcg |
| Iron | 25 mg |
| Magnesium | 500 mg |
| Manganese | 30 mg |
| Phosphorus | Obtained from food sources |
| Selenium | 400 mcg |
| Zinc | 50 mg |

R.M. is a twenty-five-year-old woman who lives and works as a secretary in the suburbs. She gets very little exercise and is overweight. She has no health complaints, and does not feel particularly stressed about anything other than her weight and her craving for sweets. Her program is:

| Supplement | Daily Dosage |
|---|---|
| Vitamin A | 5,000 IU |
| Beta-carotene | 10,000 IU |
| B complex | 25 mg |
| Vitamin C | 1,000 mg |
| Vitamin D | 400 IU |
| Vitamin E | 400 IU |

| Supplement | Daily Dosage |
| --- | --- |
| Bioflavonoids | 500 mg |
| Calcium | 1,000 mg |
| Copper | 2 mg |
| GLA | 140–240 mg |
| GTF chromium | 600 mcg |
| Iodine | 300 mcg |
| Iron | 25 mg |
| Magnesium | 500 mg |
| Manganese | 15 mg |
| Phosphorus | Obtained from food sources |
| Selenium | 100 mcg |
| Zinc | 22.5 mg |

J.S. is a thirty-five-year-old businessman who lives and works in Los Angeles. His brother and father have a history of bowel cancer, and he is quite worried that he will get it, too, especially since he has a history of spastic colitis. He does not eat an optimal diet or get regular exercise. However, he is willing to make changes. His program is:

| Supplement | Daily Dosage |
| --- | --- |
| Vitamin A | 10,000 IU |
| Beta-carotene | 50,000 IU |
| B complex | 50 mg |
| Vitamin C | 5,000 mg |
| Vitamin D | 400 IU |
| Vitamin E | 800 IU |
| Bioflavonoids | 2,500 mg |
| Calcium | 1,000 mg |
| Copper | 2 mg |
| EPA | 1,500 mg |
| GTF chromium | 200 mcg |
| Iodine | 50 mcg |

| Supplement | Daily Dosage |
|---|---|
| Iron | 15 mg |
| Magnesium | 500 mg |
| Manganese | 15 mg |
| Phosphorus | Obtained from food sources |
| Selenium | 300 mcg |
| Zinc | 50 mg |

S.S. is a sixty-seven-year-old retired teacher with osteoporosis and arthritis. She has become interested in nutrition over the years, and her diet is good. However, she cannot eat more than 1,200 calories a day because she is sedentary and is worried about gaining weight. She refuses to take drugs. Her program is:

| Supplement | Daily Dosage |
|---|---|
| Vitamin A | 10,000 IU |
| Beta-carotene | 10,000 IU |
| B complex | 100 mg |
| Vitamin C | 5,000 mg |
| Vitamin D | 800 IU |
| Vitamin E | 1,200 IU |
| Bioflavonoids | 5,000 mg |
| Boron | 6 mg |
| Calcium | 2,000 mg |
| Copper | 2 mg |
| EPA | 1,500 mg |
| GTF chromium | 200 mcg |
| Iodine | 300 mcg |
| Iron | 25 mg |
| Magnesium | 1,000 mg |
| Manganese | 30 mg |
| Phosphorus | 400 mg |
| Selenium | 200 mcg |
| Zinc | 50 mg |

E.B. is a sixteen-year-old high school student. In addition to his school work, he has daily practice and training for the basketball team. He is very stressed, always feels rushed, and often feels tired. His physician has diagnosed iron deficiency anemia. He also feels that E.B. is underweight. E.B. skips breakfast and eats school lunches. Dinner is the only good meal he eats, since his mother cooks it. His program is:

| Supplement | Daily Dosage |
|---|---|
| Vitamin A | 5,000 IU |
| Beta-carotene | 10,000 IU |
| B complex | 50 mg |
| Vitamin C | 3,000 mg |
| Vitamin D | 400 IU |
| Vitamin E | 400 IU |
| Calcium | 1,500 mg |
| Copper | 2 mg |
| GTF chromium | 400 mcg |
| Iodine | 50 mcg |
| Iron | 30 mg |
| Magnesium | 750 mg |
| Manganese | 15 mg |
| Phosphorus | 400 mg |
| Selenium | 100 mcg |
| Zinc | 30 mg |

J.Y. is twenty-seven years old and pregnant. She has quit her job and has plenty of time to cook and plan her meals. But she is concerned about excessive weight gain, and doesn't want to eat over 1,800 calories or drink more than two cups of low-fat milk a day. Her program is:

| Supplement | Daily Dosage |
|---|---|
| Vitamin A | 5,000 IU |
| Beta-carotene | 5,000 IU |
| B complex | 25 mg |
| Folic acid | 800 mg |
| Vitamin C | 1,000 mg |
| Vitamin D | 200 IU |

| Supplement | Daily Dosage |
|------------|--------------|
| Vitamin E | 400 IU |
| Bioflavonoids | 500 mg |
| Calcium | 1,000 mg |
| Copper | 2 mg |
| EPA | 560 mg |
| GTF chromium | 200 mcg |
| Iodine | 150 mcg |
| Iron | 30 mg |
| Magnesium | 500 mg |
| Manganese | 15 mg |
| Phosphorus | Obtained from food sources |
| Selenium | 100 mcg |
| Zinc | 22.5 mg |

M.R. is a thirty-eight-year-old man who lives and works in Chicago. His job as a postal worker means he has irregular hours. This has affected his eating habits, leaving him underweight. He worries about his blood pressure, which is slightly elevated. In addition to advising M.R. to reduce dietary sodium, I would recommend the following program:

| Supplement | Daily Dosage |
|------------|--------------|
| Vitamin A | 5,000 IU |
| Beta-carotene | 25,000 IU |
| B complex | 200 mg |
| Vitamin C | 3,000 mg |
| Vitamin D | 400 IU |
| Vitamin E | 400 IU |
| Bioflavonoids | 1,500 mg |
| Calcium | 1,500 mg |
| Copper | 2 mg |
| EPA | 1,500 mg |
| Garlic | 1,000 mg |
| GTF chromium | 200 mcg |
| Iodine | 150 mcg |
| Iron | 15 mg |
| Magnesium | 750 mg |

| Supplement | Daily Dosage |
| --- | --- |
| Manganese | 15 mg |
| Phosphorus | Obtained from food sources |
| Potassium | Obtained from food sources |
| Selenium | 100 mcg |
| Zinc | 2.5 mg |

J.K. is seventeen years old, and lives away from home at a college in the country. Her diet is poor, and she must rely mostly on cafeteria food. Since beginning to take birth control pills, she has noticed some water retention, mild depression, and cramps during menstruation. Her program is:

| Supplement | Daily Dosage |
| --- | --- |
| Vitamin A | 5,000 IU |
| Beta-carotene | 10,000 IU |
| B complex | 100 mg |
| Vitamin C | 3,000 mg |
| Vitamin D | 400 IU |
| Vitamin E | 400 IU |
| Bioflavonoids | 1,500 mg |
| Calcium | 1,500 mg |
| Copper | Obtained from food sources |
| GLA | 140–240 mg |
| GTF chromium | 400 mcg |
| Iodine | 150 mcg |
| Iron | 25 mg |
| Magnesium | 750 mg |
| Manganese | 30 mg |
| Phosphorus | Obtained from food sources |
| Selenium | 200 mcg |
| Zinc | 50 mg |

R.S., who lives in the suburbs, has become sedentary since his recent retirement from the police force. He is feeling depressed, and complains of joint and lower-back pain. He smokes cigarettes. His program is:

| Supplement   | Daily Dosage              |
|--------------|---------------------------|
| Vitamin A    | 10,000 IU                 |
| Beta-carotene| 50,000 IU                 |
| B complex    | 150 mg                    |
| Vitamin C    | 3,000 mg                  |
| Vitamin D    | 400 IU                    |
| Vitamin E    | 800 IU                    |
| Bioflavonoids| 1,500 mg                  |
| Boron        | 3 mg                      |
| Calcium      | 1,200 mg                  |
| Copper       | 2 mg                      |
| EPA          | 1,500 mg                  |
| GTF chromium | 200 mcg                   |
| Iodine       | 150 mcg                   |
| Iron         | 15 mg                     |
| Magnesium    | 600 mg                    |
| Manganese    | 30 mg                     |
| Phosphorus   | Obtained from food sources|
| Selenium     | 300 mcg                   |
| Zinc         | 50 mg                     |

L.L. is a thirty-five-year-old unemployed female with chronic fatigue and immune dysfunction (CFIDS). She often feels as though she is about to get the flu. Her PMS symptoms have become more intense over the past year. L.L. also has mild fibromyalgia, which causes muscle pain and weakness. Her program is:

| Supplement   | Daily Dosage |
|--------------|--------------|
| Vitamin A    | 10,000 IU    |
| Beta-carotene| 100,000 IU   |
| B complex    | 100 mg       |
| Vitamin C    | 6,000 mg     |
| Vitamin D    | 400 IU       |
| Vitamin E    | 800 IU       |

| Supplement | Daily Dosage |
|---|---|
| Calcium | 800 mg |
| Chromium | 400 mcg |
| Coenzyme Q$_{10}$ | 200 mg |
| GLA | 500 mg |
| Iodine | 150 mcg |
| Iron | 25 mg |
| L-carnitine | 1 g |
| Magnesium | 400 mg |
| Magnesium malate | 1,200 mg |
| Manganese | 20 mg |
| Quercetin | 1,000 mg |
| Selenium | 200 mcg |
| Zinc | 50 mg |

M.M. is a thirty-eight-year-old HIV-positive male. He has no symptoms and no history of infections. He refuses to take any antiviral prophylactic medications. His program includes a large amount of vitamin C, the specific dose of which was individually determined according to bowel tolerance. M.M. added 1,000 milligrams of Vitamin C to his program each week, until he reached a dosage that caused loose stools. He then cut back on the dose slightly to normalize bowel movements.

| Supplement | Daily Dosage |
|---|---|
| Vitamin A | 25,000 IU |
| Beta-carotene | 300,000 IU |
| B complex | 50 mg |
| Vitamin C | 15,000 mg |
| Vitamin D | 400 IU |
| Vitamin E | 400 IU |
| Calcium | 800 mg |
| Chromium | 200 mcg |
| Coenzyme Q$_{10}$ | 200 mg |
| EPA/DHA | 1,500 mg |

| Supplement | Daily Dosage |
| --- | --- |
| Garlic | 1,500 mg |
| Glutathione | 500 mg |
| Iodine | 150 mcg |
| Iron | 30 mg |
| Magnesium | 400 mg |
| Manganese | 20 mg |
| NAC | 1,000 mg |
| Quercetin | 1,500 mg |
| Selenium | 200 mcg |
| Zinc | 50 mg |

R.S. is a forty-five-year-old woman recently diagnosed with systemic lupus erythematosus.* She is feeling very fatigued, and has joint pains and some characteristic skin lesions on her face. Her program is:

| Supplement | Daily Dosage |
| --- | --- |
| Vitamin A | 15,000 IU |
| Beta-carotene | 100,000 IU |
| B complex | 100 mg |
| Vitamin C | 6,000 mg |
| Vitamin D | 400 IU |
| Vitamin E | 800 IU |
| Calcium | 800 mg |
| Chromium | 400 mcg |
| Coenzyme Q$_{10}$ | 50 mg |
| EPA | 2,000 mg |
| Iodine | 150 mcg |
| Iron | 25 mg |
| Magnesium | 400 mg |
| Manganese | 20 mg |
| Selenium | 200 mcg |
| Zinc | 50 mg |

*Programs for multiple sclerosis (MS) or similar autoimmune disorder would be similar. Some people with MS respond better to GLA (1,000 mg) or a combination of EPA and GLA.

## STEP 3: MATCH YOUR ODIs WITH YOUR SUPPLEMENTS

A simple way to obtain your own ODI is to start with a good multivitamin formula that combines a number of vitamins in one tablet. Generally, the multivitamin preparations currently available are your basic source of the B-complex vitamins A, D, and E. Some contain enough vitamin C for some people. They may also include negligible amounts of minerals—less than the RDIs of most, although they might contain the RDIs of iron and zinc. Therefore, I advise my patients to buy a good multimineral tablet in addition to their multivitamin tablet.

When shopping for multivitamin and -mineral tablets, look for preparations that imply high potency—for example, "extra potency," "megavitamins," or "therapeutic formula." Together, these two supplements will take care of most of the nutrients covered in this book. Depending upon their potency and your Optimum Daily Intake as specified in your program, you may need to take one, two, or more tablets of such formulas a day to get the basic amount of each nutrient that is right for you. Unfortunately, it is impossible to design a single pill that contains optimum amounts of everything you need while keeping it small enough to swallow.

An alternative to the separate multivitamin and multimineral formulas is a one-a-day multinutrient pack that has four or more different supplements in each pack. Or look for multinutrient formulas, which contain both vitamins and minerals in a single tablet or capsule. Depending on the formula and your needs, you will take four or six of these supplements a day.

Having settled on one or two basic formulas, you can further customize your program by adding to the general supplements those individual nutrients you feel you need more of. For example, your multivitamin may contain 25,000 international units of vitamin A. If you want to take a total of 50,000 international units because you have acne, you can add 25,000 international units of vitamin A. If your general multimineral supplement has 200 micrograms of chromium and you have diabetes, you might want to add 400 micrograms of chromium for a total of 600 micrograms per day. If you have a family history of heart disease, you may want to add 1,500 milligrams of EPA.

## WORKING WITH YOUR HEALTH-CARE PRACTITIONER

If you prefer to work with a nutritionist, it is important that you ask about his or her educational experience. In 1977, the National Nutrition Consortium—five nationally recognized organizations that included the American Dietetic Association and the American Institute of Nutrition—issued their report *Qualifications, Standards, and Competence in Nutrition.* According to this report, the definition of a *nutritionists* is one trained by education and experience in the science and practice of nutrition. This education involves a graduate program that includes basic science and professional courses designed to develop at least minimum competence in nutrition and allied sciences. In contrast, the definition of a *dietitian* is one who has earned a baccalaureate degree, and has met the basic academic and experience requirements needed to write the qualifying examination for professional registration in dietetics offered by the American Dietetic Association. Since entry level for the RD (Registered Dietitian) examination is an undergraduate (baccalaureate) degree, having this credential does not ensure that the individual is a nutritionist. State licensing and certification programs have furthered blurred the educational distinction between a dietitian and a nutritionist by lumping the two titles together or by credentialing dietitians as nutritionists. The only nationally recognized graduate-level certification program for nutritionists is offered by the Certification Board for Nutrition Specialists. Candidates who pass the examination receive the CNS (Certified Nutrition Specialist) credential.

Unfortunately, most physicians are not well versed in nutrition. Although this is lamentable, it is completely understandable, and is in large part due to inadequate nutritional education in medical school. Nutrition is generally offered as an elective to medical students, and the entire course usually consists of a grand total of three hours of basic nutrition. Also, medical training emphasizes the diagnosis and treatment of disease, rather than its prevention through nutrition or another means. While the situation is improving, if you have a nutritionally-oriented physician, you should consider yourself lucky.

The ideal situation is to have your physician and nutritionist work together, particularly if you have a medical problem. Many of my patients have this arrangement, and it can work out beautifully. You can't expect your physician to know and do everything. When health professionals read medical literature, we tend to read what is most relevant to our specialty. Even though much of the research in this book is from widely read and respected medical journals, your physician may not be familiar with the studies. For example, when I read *The Journal of the American Medical Association,* I naturally read the research pertaining to nutrition, rather than the latest surgical developments. There simply isn't the time to read all the research about every specialty. However, it *is* reasonable to expect your physician to be open-minded about the nutritional approach, since nutritional research is widespread throughout medical literature.

## HOW AND WHEN TO TAKE SUPPLEMENTS

Your body can absorb and use only so much of a vitamin or mineral at one time. So to increase the utilization of these nutrients, try to divide the dosage over the course of the day, especially if you are working with higher doses.

For example, if you are taking a total of 3,000 milligrams of vitamin C daily, take 1,000 milligrams three times a day. In addition, supplements are best taken at mealtime, along with your food. This increases absorption and prevents the indigestion that sometimes occurs when supplements are taken on an empty stomach. You may take supplements a few minutes before a meal, or up to a half hour after a meal.

There has been a lot of confusing information published about the interference of certain nutrients with the absorption of others. In my opinion, the evidence is not strong enough for me to advise not taking certain vitamins and minerals together, or with certain foods. As I say to my patients, nature supplies us with a variety of nutrients in each meal, so why should taking supplements together pose a problem? Life is complicated enough without your having to worry about whether your bran muffin is interfering with your absorption of calcium. In addition, studies indicate that this problem generally occurs only when you are taking a large amount of one or a few nutrients, as opposed to the full spectrum of nutrients.

## HOW WILL YOU KNOW IF YOUR SUPPLEMENTS ARE WORKING?

When people begin taking supplements for general good health and disease prevention, they usually just feel better. They feel calmer, get fewer colds, have more energy, and enjoy a general sense of well-being. Even my patients who were resistant to the idea of taking supplements have confessed this to me. These people sometimes go off their vitamins and minerals for a while, and then come back to me and say, "You know, skeptical as I was, I must admit that the supplements did make a difference in the way I felt." Because of our long life spans, there are no long-term studies that show that vitamin supplementation actually increases longevity. However, some studies show that diet and vitamin intake influences the life span of animals. In one experiment, mice that were given four times the RDAs of vitamins lived almost 20 percent longer than those given the RDAs.

If you are taking supplements to prevent a specific condition, and the condition fails to materialize, there is, of course, no way of knowing for sure whether the supplements "worked," or whether you would have remained healthy anyway. For people who take vitamins and minerals as a kind of "health insurance," no news is good news.

When you are taking supplements for a specific condition, you will know whether they are working because you will have tangible confirmation—your condition will improve. Let's suppose that you have a skin problem and you take extra vitamin A. If your skin clears up, you will know the vitamin is working. If you have high blood pressure, you might take extra calcium, magnesium, and garlic—and, hopefully, modify your diet. Then, if your blood pressure improves, again, you will know that the nutrients are working in your favor.

Vitamins and minerals do not work overnight! If you are nervous and irritable today and take a B-complex vitamin tonight, do not expect to feel calm and serene tomorrow. You must give it time—but do not wait forever. In general, you should begin to notice beneficial effects in three or four weeks. One exception is treatment for premenstrual syndrome. In this case, you will need at least two menstrual cycles to determine if supplementation is effective.

If you begin at the lower end of the ODI range and you see no results at this dose, you may increase the dose and give it another few weeks. Keep raising the dose, if necessary, until you reach the highest range of the ODI. Give that another month or so, unless you start noticing some adverse effects. For example, if you are taking beta-carotene for acne, you might start at 50,000 international units per day. If after a couple of weeks you see some improvement, but nothing spectacular, you may try going up to 75,000 international units for a while. If your skin clears up more, you might want to go up to 100,000 international units to see if this will improve it even further. If your skin begins to look slightly yellow or orange—the only adverse effect of beta-carotene—you should then cut back to 75,000 international units. If you have gone up to the maximum safe dose and have stayed there for a month or two, but have seen no results, I would suggest you cut back gradually to a more moderate level. Obviously, large doses do not work in your case, and you should investigate other means of controlling your condition.

Vitamin and mineral supplementation is an ongoing, evolving process. As your body changes with time, your need for supplements may change, too. You might, for instance, want to increase your Optimum Daily Intake of the B-complex vitamins and/or vitamin C during times of illness or extreme stress. Evaluate how you feel; see if any condition you've been treating has improved. Obviously, you want to take the smallest amount needed to correct a particular problem. Why take 75,000 international units of vitamin A if 50,000 or 25,000 works fine, or if you can get similar results with beta-carotene? Generally, you can take a supplement for a specific problem for six months. After that, try lowering the dose. If the condition returns, your body is telling you to return to the higher dose.

## CAN NUTRITIONAL SUPPLEMENTS CAUSE HARM?

Some people are afraid that they will overdose on vitamins, minerals, or other nutritional supplements and cause their bodies harm. Such caveats fall especially from the lips of nutritionally unsophisticated practitioners, and are then passed on to the public by the media. The fact is that only a few vitamins and minerals have *any* known toxicity level. Statistics gathered from the Centers for Disease Control and the National Capitol Poison Control Center over a period of seven years (1983 to 1989) revealed a total of 2,069 reported drug fatalities compared with absolutely *no* vitamin fatalities. These statistics, which appeared in a 1991 issue of the *American Journal of Emergency Medicine*, suggest that vitamins are 2,000 times safer than drugs.

Anything—even pure water—can be harmful if you take enough of it. But vitamins and minerals are among the safest substances on earth. The amounts needed to reach toxic levels are enormous. According to all available studies, none of the ODIs in this book will create any toxicity in a normal adult. By "normal," I mean that you are not on any medication and do not have a medical condition, as these factors can influence your vitamin and mineral requirements, making them higher or lower. I have included some data about these requirements. However, you should consult your physician for specifics if you have any questions.

You may fear that your body will grow dependent on large amounts of vitamins or minerals after a while. There is very little convincing evidence of this. There is some indication that certain individuals who take very high doses of vitamin C and then suddenly stop run the risk of having symptoms of rebound scurvy. While this has not been proven, common sense dictates that it is not wise to stop anything "cold turkey" if you have been ingesting it for a prolonged period of time. This holds true both for drugs—Valid, hormones such as cortisone, and many psychiatric drugs—and for vitamins. If your body has been finely tuned and is accustomed to having an optimal amount of a certain nutrient, it naturally will have to adjust when you change the way you are feeding it.

Therefore, if you want to cut back for any reason, it is logical to "wean" yourself away from supplements gradually. I generally recommend stepping down every two weeks until you reach your desired new level. For instance, many people increase their intake of vitamin C during the cold and flu season. If you have been taking 5,000 milligrams of vitamin C every day during the winter, you may cut down to 4,000 milligrams for two weeks, then to 3,000 milligrams for the next two weeks, then to 2,000 milligrams, and so on.

If you're traveling and want to reduce your dosages because of the inconvenience, it is generally safe to cut your doses in half during this time. Nothing dramatic will happen if you forget to take your vitamins for a day every once in a while, either. Even the water-soluble vitamins remain in the body for about two days, so you do have a margin of safety.

## A GUIDE TO BUYING SUPPLEMENTS

One of the most common questions my patients ask me is: "Should I buy

# Getting the Most From Your Supplementation Plan

- *Never take just one nutritional supplement, or just a select few. An imbalanced program can actually cause deficiencies. Also, nutrients work best when they're part of a balanced regimen.*

- *Divide your doses over the course of the day. This will allow your body to absorb more of each nutrient.*

- *Take your supplements with meals—up to 10 minutes before eating, or up to 30 minutes afterwards. This will both enhance absorption and prevent the indigestion that can occur when supplements are taken on an empty stomach.*

- *Increase or decrease your doses slowly over time.*

- *Buy "natural" supplements—ones that don't contain coal tars, artificial coloring, preservatives, and other additives that are unnecessary or even harmful.*

- *Store your supplements in a cool, dark, dry place, and periodically check the expiration dates to ensure potency.*

'natural' or 'synthetic' vitamins?" As far as I know, there doesn't seem to be much difference between a vitamin found in food and one made in the laboratory. They are essentially the same chemical, made of the same molecules. The fat-soluble vitamins may be the exception: Studies have shown that the naturally occurring form of vitamin E is more absorbable and biologically active than its synthetic counterpart.

However, the word "natural" on the label does not necessarily mean that all the vitamin in the bottle is simply extracted from a natural food source. In fact, most so-called natural vitamins actually contain a large amount of synthetic vitamins. The reason for this is primarily economic: If vitamin C supplements, for example, were derived solely from rose hips, the cost would be enormous.

The term "natural" really refers to the fact that the supplement does not contain other unnatural ingredients. Here, there is a difference. Supplements that are not labeled "natural" may also include coal tars, artificial coloring, preservatives, sugars, starch, and sometimes other additives. This is why I generally recommend "natural" vitamins. Why take potentially harmful substances into the body when you don't have to?

Mineral supplements may be chelated, meaning that they are surrounded by a carrier protein that transports the mineral to the bloodstream in an attempt to enhance absorption. Because studies on the absorbability of the various forms of mineral supplements are rather sparse at this time, I cannot recommend chelated minerals across the board. However, some combinations have been shown to be more absorbable. Unfortunately, they are often more expensive and may not be cost effective. If the difference in price is not enormous, you may prefer to buy chelated minerals for possible enhanced absorption. Keep in mind, though, that if you take supplements with a meal, they are usually automatically chelated in your stomach during digestion.

Some supplements are offered in a time-release formula in an attempt to release the nutrients gradually. While this sounds fine in theory, in practice, it may actually decrease absorption. Studies have shown, for instance, that time-release or sustained release vitamin C does not raise blood levels of vitamin C as effectively as nontime-release supplements. For this reason, I do not generally recommend time-release over regular formulas.

In the following chapters, I have listed the most common forms of supplements available. New and innovative forms are being created all the time in an effort to find a form that is easily absorbed by the body, bioavailable (usable by the body once it has been absorbed), and able to enter the enzyme system more quickly. But without good studies, it's difficult to decide whether these claims are valid. Check with your health food store or your nutritional professional to see if there is any literature about the new forms of any nutrient you are considering taking.

## A GUIDE TO STORING SUPPLEMENTS

Supplements do not last forever; their potency gradually diminishes over a period of time. Unopened, vitamins generally last for two to three years. Opened, they generally last for about one year. Mineral supplements last longer, and usually it is not the minerals themselves that go bad—it is the other substances in the supplement, such as the chelating agents, which spoil. As a safeguard, it's best to buy supplements with an expiration date.

Supplements should be stored in a cool, dry, dark place. The refrigerator usually has a lot of moisture in it, and is quite cold, which could affect certain vitamins, so I don't recommend this as a storage place. Many people keep their supplements on top of the refrigerator; however, this location is generally too warm. A room-temperature closet is usually fine.

Many people transfer their supplements to smaller, more convenient containers for work and travel. If the container is opaque and closes tightly, supplements can be stored in them for several months without losing much of their potency.

# Chapter 5

---

# YOUR TOTAL HEALTH PLAN

T aking supplements does not give you carte blanche to eat and drink anything you want, nor is it a panacea for all your ills. Nutritional supplements are just that—supplements. They work best when they are part of a well-rounded plan for optimum health. Along with your supplements, it is important for you to also eat wholesome foods, get a reasonable amount of exercise, and maintain a healthy, wholesome lifestyle that includes no smoking, a minimum of alcohol and other drugs, and stress management.

## THE BASIC INTELLIGENT DIET

For all their value, nutritional supplements do not take the place of good fresh food. In the first place, you still need a balanced amount of carbohydrates, fats, and proteins—nutrients not found in supplement capsules. In the second place, by eating nutritious foods, you are assured of getting at least some vitamins and minerals in their natural form. This is important, because when nutrients are ingested as part of the food in which they are naturally found, they are generally absorbed and utilized better. Then, by taking supplements along with nutritious foods, you will enhance the absorption of the nutrients contained in the supplements, as well. Taking supplements after eating a bowl of low-fat yogurt mixed with fresh fruit would probably result in better nutrient absorption than would taking them after a snack of potato chips or cookies.

Finally, there is so much we still don't know about the many beneficial components of certain foods. Plants—fruits, vegetables, and herbs—contain an enormous number of compounds, collectively known as phytochemicals (*phyto* means "plant"). Unlike vitamins and minerals, phytochemicals are not classified as essential nutrients; yet they appear to have many benefits. Those which protect against cancer have been the most studied, but there are many other biological actions that may prove helpful as well, and which may or may not be due to antioxidant properties. For instance, genistein, found in soybeans and vegetables in the cabbage family, appears to deter the growth of blood vessels that nourish cancerous tumors. Indoles—substances found in cabbage, Brussels sprouts, and kale—also seem to protect against cancer. Carotenoids, present in the same foods that contain beta-carotene, are antioxidants, and thus protect against many diseases and conditions associated with aging. Quercetin, found in citrus fruits, has antioxidant, antihistamine, and anti-inflammatory activities. Phytosterols, contained in plants such as yams and alfalfa sprouts, play a role in maintaining the hormone balance in the body. We can only guess at the many other undiscovered substances, let alone put them in a pill.

My Basic Intelligent Diet, which I recommend for most of my patients in addition to their Optimum Daily Intake of vitamins and minerals, is high in fiber, low in fat and sugar, and moderate in protein. Below, you will find some dietary guidelines designed to help you choose and prepare the foods on this diet. Following this, you'll find two Daily Food Guides and two sample menus—customized for men and women—that illustrate how these guidelines can be followed to make meals that are wholesome and enjoyable.

### Healthy Eating Guidelines

Eating wisely involves the selection of healthful foods, and the avoidance of foods that are low in nutrients and high in harmful substances like salt and sugar. The following tips should help you choose the best possible foods and prepare them in a way that maximizes their nutritional value.

❑ Avoid processed foods such as white flour.

❑ Eat an abundant amount of brown rice and other whole grains, as well as whole-grain breads and cereals.

❑ Eat whole fresh foods rather than canned, frozen, or commercially prepared foods. Try to use organic foods whenever possible.

❑ Use low-fat or fat-free dairy products, soymilk, rice milk, tofu, or soy cheese.

❑ Minimize your consumption of high-fat meats such as pork, lamb, and beef. If you choose to eat red meat, use leaner cuts. Preferable to beef and pork are white meat chicken and turkey, seafood, and organic eggs.

❑ Use butter and oil very sparingly. Do not use margarine, which contains oil that has been hydrogenated. Hydrogenated vegetable oils contain trans-fatty acids, which may increase low-density lipoproteins (LDLs, often referred to as "bad cholesterol") as much as saturated fats do, and also decrease high-density lipoproteins (HDLs, often referred to as "good cholesterol"), which saturated fats do not do. (For more information on LDLs and HDLs, see the inset "Understanding Cholesterol" on page 32.) Instead, use vegetable or chicken broth or apple juice for sautéing and flavoring dishes.

❏ Minimize your use of salt. Many foods naturally contain some salt, so try not to add any extra. Substitute salt-free spices and herbs such as garlic, ginger, oregano, rosemary, pepper, and lemon juice.

❏ Avoid using sugar. You may substitute honey, maple syrup, or blackstrap molasses, but use these sparingly. Many people consume too much fruit, and consequently too much sugar. Keep in mind that fruit is a major source of sugar, and eat it in moderation.

❏ Minimize your consumption of coffee, tea, sodas, other caffeine- and sugar-containing beverages, and chocolate. Club soda or seltzer, herbal teas, grain-type coffee substitute, and filtered or bottled water are preferable. Natural fruit juices are good, too, but drink them only in moderation. Remember that one glass of natural, unsweetened juice contains the equivalent of three to four fruits. Try mixing juice with salt-free club soda or water to make it less sweet and concentrated.

❏ To preserve as many nutrients as possible, cook food quickly, using a minimum of fat or water. Eat vegetables raw, steamed, or quickly stir-fried in a small amount of oil, apple juice, or vegetable broth.

❏ Eat slowly, and enjoy your food! The slower you eat, the less you eat.

### Daily Food Guides and Menus

The Basic Intelligent Diet is both well-balanced and satisfying, and will help you maintain or achieve a lower, healthier, more attractive level of body fat. Below you will find Daily Food Guides for men and women. Each guide shows exactly how much of each type of food should be eaten each day. For specific menus, see pages 60 and 61.

### *The Daily Food Guide for Women*

The following Daily Food Guide is for women five feet three inches to five feet nine inches tall. If you are over five feet nine inches, add one portion each of vegetables and fiber foods. If you are under five feet three inches, subtract one portion each of vegetables and fiber foods.

❏ 8 ounces of nonfat milk or yogurt, or ½ cup nonfat cottage cheese. (If you have a problem digesting dairy products, substitute soy products such as low-fat or nonfat soymilk, soy yogurt, and tofu, or try rice milk. Do not use nut milks, which are generally high in fat, unless you can find low-fat—1-percent fat—or fat-free products.)

❏ 3 cups of nonstarchy vegetables: lettuce, zucchini, tomatoes, broccoli, cucumber, cabbage, etc.

❑  2 fresh fruits or 1–2 cups of diced fresh fruit.

❑  4–6 fiber food servings. (For fiber food equivalents, see Table 5.1.)

❑  2–3 ounces of lean protein food at each meal: seafood, eggs, fat-free cheese, nonfat yogurt, nonfat milk, chicken, turkey, fat-free or low-fat soy products, or other vegetable-protein products, such as veggie-burgers.

### The Daily Food Guide for Men

The following Daily Food Guide is for men five feet ten inches tall and up. If you are under five feet ten inches tall, subtract one serving each of vegetables and fiber foods.

❑  8 ounces of nonfat milk or yogurt, or ½ cup nonfat cottage cheese. (If you have a problem digesting dairy products, substitute soy products such as low-fat or nonfat soymilk, soy yogurt, and tofu, or try rice milk. Do not use nut milks, which are generally high in fat, unless you can find low-fat—1-percent fat—or fat-free products.)

❑  5 cups of nonstarchy vegetables: lettuce, zucchini, tomatoes, broccoli, etc.

❑  3–4 fresh fruits or 2–3 cups diced fresh fruit.

❑  7–8 fiber food servings. (For Fiber Equivalents, see Table 5.1.)

❑  4–5 ounces of lean protein food at each meal: seafood, eggs, fat-free cheese, nonfat yogurt, nonfat milk, chicken, turkey, fat-free or low-fat soy products, or other vegetable-protein products, such as veggie-burgers.

### Table 5.1. Fiber Food Equivalents

| *One Fiber Food Serving* |
|:---:|
| ½ cup whole-grain pasta, brown rice, or other grain |
| 1 slice whole-grain bread |
| 1 small potato or ear of corn |
| ½ cup low-fat, sugar-free granola |
| ½ cup winter squash |
| ½ yam, sweet potato, or Idaho potato |
| ½ cup cooked peas, beans, or lentils |
| 1 cup puffed rice cereal |
| 1½ tablespoons nut butter, or 20 nuts* |

*Have no more than one serving per day. Omit if you want to reduce body fat.

## The Sample Menus

The following sample menus show you how the Daily Food Guides translate into a typical day's meals. If you are physically active, you may eat more by increasing your intake of nonfat or low-fat protein and high-fiber foods by two to three servings. If butter, oil, or dressings are used, remember to add them only sparingly. I recommend putting the oil in a spray bottle and using only one or two squirts. You may also have additional fruit juice diluted with water or club soda. But don't drink too much juice! Women should not exceed one cup per day, and men should not exceed two cups.

### Sample Menu 1

| Women: 1,200 Calories | Men: 1,800 Calories |
| --- | --- |
| *Breakfast:* | |
| • 1 cup puffed rice cereal | • 1½ cups puffed rice cereal |
| • ½ banana | • 1 banana |
| • ½ cup nonfat milk or yogurt | • 1 cup low-fat milk or yogurt |
| *Lunch:* | |
| • 2–3 cups salad or fresh vegetables | • 3–4 cups salad or fresh vegetables |
| • 3–4 ounces chicken on 2 slices whole wheat bread | • 4–5 ounces chicken on 2 slices whole wheat bread |
| | • 1 cup lentil soup |
| *Dinner:* | |
| • 1½ cups pasta with tomato sauce | • 2 cups pasta with tomato sauce |
| • 3–4 ounces broiled filet of sole | • 4–5 ounces broiled filet of sole |
| • 2–3 cups salad or fresh vegetables | • 3–4 cups salad or fresh vegetables |
| *Snack:* | |
| • ½–1 cup nonfat yogurt | • 1–2 cups low-fat yogurt |
| • 1 medium apple | • 1 medium apple |
| • 1 teaspoon oat bran | • 1 tablespoon oat bran |

**Sample Menu 2**

| Women: 1,200 Calories | Men: 1,800 Calories |
| --- | --- |
| *Breakfast:* | |
| • 2 slices whole wheat bread | • 3 slices whole wheat bread |
| • 3 ounces low-fat cottage cheese | • 4 ounces nonfat soy Jarlsberg cheese |
| • 2 slices tomato | • 3 slices tomato |
| *Lunch:* | |
| • 2–3 cups salad or fresh vegetables | • 3–4 cups salad or fresh vegetables |
| • 3–4 ounces baked fish | • 4–5 ounces baked fish |
| • 1 medium baked potato | • 1 medium baked potato or yam |
| | • 1 ear of corn |
| *Dinner:* | |
| • 3–4 ounces broiled chicken | • 4–5 ounces broiled chicken |
| • 2–3 cups salad or vegetables | • 2 cups salad or vegetables |
| • 1 cup brown rice | • 2 cups brown rice |
| • 1 baked or fresh apple | • 1 baked or fresh apple |
| *Snack:* | |
| • ½–1 cup low-fat cottage cheese | • 1 cup low-fat cottage cheese |
| • 1 medium pear | • 1 medium pear |
| • 1 teaspoon oat bran or wheat germ | • 1 tablespoon oat bran or wheat germ |

## THE EXERCISE PRESCRIPTION

The benefits of exercise are almost endless. Exercise lowers your risk of heart disease, diabetes, osteoporosis, colon cancer, and breast cancer. It enhances energy, helps you handle stress better, and gives you a psychological lift and a general sense of well-being. And it helps you normalize your weight by burning calories, speeding up your metabolism, and controlling appetite. As if these aren't enough reasons to exercise, in 1996, the continuing Aerobics Center Longitudinal Study, designed to examine the effects of different fitness levels, showed that low fitness may actually pose as great a risk to health as smoking, and a *greater* risk than high cholesterol, high blood pressure, and obesity. This report, published in the *Journal of the American Medical Association,* underscores the importance of exercise in a healthy lifestyle.

Aerobic exercise is the best form of activity for your cardiovascular system. It enhances circulation, and exercises your heart, lungs, and major muscles. To reap the greatest rewards from your aerobic exercise sessions, move at an intensity sufficient to raise your heart rate, exercise continuously for at least twenty to thirty minutes, and exercise at least three times a week. Examples of aerobic exercise include brisk walking, jogging; running, stair climbing, bicycling, aerobic dancing, skating, swimming, jumping rope, and rowing or cross-country skiing—either the actual sports or use of a rowing or skiing machine.

For many people, walking is the easiest way to begin and maintain a more active lifestyle. If you are out of shape, start with just five minutes. Then add one minute each week until you can sustain twenty to thirty minutes of continuous walking.

By varying your exercises, you will ensure that you exercise all parts of your body, reduce your chance of injury, and help keep boredom at bay. I recommend that you add at least a light weight-training program to your aerobic sessions to condition and strengthen many different muscle groups. Be sure to also include some stretching exercises, such as yoga, to keep your joints limber and your muscles long and lithe.

At least initially, I suggest that you work with a professional who can design a program for you and make sure you are doing the exercises properly. Most health clubs have such trainers. There are many books and videotapes that can assist you, as well. Also, look for ways to add more activity to your daily life. For instance, whenever possible, walk instead of drive, and take the stairs instead of the elevator.

A word of caution is in order. If you are over thirty-five, have been sedentary for some time, or have any health problems, it is important to consult with your health-care provider before starting any exercise program.

While even a well-rounded diet cannot provide you with everything you need to be at your best, it is a vital first step toward optimal nutrition. Couple it with the proper supplement program and adequate exercise, as well as other wholesome lifestyle choices, and you have the perfect formula for good health.

# Part Two

## THE VITAMINS

# FAT-SOLUBLE VITAMINS

- ❏ Vitamin A and Beta-Carotene
- ❏ Vitamin D
- ❏ Vitamin E
- ❏ Vitamin K

# Chapter 6

# VITAMIN A
# AND BETA-CAROTENE

V itamin A has a number of important functions in the body. It plays an important role in immune system function; it helps protect the body from cardiovascular disease and cancer; it is needed for the growth and maintenance of the skin; and it is essential for the proper function of the eye.

The compounds that form this nutrient fall into two groups: the retinoids (preformed vitamin A), and the carotenoids (precursors of vitamin A that the body converts into active vitamin A). Among the carotenoids is beta-carotene. Originally, researchers began using beta-carotene as a supplement because it is readily converted into vitamin A in the body and, unlike the preformed vitamin, it is nontoxic. Since then, beta-carotene has been found to have its own unique antioxidant actions. While there are several hundred other carotenoids that also have important biological effects, the research we have thus far is based on supplements of vitamin A and beta-carotene.

## FUNCTIONS AND USES

### Infections and Immunity

In many animal studies, vitamin A has been shown to improve resistance to infections, and to be especially useful in preventing both infectious and noninfectious diseases of the respiratory system. In my clinical experience, I have found that vitamin A supplementation is a safe and effective immune system booster. Chronic infections and illnesses can reduce the body's levels of vitamin A, thereby weakening the mucous membranes and making them more susceptible to viral infection. Patients who get frequent sore throats, colds, flu, sinusitis, or bronchitis have experienced a marked decrease in the frequency and severity of these respiratory infections when given optimal amounts of vitamin A. I have also found that vitamin A supplementation is effective in decreasing the symptoms associated with allergic reactions, emphysema, and asthma.

### Cardiovascular Disease

While most of the research on the prevention of coronary heart disease has focused on vitamin E (see Chapter 8), human studies have shown that beta-carotene, as well as other carotenoids, may have various protective and therapeutic effects regarding cardiovascular disease.

Like vitamin E, beta-carotene is incorporated into low-density lipoproteins (LDLs), and may work synergistically with other nutrients, including vitamin A, to prevent LDL oxidation, a major culprit in the development of coronary heart disease.

In the ongoing Physicians' Health Study, Harvard researchers have been studying a total of over 22,000 male physicians over the long term. Ten years into this study, the researchers evaluated a subgroup of 333 men who had histories of cardiovascular disease. The data showed that the physicians in this group who took 50 milligrams (approximately 85,000 international units) of beta-carotene every other day had half as many heart attacks, strokes, and deaths due to heart disease as those who did not take the supplements. The beneficial effects of the supplements did not appear until the second year of the study. Interestingly, the reduction of all aspects of cardiovascular disease appeared to be greater with beta-carotene than with aspirin, which is commonly recommended to prevent heart attacks.

Yet another study conducted in India looked at the effects of a combined antioxidant treatment, including 50,000 international units of vitamin A, 1,000 milligrams of vitamin C, 400 international units of vitamin E, and 25 milligrams of beta-carotene. In this double-blind study, sixty-three patients received the supplements, while sixty-two received the placebo. All subjects were suspected of having acute myocardial infarction (heart attack). The results of this study reveal that such a combined antioxidant treatment in patients with recent heart attacks may be protective against cardiac necrosis (tissue death) and oxidative stress, and could be beneficial in preventing complication and future heart attacks.

### Cancer

There is growing evidence that vitamin A and beta-carotene can provide some protection against certain forms of cancer. In many countries of the world, investigations of dietary intake and blood levels of beta-carotene and vitamin A have generally found that lower levels of the nutrients are associated with an increased incidence of certain cancers, including cancers of the bronchus, mouth, larynx, esophagus, endometrium, bladder, breast, prostate, cervix, colon, rectum, and stomach, as well as melanoma, a deadly form of skin cancer. On the other hand, *increased* levels of beta-carotene and vitamin A have been correlated with a lower risk of cancer, with results including a threefold decrease in lung cancer and an 80-percent decrease in cancer of the cervix. There is also evidence that these nutrients may offer protection from gastrointestinal ulcers. Since people with ulcers are more prone to gastrointestinal cancer, it is possible that this nutrient may also protect against the latter disorder.

Numerous studies have also shown that vitamin A and beta-carotene are useful in the treatment of existing cancers or precancers. Human studies have shown that high doses of vitamin A and beta-carotene supplements can cause a regression of a precancerous condition of the mouth called leukoplakia. Preliminary studies using high-dose vitamin A and/or beta-carotene in the treatment of cervical cancer have also been encouraging. In another study, performed in Italy and published in 1993, 307 patients with lung cancer had the cancerous lesions removed surgically. One group of patients was then given daily doses of 300,000 international units of vitamin A for one year, while the other group received no supplements. After a forty-six-month follow-up, 37 percent of those who took the supplements had a recurrence of the cancer, while 48 percent of the unsupplemented group had a recurrence.

Vitamin A and beta-carotene therapy have also been valuable adjuncts in the treatment of breast cancer. In animal studies, vitamin A has been shown to slow the spread of breast cancer to other parts of the body. In a study of women with breast cancer undergoing chemotherapy, women with higher blood levels of vitamin A responded twice as well to the therapy as did women with lower levels. There are two theories as to why these results were obtained. Vitamin A may have helped protect the women from the toxicity of the drugs, or it may have interacted with the drugs in a way that increased their effectiveness. In another study, Vitamin E and A levels were measured in women with breast cancer who were to undergo chemotherapy. These levels were then compared with those of healthy control subjects. Among the patients with vitamin A levels equal to or higher than those of the control subjects, 83 percent responded favorably to chemotherapy, and none experienced a progression of the cancer. Among patients with vitamin A levels below those of the control subjects, only 36 percent responded favorably to chemotherapy, and 40 percent experienced a progression of the cancer.

Other human studies have shown similar results with other cancers. Scottish researchers reported that patients with melanoma (skin cancer), breast cancer, and bowel cancer all responded better to chemotherapy when their vitamin A levels were higher. In Finland, researchers treated cancer patients with both chemotherapy and a wide variety of vitamin and mineral supplements, including 15,000 to 40,000 international units of vitamin A, and 10,000 to 20,000 international units of beta-carotene. These patients lived longer and suffered fewer side effects than did unsupplemented patients.

In yet another study, one group of patients receiving conventional chemotherapy for metastatic gastric cancer also received antioxidant supplements containing vitamins A and E, while another group received only the chemotherapy. The supplemented group was found to have a significantly better response rate to their treatment and a prolonged survival time when compared with the unsupplemented group. At Cancer Treatment Centers of America's 1995 symposium, "Adjuvant Nutrition in Cancer Treatment," Dr. Jae Ho Kim, Professor of Radiology at Case Western Reserve University, explained that vitamin A works synergistically with chemotherapy and radiation. It appears to make the treatment more selective and, at the same time, it offers some protection against the toxic effects of the therapy.

The co-author of this book, Nancy Bruning, experienced similar results during her cancer treatment. Luckily, Nancy's doctor recommended that she take vitamin A and other supplements during chemotherapy for breast cancer. I find it interesting that her side effects were relatively minor, and that sixteen years after her diagnosis, she has no evidence of cancer.

Since 1994, a debate has raged concerning the use of beta-carotene as a cancer preventive. In that year, a study conducted in Finland obtained negative results when using beta-carotene in long-term smokers. Toward the end of 1995, another study, CARET (Beta-carotene and Retinol Efficacy Trial), reported similar results—that beta-carotene might actually *increase* the risk of lung cancer in long-term smokers, as well as in asbestos workers.

Why were the results of these studies so different from those of previous studies? Some of the issues raised by the scientific community include the fact that the dose of beta-carotene used may have been too low. The CARET study, for instance, used about 55,000 international units of beta-carotene, rather than the 300,000 to 500,000 international units that have met with favorable results in other cancer studies. In addition, most scientists agree that antioxidant nutrients are more effective when taken together, rather than individually. Most important, perhaps, is the finding of the Finnish and CARET studies that was *not* highly publicized—that those individuals who had high beta-carotene intakes prior to the start of the studies were protected against lung cancer.

Studies like the CARET and Finnish studies should not simply be dismissed, since they do raise questions that need to be answered. Nevertheless, there are numerous human studies demonstrating the beneficial effects of beta-carotene on the incidence of oral, lung, and cervical cancers. At this time, the research, on balance, seems to support the merits of beta-carotene not only as a cancer fighter, but also as a powerful weapon against a variety of other disorders.

## Skin

Studies indicate that vitamin A is useful in promoting healthy cell growth, and is vital for healthy skin. As such, it has been found to be an effective means of treating acne. The type of vitamin A prescribed to treat severe forms of acne medically is a synthetic form of vitamin A called *cis-retinoic acid*. This form is available only by prescription, and was developed so that the vitamin could be administered in very high oral doses—200,000 to 300,000 international units—without the level of toxicity that might occur if other active forms of vitamin A were used. Although this treatment is quite successful, there are toxicity problems even with this form of the vitamin. Beta-carotene, however, is nontoxic. When using beta-carotene, I have had excellent results without ever exceeding 100,000 international units per day. I must point out that beta-carotene works even for patients with severe acne that has not improved significantly with medical treatment, including antibiotics. I have also found beta-carotene to be a useful nontoxic treatment for dry skin, eczema, and psoriasis.

In addition to its use in the treatment of a variety of existing skin disorders, beta-carotene appears to offer protection from skin cancer and age-associated damage. Studies show that oral and topical applications of the antioxidants—including beta-carotene—can diminish ultraviolet-light-induced free radical tissue damage, which is implicated in both skin cancer and aging. Researchers working in this field recommend that the products be used daily throughout the year for best protection. When taken orally, 50,000 international units of beta-carotene were found to protect against suppression of immune function caused by exposure to ultraviolet (UV) light. This immune suppression is thought to be a culprit in the development of skin cancers.

## HIV Infection and AIDS

Beta-carotene may also offer hope to people infected with the human immunodeficiency virus (HIV). In a study by Dr. Greg Coodley, HIV-infected patients, many of whom were taking the drug AZT (azidothymidine), were given either 180 milligrams (300,000 international units) per day of beta-carotene or a placebo for four weeks. Then treatments were switched, so that the beta-carotene group received placebos, and vice versa. It was found that CD4 cells and white blood cells—both of which are important for immune function—increased only during beta-carotene supplementation. Considering the immune system-enhancing effect of beta-carotene supplementation, as well as its lack of side effects, there is a possibility that the supplemented patients would not be as susceptible to opportunistic infection as would patients not receiving supplements, and that progression to AIDS (acquired immune deficiency syndrome) would also be delayed.

## Other Functions

Vitamin A is known to be essential for healthy eyes. High dietary and supplemental intake of this nutrient, as well as high plasma levels of beta-carotene, have been associated with a decreased risk of cataracts and macular degeneration, a leading cause of blindness in the elderly.

## RDIs AND CLASSIC DEFICIENCY SYMPTOMS

The traditionally recognized deficiency symptoms of vitamin A are night blindness and other eye problems, skin disorders, suboptimal growth, and reproductive failure. Low-level night blindness is becoming more common in the United States, and in some cases may represent a subclinical deficiency. To prevent these severe deficiencies, the RDI is 5,000 international units for men and women, and 8,000 international units for pregnant and lactating women.

*Food Sources:* Active vitamin A is found only in animal sources. It is especially high in the fish liver oil from cod, halibut, salmon, and shark. It is also found in beef and chicken liver, and in eggs and dairy products. Beta-carotene, the vitamin A precursor, is found only in green and yellow-orange fruits and vegetables, such as carrots, kale, kohlrabi, parsley, spinach, turnip greens, dandelion greens, apricots, and cantaloupe.

When relying on food sources, be aware that vitamin A and beta-carotene can be destroyed by heat; by alkalis such as baking soda, which is sometimes added to cooking vegetables to keep them green; by light; and by air. Because beta-carotene is especially susceptible to oxidation, carrot juice is rich in this substance only if it is consumed directly after pressing.

## SUPPLEMENTS

Studies of the effects of vitamin A and beta-carotene on cancer have correlated a decreased risk of cancer more often with a high beta-carotene intake than with a high intake of the vitamin A in fish liver oil. Since active vitamin A (from fish liver oil) and beta-carotene may have slightly different functions in the body, I recommend that my patients take a combination of beta-carotene and active vitamin A. My clinical experience has shown this combination to be most effective. Palmitate, the synthetic form of vitamin A, is water miscible (water soluble), and is therefore preferable for people who have difficulty absorbing fats.

There are over 400 carotenoids, the best known of which are beta-carotene, lutein, canthaxanthin, zeaxanthin, lycopene, alpha-carotene, and cryptoxanthin. Although not all of them have vitamin A activity, many have powerful antioxidant properties and specific anticancer and cardiovascular-protective effects. Therefore, I now recommend a natural beta-carotene supplement with mixed carotenoids.

## OPTIMUM DAILY INTAKE—ODI

For optimum general health, the basic Optimum Daily Intake for vitamin A (at least half of which should be in the form of beta-carotene) is:

### 5,000–50,000 IU for men and women

Vitamin A is always measured in terms of international units (IU). Beta-carotene may be measured in terms of milligrams (mg) or international units. For simplicity's sake, in this book we use only international units.

Based on a thorough scientific review of Vitamin A and beta-carotene, and on my clinical experience, the following amounts of vitamin A and beta-carotene appear to be valuable for:

| Condition | Suggested Dosage* Vitamin A | Suggested Dosage* Beta-Carotene |
|---|---|---|
| Acne, eczema, psoriasis | 10,000–50,000 IU | 50,000–200,000 IU |
| Cancer prevention | 10,000–50,000 IU | 100,000–200,000 IU |
| Dry skin | 10,000–25,000 IU | 25,000–50,000 IU |
| Enhancing immunity | 10,000–25,000 IU | 50,000–100,000 IU |
| Gastrointestinal ulcers | 10,000–50,000 IU | 25,000–50,000 IU |
| HIV/AIDS | 5,000–25,000 IU | 300,000–500,000 IU |
| Polluted air | 5,000–25,000 IU | 25,000–50,000 IU |
| Respiratory problems: allergies, asthma, bronchitis, emphysema, sinusitis | 15,000–50,000 IU | 100,000–200,000 IU |

*Note that for each condition, you can use the lowest listed amount of vitamin A and the highest listed amount of beta-carotene, as I generally do, with excellent results.

*Remember:* If you have a medical condition, please consult with your physician before taking supplements. If you are pregnant or lactating, do not exceed 8,000 international units of vitamin A per day, as vitamin A may cause birth defects or be toxic to the infant.

## TOXICITY AND ADVERSE EFFECTS

All forms of active vitamin A—both fat- and water-soluble—are stored in the liver. This supplement can, therefore, be toxic in large amounts. In general, a normal healthy adult must take at least 100,000 IU of vitamin A daily for a period of months in order to display any signs of toxicity. Early signs of toxicity are fatigue, nausea, vomiting, headache, vertigo, blurred vision, muscular incoordination, and loss of body hair. Although all of these symptoms are reversible when vitamin A supplementation is stopped, I would not recommend this dose unless you are under professional guidance.

Beta-carotene, on the other hand, can be given for long periods of time virtually without risk of toxicity. Since beta-carotene is a naturally occurring pigment, the only adverse effect of taking too much beta-carotene is the possibility of *carotenemia*, a harmless condition in which the skin turns a slight orange color. This is a signal that the body has converted as much beta-carotene to active A as it can, leaving the excess as an orange-yellow pigment. I often tell my patients that if they get carotenemia, they can cut back on their beta-carotene intake. On the other hand, such pigments are often given to sun-sensitive individuals, since the tinting of the skin affords some additional protection against sunburn. Carotene preparations are also used by some people for a cosmetic effect. The slight tint looks like a suntan, and also allows them to tan more easily and keep the tan longer. And, as we have seen, high levels of carotenoids may also be protective against skin cancer.

# Chapter 7

# VITAMIN D

Vitamin D is not truly a vitamin for two reasons. First, our bodies can make it upon exposure to sunlight. Second, in its active form, it is considered to be a hormone. Specifically, it has hormone-like effects on mineral absorption, bone mineralization, and some secretions.

## FUNCTIONS AND USES

Because of vitamin D's role in mineral absorption and bone mineralization, it is an extremely important vitamin in maintaining bone density. While this is vitamin D's best-known function, studies have revealed other possible roles that vitamin D might play. For example, vitamin D combined with calcium has been found to possess anticancer properties. In some people, low levels of vitamin D may increase blood pressure, suggesting that therapeutic levels may help regulate it. Vitamin D has also been found to play a role in the treatment of some immunological disorders such as multiple sclerosis and psoriasis. In addition, vitamin D has been found to improve psoriasis, as well as to affect biological rhythms, mood, and behavior. It may also improve muscle strength.

## RDIs AND CLASSIC DEFICIENCY SYMPTOMS

In children, rickets is the classic deficiency disease of this vitamin. The symptoms of rickets include stunted growth, delayed tooth development, weakness, softened skull (in infants), and irreversible bone deformities.

In adults, *hypocalcemia* (low level of calcium in the bloodstream), *osteomalacia* (reduction of the mineral content of the bone), and *osteoporosis* (reduction in total bone mass) are associated with vitamin D deficiencies. Thinning bones that fracture easily—a classic sign of osteoporosis—have recently been recognized as a growing problem in postmenopausal women, whose hormone production has changed from its premenopausal state. (Men can suffer, too, but are usually protected against bone loss by their higher testosterone levels.)

Additionally, women with a history of vitamin D deficiency may have irregularities in the pelvic bones, making it difficult to give birth. Calcium and magnesium, as well as other minerals and vitamins, should be taken along with vitamin D for these conditions, as these nutrients all work hand in hand in the body to form and maintain bone mass. In fact, when calcium supplements are taken alone—without vitamin D or other minerals—by postmenopausal women, the rate of bone loss is only slowed. The same is true of estrogen-replacement therapy.

The RDI for vitamin D is 400 international units. Surprisingly, the amount generally agreed upon by most professionals is 400 international units per day.

*Food Sources:* Foods are generally low in this vitamin. The richest sources of vitamin D are fish liver oils and fatty saltwater fish such as sea bass, halibut, swordfish, herring, tuna, cod, and sable. Because milk is usually fortified with vitamin D, milk and dairy products are also a good source of this vitamin.

### SUPPLEMENTS

There are two forms of vitamin D: Vitamin $D_2$ (ergocalciferol) and $D_3$ (chole-calciferol). Vitamin $D_3$ is the preferred form, since it is the naturally occurring form. But both $D_3$ and $D_2$ become the active hormone vitamin D after passing through the liver and kidney. Special "active" forms are available by prescription for patients who have a chronic liver or kidney disease that may impair their ability to convert the vitamin to its active form.

### OPTIMUM DAILY INTAKE—ODI

For optimum general health, the basic Optimum Daily Intake for vitamin D is:

### 400–800 IU for men and women

Based on a thorough scientific review of vitamin D, and on my clinical experience, the following amounts of vitamin D appear to be valuable for:

| Condition | Suggested Dosage |
|---|---|
| High blood pressure | 400–800 IU |
| Osteoporosis | 400–800 IU |

Lifestyle, skin color, degree of air pollution, and geographical latitude all affect the degree of exposure to the sun, and therefore the amount of vitamin D that can be made by the body. It is also questionable whether any vitamin

D is synthesized during the winter months, and whether the body's stores of this vitamin are able to meet the daily requirements during this period. Therefore, if you rarely spend time in the sun, have dark skin, live in the northern latitudes, avoid fortified dairy products, or have liver or kidney disease, you may be marginally deficient in this vitamin.

Recent research indicates that elderly people, also, may be at high risk for vitamin D deficiency. Anyone with osteoporosis who has not responded to calcium supplementation may be advised to add moderate vitamin D and magnesium supplementation to his or her regimen, and to increase sunlight exposure. One study suggested that elderly women may actually require 600 to 800 international units, rather than 400 international units, per day. Most patients with Crohn's disease have low levels of vitamin D, and should be supplemented with this nutrient to prevent osteomalacia.

*Remember:* If you have a medical condition, please consult your physician before taking supplements.

## TOXICITY AND ADVERSE EFFECTS

According to several studies, amounts of up to 1,000 international units per day of vitamin D appear to be safe for adults. Both the beneficial and adverse effects of exceeding this amount are controversial. Symptoms of too much vitamin D are nausea, loss of appetite, headache, diarrhea, fatigue, and restlessness. Mild cases of hypervitaminosis—a condition caused by vitamin overdose—are treatable. However, doses of more than 1,000 international units can cause hypercalcemia (high levels of calcium in the blood). This can lead to calcium deposits in soft tissues, such as those of the kidneys, heart, lungs, and vascular system—deposits that may be irreversible.

There is evidence that the synthetic active forms of vitamin D, available by prescription, may be a better treatment in individuals with malabsorption since smaller doses can be used, thus decreasing the risk of toxicity. These forms also act much more quickly to reverse deficiency symptoms.

# Chapter 8

# VITAMIN E

Next to vitamin C, vitamin E is America's most popular vitamin supplement. And its popularity seems well deserved, as recent studies suggest that this nutrient plays a vital role in the prevention of aging-related degenerative diseases, such as cancer and cardiovascular disease. In addition, vitamin E plays other important roles in the body. By some estimates, if we all took adequate vitamin E supplements, we could reduce our health-care costs by $8 billion.

## FUNCTIONS AND USES

### Vitamin E's Antioxidant Powers

Studies indicate that Vitamin E may slow the aging process and prevent premature aging by prolonging the useful life of our cells, thus maintaining the function of our organs. For example, it has been shown that the red blood cells of healthy people who receive vitamin E supplements age far less than do the red blood cells of those who receive no supplements. Human cells grown in a medium enriched with extra amounts of vitamin E divided and lived much longer than did cells grown in ordinary culture mediums. Further studies are needed, but the results of such experiments do indicate exciting possibilities.

What holds true for the cells in these experiments may hold true for other cells of the body, since vitamin E is utilized by practically all of our tissues. The bulk of it is stored in the muscles and fat tissue, but the highest concentrations are found in the pituitary gland, adrenal gland, and testes. In animal studies, vitamin E deficiency has been implicated in widely diverse conditions, including cataracts, muscular and neuromuscular disease, and the weakening of the cells of the lungs, liver, heart, and blood. In some studies, a deficiency of this nutrient also caused testicular degeneration and sterility in animals—a fact that resulted in vitamin E's reputed powers to improve your sex life.

Much of vitamin E's usefulness seems to stem from its role as a powerful antioxidant and anticarcinogen. (For more information on antioxidants, see

Chapter 3.) There is a large body of evidence to support both this role and the synergy of vitamin E with selenium, another antioxidant. Part of vitamin E's benefits may be due to its ability to protect vitamins A and C from oxidation, thus keeping them potent. In addition, vitamin E helps to increase the body's level of superoxide dismutase, an enzyme that, like vitamin E itself, is a powerful free radical scavenger. Vitamin E is also able to prevent the rancidity caused by the oxidation of polyunsaturated fats (PUFA), and thus prevent the free radical damage that can result from ingesting these fats.

Because of its antioxidant capabilities, vitamin E helps protect the body from mercury, lead, carbon tetrachloride, benzene, ozone, nitrous oxide, and a variety of other carcinogens and toxins that bring about harm through their ability to act as free radicals. Similarly, vitamin E has been shown to prevent the formation of nitrosamines from nitrites and nitrates found in cured meats, cigarette smoke, and polluted air.

### Cancer

Over fifty human studies have been conducted on the role of vitamins in the prevention of cancer. These studies showed that vitamin E appears to protect us from lung, esophageal, and colorectal cancer, and possibly from cancer of the cervix and breast, as well. Animal studies indicate that the vitamin may protect against additional cancers, too. When vitamin E was given to animals who were exposed to potent carcinogens, it was found that the supplement reduced the incidence of cancer of the skin, mouth, colon, and breast. Additionally, topical vitamin E has been shown to protect the skin of animals against free radical damage caused by ultraviolet (UV) light.

Evidence indicates that vitamin E is also useful in the treatment of existing cancers. In animal studies, vitamin E has enhanced the ability of radiation treatments to shrink implanted cancerous tumors. In human studies, when vitamin E was given to cancer patients, the supplement appeared to protect normal cells from the damaging effects of chemotherapy drugs without protecting the cancer cells. Thus, it reduced some of the drugs' side effects without reducing their effectiveness.

### Cardiovascular Disease

Although studies examining the effects of vitamin E on circulation remain inconclusive and conflicting, this research has nevertheless yielded tantalizing results. These studies aside, practitioners, myself included, have found that vitamin E does improve blood flow to the extremities. Some practitioners have reported positive results in treating circulatory problems such as angina, arteriosclerosis, and thrombophlebitis. Others have reported that supplementation helps relieve intermittent claudication—leg weakness and pain caused by poor circulation. This condition is often found in the elderly, and is usually treated with drugs that thin the blood and widen the blood vessels to encourage normal blood flow. Vitamin E appears to relieve the condition through the same mechanisms, without the accompanying side effects.

Some data indicates that vitamin E has the ability to increase the level of high-density lipoproteins (HDLs, the "good" cholesterol) in men and women with initially low levels of this substance. HDL is a substance recently discovered to be very protective against heart disease. (For more information about cholesterol, see page 32.) Some studies have also shown that vitamin E lowers cholesterol levels in the blood. In several studies, it was suggested that vitamin E plays an important role in the metabolism of fats in the arterial wall.

Early studies linking vitamin E with possible heart disease prevention were often conflicting or inconclusive. Then, in 1993, two large-scale Harvard studies hit the scientific community like a bombshell. The Nurses' Health Study followed 87,000 female nurses for eight years, during which subjects regularly filled out questionnaires about their lifestyles and diets. After adjusting for factors such as age and the use of other antioxidant vitamins, researchers found that women who had the highest intake of vitamin E—most of which was attributable to supplements—had a 36-percent lower risk of major coronary disease than did those with the lowest intake. Only women who took the supplements for at least two years showed any benefit.

The similarly designed Physicians' Health Study followed 22,000 male physicians for four years. Researchers found that men who consumed at least 100 international units of vitamin E for at least two years enjoyed a 40-percent reduction in risk of heart disease. These benefits occurred even when blood cholesterol levels did not change. It is interesting to note that the greatest protective effects were found in people who consumed between 100 and 249 international units of vitamin E per day, an amount impossible to get from food alone.

Another landmark study, from the Center of Human Nutrition of the University of Texas Southwestern Medical Center, gave subjects either 60, 200, 400, 800, or 12,000 international units of vitamin E over the course of eight weeks. Researchers found that only those groups of subjects who received at least 400 international units of vitamin E per day experienced a decrease in the susceptibility of LDL cholesterol to oxidation from free radicals.

These studies have strengthened the conviction of physicians who believe that there is ample evidence supporting the use of vitamin E supplements in the prevention of heart disease. However, many physicians are still reluctant to recommend supplementation to the general public, even though a growing number of practitioners are supplementing their own diets with vitamin E. There have been numerous editorials concerning this dichotomy.

Yet another study concerning coronary disease also showed the benefits of vitamin E supplementation. In this 1987 study, vitamin E supplementation was found to minimize the tendency of blood platelets to stick together (aggregate) in women taking oral contraceptives. This was an important finding, since stroke, which can result from platelet aggregation, is a disturbing side effect of taking the pill.

## Wound Healing

Vitamin E may also play a role in the healing of wounds and the reduction of scar formation. Several studies have been performed to date, and many practitioners, myself included, recommend the topical application of vitamin E for these purposes. Some physicians prescribe oral vitamin E to lessen the risk of internal scar formation in women who have had breast implants following surgery for breast cancer. This is significant, as scar formation may lead to the hardening of the implants. Other practitioners recommend puncturing vitamin E capsules and applying the oil topically to any injury *after a scab has formed* to promote healing and reduce scarring.

## The Immune System

Animal studies have clearly shown that excesses of vitamin E enhance resistance to disease, and many human studies support these findings. Two studies of people with the autoimmune disease discoid lupus erythematosus showed that large doses of vitamin E had a beneficial effect, and some subjects experienced a complete clearing of symptoms. Patients suffering from rheumatoid arthritis, another autoimmune disease, have also benefited from vitamin E supplementation. In a study of seven patients who were given vitamin E and selenium along with their usual treatment, which was no longer effective, joint pain either diminished or disappeared completely.

## The Nervous System

Vitamin E may also be important for normal functioning of the nervous system. Certain children with progressive neuromuscular disease were shown to have a vitamin E deficiency. Their symptoms—which included difficulty walking, frequent falling, and abnormal reflexes—improved after vitamin E supplementation. Studies have also shown promising results in slowing neurological problems in older patients, in preventing these problems in children, and in treating Parkinson's disease.

## Women's Health

Some studies have shown that vitamin E helps lessen fibrocystic breast disease—benign lumps in the breast. In one study, 85 percent of the supplemented group responded to treatment, with a total disappearance of cysts and tenderness in 38 percent of the patients. My patients with fibrocystic disease have responded beautifully when vitamin E supplements were included in their health program.

Vitamin E also helps alleviate the symptoms associated with premenstrual syndrome (PMS). Many of my female patients have enjoyed marked improvement in their PMS symptoms in as short a period of time as two months. Studies also indicate that vitamin E supplementation may be useful for treating excess bleeding due to insertion of an intrauterine device. Many practicioners, myself included, have also had excellent results using vitamin E supplementation to reduce the incidence of "hot flashes" in menopausal women.

## Other Uses

New functions and uses of vitamin E are being discovered all the time. In two studies, vitamin E has been shown to reduce the need for insulin in diabetes by improving insulin function and reducing the oxidative stress that leads to many of the side effects of diabetes, including vascular disease and atherosclerosis. Vitamin E, along with vitamin C and beta-carotene, may also protect against cataracts. A 1991 study of 350 men and women found that people who took daily supplements of more than 400 international units of vitamin E per day had less than half the risk of developing cataracts than did people who took no supplements. Finally, there is some evidence that vitamin E may be helpful in the treatment of lipofuscin—"age" or "liver" spots.

## RDIs AND CLASSIC DEFICIENCY SYMPTOMS

Classic vitamin E deficiency symptoms include anemia caused by the premature aging and death of red blood cells, neurological disturbances such as difficulty in walking, and fragile capillaries. These symptoms generally appear only when there is the severe fat malabsorption that occurs in premature infants, or in people with disorders of the pancreas, tropical sprue, celiac disease, and cystic fibrosis. Vitamin E-deficient premature infants may also suffer from disorders of the retina, which can lead to blindness. The RDI to prevent these overt deficiencies is approximately 30 international units for men and women.

New data suggests that many people without severe fat malabsorption problems are at risk for prolonged marginal vitamin E intake, which may influence aging, cancer, and heart disease. In recent years, we've all been told to reduce our consumption of saturated fats, such as butter, and to increase our consumption of polyunsaturated fats, such as vegetable oil and margarine. This increase in PUFA is supposed to reduce the risk of coronary disease, but it also increases our need for protective vitamin E. Since the vegetable oils that are high in PUFA are also naturally high in protective vitamin E, this would seem to pose no problem. However, *most of the commercial polyunsaturated oils are so highly processed, there is very little vitamin E left.* So while we are increasing our PUFA consumption, we are not correspondingly increasing our intake of vitamin E, a situation that has many implications. For example, some studies have suggested that people who ingest high amounts of processed polyunsaturated vegetable oils with inadequate amounts of vitamin E may have a higher risk of cancer in general, and of breast cancer in particular.

*Food Sources:* Vitamin E generally occurs in the fats of vegetable foods. Natural (unprocessed) vegetable oils are a particularly rich source of vitamin E, with cottonseed, corn, soybean, safflower, and wheat germ oil having the highest concentrations. Smaller amounts of vitamin E are found in whole grains, dark green leafy vegetables, nuts, and legumes. Animal foods, such as meat and dairy products, have some vitamin E, but generally are low in this nutrient.

Cooking and processing cause foods to lose their vitamin E, since it is destroyed by heat, alkalis, light, air, and freezing. The milling of grains, for example, causes a loss of about 80 percent of the grain's vitamin E. As mentioned earlier, commercially processed vegetable oils are also low in vitamin E. In fact, the by-products of processed oils have become important sources for the production of vitamin E supplements! If you depend on vegetable oils for your vitamin E, choose cold-pressed or unrefined oils.

## SUPPLEMENTS

Vitamin E actually consists of eight substances, of which alpha-, beta-, delta-, and gamma-tocopherol are the most active. There are natural and synthetic forms of all the tocopherols. The naturally occurring form of vitamin E is the "D" form, as in D-alpha tocopherol. The synthetic form is the "DL" form, as in D,L-alpha tocopherol, which contains only a small proportion of natural vitamin E. The natural form appears to be the most absorbable, and recent studies indicate that it is also the most potent (bioavailable). A supplement containing D,L tocopherol supplies only an eighth to a half of the bioavailable vitamin E found in a comparable natural supplement.

Vitamin E supplements often contain alpha-tocopherols alone, because that has been shown to be the most active form. However, many nutritionists recommend that you buy your tocopherols "mixed," since that is how they exist in food.

Vitamin E succinate is a synthetic vitamin that comes in a dry, oil-free powder. Since it is the water miscible (water soluble) form of vitamin E, it can be tolerated by people who have a problem with fat malabsorption. Vitamin

E is measured in either international units (IU) or milligrams (mg). One milligram is equal to approximately 1.5 international units.

## OPTIMUM DAILY INTAKE—ODI

For optimum general health, the basic Optimum Daily Intake for vitamin E is:

400–1,200 IU for men and women

Based on a thorough scientific review of vitamin E, and on my clinical experience, the following amounts of vitamin E appear to be valuable for:

| Condition | Suggested Dosage |
| --- | --- |
| Aging | 400–800 IU |
| Cancer prevention | 400–800 IU |
| Cardiovascular disease prevention | 400–800 IU |
| Diabetes | 800–1,200 IU |
| Fibrocystic breast disease | 400–1,200 IU |
| Menopausal "hot flashes" | 400–1,200 IU |
| Poor circulation | 600–1,200 IU |
| Premenstrual syndrome | 400–1,200 IU |
| Prevention of excessive bleeding with IUDs | 100–400 IU |
| Wound healing | 400–800 IU |

*Remember:* If you have a medical condition, please consult your physician before taking supplements.

*Warning:* If you have high blood pressure, you should not take large amounts of vitamin E (over 400 international units) unless you are being monitored by a professional. At the onset of vitamin therapy, blood pressure may actually rise temporarily. In addition, you should start with a low dose of 200 international units and increase it gradually. If you are on anticoagulants, do not take large amounts of vitamin E (above 400 international units) without professional supervision.

## TOXICITY AND ADVERSE EFFECTS

There is no well-documented toxicity of vitamin E in doses of 800 to 1,200 international units per day. However, with *very* high doses—over 1,200 international units per day—some adverse effects, such as nausea, flatulence, diarrhea, headache, heart palpitations, and fainting, have been reported. These are completely reversible upon reduction of the dose. For greatest safety, begin with a lower dose of vitamin E, and increase the dose gradually to minimize the possibility of adverse effects.

# Chapter 9

# VITAMIN K

Vitamin K is found in food, but is also created by the bacteria in our intestines. For this reason, vitamin K is not strictly considered a vitamin.

## FUNCTIONS AND USES

### Blood Clotting

Vitamin K's most important function is the role it plays in the production of coagulation (blood-clotting) factors in the body. It is required to make a substance called prothrombin, which is then converted to thrombin. Thrombin, in turn, converts fibrinogen to fibrin, which then creates the blood clot. (By the way, many rodent poisons work by counteracting vitamin K, and thus causing the rodents to bleed to death.)

### Other Uses

Recent studies have revealed other possible roles for vitamin K. For example, low levels of vitamin K may be related to the development of osteoporosis (loss of bone density), and may also adversely affect behavior. Anticoagulant drugs have been shown to reduce the metastasis (spread) of cancer, improving the survival of cancer patients. Since vitamin K is involved in coagulation, one would think it might be contraindicated in cancer patients. However, vitamin K not only has unique antineoplastic (anti tumor growth) properties when used alone, but also augments patient survival when used in conjunction with radiation therapy. Paradoxically, vitamin K also increases the antimetastatic capacity of anticoagulant therapy.

## RDIs AND DEFICIENCIES

Since vitamin K is easily obtained from the diet and synthesized in the body, deficiencies are rare, and usually occur only when there is malabsorption due to bowel obstruction, sprue, bowel shunts, regional ileitis, ulcerative colitis, or chronic liver disease. Vitamin K is given prophylactically to infants at birth to prevent hemorrhage, and presurgically to people who have bleeding and clotting disorders. The RDI for vitamin K is 80 micrograms for men and women.

*Food Sources:* Vitamin K is found in a wide range of foods, with the highest amounts found in spinach, turnip greens, broccoli, green cabbage, tomatoes, and liver. Smaller amounts are found in egg yolks, whole wheat, fruits, cheese, ham, and beef.

## SUPPLEMENTS

Vitamin K is a general term used to describe a group of similar compounds, including $K_1$, which is found in foods; $K_2$, which is made by our intestinal bacteria; and $K_3$, a synthetic form that is available only by prescription. Since vitamin K is widely available in foods and made in our bodies, supplements are necessary only in cases of malabsorption or medical disorders, or at birth to prevent hemorrhaging in newborns.

## OPTIMUM DAILY INTAKE—ODI

The ODI for vitamin K is the same as the RDI:

$$80 \text{ mcg for and women}$$

*Remember:* If you have a medical condition, please consult with your physician before taking supplements, especially if you are on anticoagulant therapy.

## TOXICITY AND ADVERSE EFFECTS

Only the $K_3$ form of vitamin K—the synthetic form—is known to have any degree of toxicity. The major symptom of vitamin K overdose is hemolytic anemia, in which the red blood cells die more quickly than the body can replace them.

# WATER-SOLUBLE VITAMINS

❏ Vitamin B Complex
❏ Vitamin C

# Chapter 10

# Vitamin B Complex

The vitamins that belong in the B-complex group are $B_1$ (thiamin), $B_2$ (riboflavin), $B_3$ (niacin and niacinamide), $B_6$ (pyridoxine), $B_{12}$ (cobalamin), folic acid, pantothenic acid, biotin, choline, inositol, and PABA (para-aminobenzoic acid). Although each B vitamin has its own unique biological role to play and its own individual properties, as a group, these nutrients have so much in common that they are often thought of as a single entity. In addition, the B vitamins work together in the body, and many of them are found in the same foods.

This chapter will give you an overview of the group of vitamins known as B complex. It will provide you with a general understanding of their uses, sources, RDIs, and ODIs. The following chapters will then deal with each B vitamin individually.

## FUNCTIONS AND USES

The B vitamins are utilized as coenzymes—components of enzymes—in almost all parts of the body. They are essential for maintaining healthy nerves, skin, hair, eyes, liver, and mouth; and for preserving good muscle tone in the gastrointestinal tract. The B vitamins also give us energy, as they are necessary for the metabolism of carbohydrates, fats, and proteins.

Research is always finding new functions of the B vitamins, as well as more clinical uses for B-vitamin supplementation. For example, the B complex's well-documented role in nervous system function has led many practitioners to use high doses to alleviate psychiatric symptoms such as mild depression, anxiety, nervousness, and poor memory. Additionally, specific vitamin B deficiencies have been found to be associated with psychiatric disorders such as schizophrenia, depression, delirium, and anxiety. In many cases, when B vitamin doses moderately above the RDAs were used to correct these deficiencies, the symptoms disappeared. In some instances, practitioners of orthomolecular medicine, such as Dr. Abram Hoffer, treated schizophrenia and other psychiatric disorders with B vitamins in ranges far above the RDA. This, too, resulted in many positive case reports. Considering the low toxicity of even high B-complex doses, supplementation certainly seems worth a try.

Although the B vitamins are not antiaging nutrients per se, they are involved in preventing a variety of aging-related problems. B vitamins have also been linked with stress of many kinds. When you are under emotional stress; when you undergo surgery; and when you are sick, pregnant, or breastfeeding, your requirements for the B vitamins automatically increase. And yet it is a far from common practice to give hospital patients even RDI-level doses of the B vitamins—or of any other vitamins, for that matter. Nor is it common practice to give such supplements to elderly nursing-home patients, who are known to be at risk for nutrient deficiencies.

The B vitamins may also play a role in supporting your immune system. According to animal studies, all of the B vitamins enhance the immune system in some way when given in excess of the RDI. This is not because B vitamins themselves make white blood cells or antibodies, but because they are part of the enzymes that make these components of our immune system.

Considerable recent research has focused on the use of vitamins $B_6$, $B_{12}$, and folic acid in the treatment of homocysteinemia, a condition in which there are elevated amounts of the amino acid homocysteine in the blood. This disorder, which is sometimes found in the elderly due to deficiencies of these vitamins, is a risk factor for stroke. A similar condition, homocystinuria, is a hereditary disorder of metabolism that, if untreated, can cause death in late childhood or early adolescence. Again, high-dose therapy with vitamins $B_6$, $B_{12}$, and folic acid is being used to treat this condition.

## RDIs AND DEFICIENCY SYMPTOMS

The classically recognized deficiency diseases of the individual B vitamins include beriberi (thiamin) and pellagra (niacin). However, deficiency in a single B vitamin is rare; rather, people tend to have multiple deficiencies, making subtle deficiency symptoms more difficult to diagnose, yet more likely to be present. Researchers have found that activity originally attributed to individual B vitamins actually seems to depend on several vitamins acting in concert. The RDIs for the B vitamins vary (see the following chapters), but in general are quite low—around 2 milligrams each, or less.

*Food Sources:* The B vitamins are most plentiful in whole grains such as wheat, rice, oats, and rye; and in liver. They are also found in green leafy vegetables, meats, poultry, fish, eggs, nuts, and beans. Most of the B vitamins—and many other nutrients, as well—are removed when grains are highly refined. Although such products may have gone through the so-called "enrichment" process, this replaces only a few nutrients, leaving what was a nicely balanced source of B-complex vitamins sadly lacking.

## SUPPLEMENTS

B complex is widely available as a supplement. Individual supplements of each B vitamin are also available. Brewer's yeast is a low-potency food supplement for a variety of B vitamins.

## OPTIMUM DAILY INTAKE—ODI

As you will see from the chapters on the individual B vitamins, the approximate basic Optimum Daily Intake for B complex is:

50–300 mg in men and women
(and 25–300 mcg for $B_{12}$, folic acid, and biotin)

The entire B complex is generally available in B-complex supplements and multivitamin formulas. If you buy a "B complex 50," for example, it usually contains 50 milligrams of all the B vitamins measured in milligrams ($B_1$, $B_2$, $B_3$, $B_6$, choline, inositol, and PABA), and 50 micrograms of all those measured in micrograms ($B_{12}$, folic acid, and biotin).

There are many physicians and other practitioners who prescribe as much as 2,000 milligrams (or micrograms) of a B vitamin. However, it is not recommended that you take this amount without professional supervision. And if you have a medical condition, it is not recommended that you take any amount without consulting your physician.

The ratio of one B vitamin to another in supplements is generally 1:1. *Never take high doses of a single B vitamin without increasing the amount you take of all the others.* This is an important rule not just because the B vitamins tend to work together, but also because B vitamins compete in the intestines for absorption by the body. Thus, if you take an enormous amount of $B_1$, for instance, you might decrease the amount of $B_3$ being absorbed, and, ironically, wind up with a B-vitamin imbalance. Many well-meaning but insufficiently educated professionals mistakenly prescribe supplements of a single member of the B-vitamin complex. For example, professionals have often prescribed $B_6$ for carpal tunnel syndrome. In my opinion, some of the side effects ascribed to $B_6$ supplementation (see Chapter 14) may be due to the fact that other B vitamins were not given along with the $B_6$. This seems especially likely when massive doses of $B_6$—2,000 milligrams or more—have been taken.

To simplify matters, many people buy a B-complex or multivitamin supplement that contains all the B vitamins. Once you have established your basic ODI of the B vitamins, you can then add additional amounts of one or two individual B vitamins to suit your particular needs. In general, it is safe to take up to about two to three times the amount of the other B's you are taking. For instance, if you take 100 milligrams of the entire B complex, you can then safely take a total of up to 200 to 300 milligrams of vitamin $B_6$.

## TOXICITY AND ADVERSE EFFECTS

In general, no toxicity of the B vitamins has been reported.

# Chapter 11

# VITAMIN B₁ (THIAMIN)

Vitamin $B_1$, also known as thiamin, was the first B vitamin to be discovered, having been first isolated in the 1920s. Today we know that this nutrient has several important functions that contribute to good health.

## FUNCTIONS AND USES

Vitamin $B_1$ plays an essential role in the metabolism of carbohydrates, a major source of energy in our cells. This probably explains why the cells of the brain and the nervous system—which are extremely sensitive to carbohydrate metabolism—are the first to show signs of thiamin deficiency. Thiamin is also involved in converting fatty acids into steroid hormones such as cortisone and progesterone. It is also necessary for proper growth and for the maintenance of healthy skin. Finally, there is some indication that thiamin, like all the B vitamins, plays a role in our resistance to disease.

Since thiamin is needed as a catalyst in the burning of carbohydrates, it should come as no surprise that if you increase your daily intake of either complex or simple carbohydrates, your need for thiamin increases, as the extra carbohydrates utilize more $B_1$. This affects both junk-food junkies and health-conscious people who have switched to high complex-carbohydrate diets. In fact, in one study, 28 percent of the subjects were deficient in thiamin, although they did not show classic symptoms of thiamin deficiency. The authors commented that this subclinical condition may be due to the placement of excess stress on the metabolism by a high-carbohydrate diet.

Thiamin requirements also rise during periods of increased metabolism, including times of fever, muscular activity, an overactive thyroid, pregnancy, and lactation, as well as during all forms of physical or emotional stress. In one study, surgical patients showed a significant fall in their thiamin levels forty-eight hours after surgery, indicating a higher rate of use. Oral contraceptives have been found to lower body levels of thiamin, too. Kidney patients undergoing long-term dialysis and patients being fed intravenously are also at risk of becoming thiamin deficient. Moreover, the consumption of large amounts of tea and coffee—whether decaffeinated or not—hinders thiamin absorption, and therefore also increases the risk of deficiency. In fact, it is believed that many heavy tea and coffee drinkers have symptoms of nervous disorders associated with thiamin deficiency, but either have been misdiagnosed or have failed to seek medical help. Other foods with antithiamin activity are blueberries, red chicory, black currants, Brussels sprouts, red cabbage, and raw seafood. (Ascorbic acid, however, has been shown to protect against thiamin destruction in some of these foods.)

Schizophrenics are yet another group that tends to have low levels of thiamin. One survey of psychiatric patients showed 47 percent to be deficient in at least one of the three vitamins assessed. Thiamin deficiency was detected in 30 percent of the patients—although only *one* patient showed clinical symptoms of deficiency. In the mentally ill, the elderly, and people with poor diets, subclinical thiamin deficiency is common. Understandably, it has been found that an inadequate intake of vitamins, particularly of $B_1$, may result in mental illness. Some psychiatrists use $B_1$ in combination with other B vitamins to treat various emotional and psychiatric illnesses, often in conjunction with medication.

## RDIs AND CLASSIC DEFICIENCY SYMPTOMS

The classic deficiency disease for $B_1$ is beriberi, a disease that affects the gastrointestinal, cardiovascular, and peripheral nervous systems. Advanced symptoms include indigestion, constipation, headaches, insomnia, a heaviness and weakness in the legs often followed by the cramping of leg muscles, and the burning and numbness of feet. In addition, the heart may become damaged or enlarged, or beat rapidly and irregularly. Severe vitamin $B_1$ deficiency also causes Korsakoff's syndrome, characterized by confusion, loss of memory, delusions, and amnesia; and Wernicke's disease, characterized by apathy, confusion, and delirium.

In this country, beriberi is usually confined to alcoholics. However, as we have seen, there are many other groups of people who are at risk of being deficient in this nutrient to a lesser extent, and so may suffer more subtle effects on the nervous system, digestive system, and heart. As a result, many people may in fact be experiencing early subclinical symptoms of beriberi, including fatigue, apathy, mental confusion, the inability to concentrate, poor memory, insomnia, anorexia (loss of appetite), loss of weight and strength, emotional instability, irritability, depression, and irrational fears. To prevent these symptoms of thiamin deficiency, the RDI for vitamin $B_1$ is 1.5 milligrams for men and women, and 1.7 milligrams for pregnant and lactating women.

*Food Sources:* The richest sources of thiamin are organ meats (especially liver), pork, dried beans, peas, soybeans, peanuts, whole grains such as brown rice, wheat germ, rice bran, egg yolks, poultry, and fish. Sources of moderate amounts include plums, prunes, raisins, asparagus, beans, broccoli, oatmeal, Brussels sprouts, and a wide variety of nuts. In addition, many foods are fortified with this vitamin to prevent overt deficiency symptoms.

Foods lose their thiamin content if exposed to ultraviolet light, sulfites, nitrites, and live yeast. Cooking, too, destroys at least a portion of the nutrient. Baking, for instance, reduces the thiamin content of flour by 15 to 20 percent; broiling and roasting reduces the thiamin content of meat by 25 percent; and boiling reduces the thiamin in meat by 50 percent. Vitamin $B_1$ is also destroyed by thiaminase, an enzyme found in raw seafood, as well as by the tannins present in tea and coffee.

## SUPPLEMENTS

$B_1$ (as thiamin hydrochloride or thiamin mononitrate) is available in individual supplements, and in B-complex supplements, in a wide range of potencies.

## OPTIMUM DAILY INTAKE—ODI

For optimum general health, the basic Optimum Daily Intake for thiamin is:

25–300 mg for men and women

Based on a thorough scientific review of vitamin $B_1$, and on my clinical experience, the following amounts of thiamin appear to be valuable for:

| Condition | Suggested Dosage |
|---|---|
| Anxiety, depression | 100–500 mg |
| Emotional or physical stress | 100–500 mg |
| High complex-carbohydrate diet | 50–100 mg |

*Remember:* If you have a medical condition or psychiatric disorder, please consult with your physician before taking supplements.

## TOXICITY AND ADVERSE EFFECTS

Thiamin has no known toxicity.

# Chapter 12

# VITAMIN B$_2$ (RIBOFLAVIN)

Vitamin B$_2$—commonly known as riboflavin—was first isolated from milk in 1935. Although its function in the body was not at first understood, we now know that it is a vital component in the process of energy production, and plays a role in many other processes as well.

## FUNCTIONS AND USES

### Energy Production and Tissue Repair

Riboflavin is important in the oxidation of amino acids, the synthesis and oxidation of fatty acids, and the oxidation of glucose—three processes involved in energy production. This vitamin also plays a role in thyroid hormone metabolism, which influences our metabolism and energy production.

In order for tissue repair to take place, the cells must be fueled by energy. Thus, an increased need for riboflavin is associated with many types of tissue damage, including that which occurs with burns, surgery, injuries, fever, and malignancies, as well as disorders such as tuberculosis, hypothyroidism, acute diabetes, and alcoholism.

### The Blood

The blood, too, requires riboflavin, a deficiency of which can lead to vitamin B$_2$ anemia. It is thought that this disorder occurs either because the deficiency inhibits red blood cell production, or because it causes the cells to die too early. There is also evidence that riboflavin may work in conjunction with iron to correct iron-deficiency anemia. Researchers have discovered that some sickle-cell anemia patients are deficient in B$_2$, and thus may have an increased need for this vitamin.

### The Immune System

Riboflavin may also play a role in the immune system, since animal studies have indicated that riboflavin deficiency reduces the body's ability to produce antibodies. Animal experimentation also suggests that riboflavin deficiency may increase the susceptibility of the tissues of the esophagus to cancer.

## The Eyes

Riboflavin is essential for healthy eyes. Found in the pigment of the retina, this vitamin enables the eyes to adapt to light. Thus, $B_2$ deficiencies can manifest themselves as photophobia, an excessive sensitivity to light that causes the eyes to water and become inflamed and bloodshot. Vision may become blurred, and the eyes may easily become tired. Animal studies have shown that there is also a correlation between cataracts and a lack of $B_2$, leading many practitioners to treat the early stages of cataracts in humans with the vitamin. The encouraging results indicate that this vitamin may either prevent cataracts or delay their progress.

## The Nervous System

Like $B_1$ and the other B vitamins, $B_2$ is often found to be deficient in patients with psychiatric disorders, and is sometimes given to these patients along with their medication. Another indication that $B_2$ is useful for neurological problems is its beneficial effect on carpal tunnel syndrome. Practitioners, including myself, have had success with carpal tunnel patients using this nutrient and vitamin $B_6$, and even $B_3$ (niacin).

## RDIs AND CLASSIC DEFICIENCY SYMPTOMS

The classic deficiency symptoms of vitamin $B_2$ involve the lips, tongue, eyes, skin, and nervous system. Early signs of deficiency include changes in the eyes, such as increased light sensitivity, tearing, burning and itching, eye fatigue, and decrease in the sharpness of vision. Cheilosis—tiny lesions in the mouth or cracks in the corner of the mouth—is another early warning sign, as are sore or burning lips, an inflamed or purple tongue, and discomfort in eating and swallowing. There may also be flaking of the skin around the nose, eyebrows, chin, cheeks, earlobes, or hairline. Additionally, dermatitis and sores may occur on the vulva and scrotum. Behavioral changes, too, are common, and include depression, moodiness, nervousness, and irritability.

To prevent these overt deficiencies, the RDI for vitamin $B_2$ is 1.7 milligrams per day for both men and women, and 2 milligrams for pregnant and lactating women. Many people may be marginally deficient in $B_2$ as the result of taking antibiotics, oral contraceptives, or other medications; or as the result of alcohol consumption. These substances deplete or interfere with the absorption or utilization of riboflavin. In addition, exercise may increase the need for $B_2$, as can a weight-loss diet. As we have learned, requirements also increase during any kinds of stress, including pregnancy and lactation.

*Food Sources:* Foods naturally high in $B_2$ are cheese, yogurt, and eggs; meat, poultry, and fish, especially kidney and liver; beans; and spinach. Other good sources are avocados, currants, asparagus, broccoli, Brussels sprouts, and nuts. Unless they are made with whole grains, cereals and grains are ordinarily low in riboflavin; however, they are often enriched with $B_2$. Milk, which begins as a good source of $B_2$, loses 10 to 12 percent of this nutrient when it is pasteurized, irradiated, evaporated, or dried. Storing it in clear glass bottles leads to losses of up to 75 percent in three and a half hours. Cooking causes meat to lose about 25 percent of its $B_2$. Adding sodium bicarbonate to preserve the green color of vegetables during cooking also destroys riboflavin.

## SUPPLEMENTS

Riboflavin is available in many potencies, both individually and in B-complex supplements.

## OPTIMUM DAILY INTAKE—ODI

To maintain and achieve optimum general health, the basic Optimum Daily Intake for $B_2$ is:

25–300 mg for men and women

Based on a thorough scientific review of vitamin $B_2$, and on my clinical experience, the following amounts of riboflavin appear to be valuable for:

| Condition | Suggested Dosage |
| --- | --- |
| Anxiety, depression | 100–500 mg |
| Carpal tunnel syndrome | 100–500 mg (with an equal amount of $B_6$) |
| Cataract prevention | 100–500 mg |
| Emotional or physical stress | 25–200 mg |
| Oral contraceptive use | 100–300 mg |
| Strenuous exercise | 50–100 mg |

*Remember:* If you have a medical condition or psychiatric disorder, please consult with your physician before taking supplements.

## TOXICITY AND ADVERSE EFFECTS

Riboflavin has no known toxicity.

# Chapter 13

# VITAMIN B₃ (NIACIN AND NIACINAMIDE)

V itamin B3 comes in two forms: niacin (or nicotinic acid) and niacinamide. Our bodies can make niacinamide from tryptophan, an
amino acid found in animal foods, but this accounts for only a small
fraction of our needs. We also convert niacin into niacinamide.

Vitamin B3 is a coenzyme in several important biochemical functions,
particularly those needed to maintain healthy skin, and a properly functioning gastrointestinal tract and nervous system. This nutrient is involved in
other important processes, as well, including the metabolism of lipids (fats).

## FUNCTIONS AND USES

### Cardiovascular Disease

Because of niacin's role in metabolizing fats, much of the therapeutic use of
niacin (not niacinamide) involves the treatment of high levels of cholesterol.
An overwhelming number of studies have shown that niacin is effective in
reducing both cholesterol and triglyceride levels in the blood. For example,
one study compared the efficacy of niacin with that of clofibrate, a widely
prescribed cholesterol-lowering drug. Niacin was much more effective than
the drug in lowering serum cholesterol, very-low-density lipoproteins
(VLDLs), and triglycerides. It also significantly increased high-density lipoproteins (HDL, or the "good" cholesterol). (For more information on cholesterol, see "Understanding Cholesterol" on page 32.) The authors of this study
and others concluded that because of these effects, as well as niacin's low cost
and low toxicity, niacin should be considered the treatment of choice for many
patients with elevated cholesterol levels. The option of using niacin seems
particularly attractive when one considers that many of the medications used
to treat this condition can have serious side effects, including a higher incidence of gastrointestinal cancer and an increased risk of gallbladder disease.

In my clinical practice, I have found niacin to be extremely effective in
lowering cholesterol and triglycerides. When patients using niacin returned

to their physicians for follow-up exams, the doctors were delighted with the results. When I gave one particular patient niacin supplements as part of his overall health program, he was able to reduce his cholesterol from 350 to 225 and his triglycerides from 225 to 90.

Niacin is especially useful for people who, like me, have a stubborn hereditary predisposition to high cholesterol. By following a strict diet and exercise regimen, I was able to lower my cholesterol from 270 to 245. This reflected an improvement, but not an adequate improvement. Now that I have added extra niacin to my plan, my cholesterol stays around or below 200, and my HDLs at 90 or above.

Vitamin B3 has other cardiovascular functions, as well. In the form of niacin, it is a vasodilator—an agent that relaxes and widens the blood vessels. Thus, niacin is also used in the treatment of various circulatory problems.

### The Nervous System

Some of the early symptoms of niacin deficiency include apprehension, irritability, depression, weakness, and loss of memory—all nervous system-related disorders. These symptoms may be followed by disorientation, confusion, and hysteria. Because of the importance of niacin to the nervous system, many practitioners use niacin and/or niacinamide alone or in conjunction with other medications in the treatment of mental disorders such as anxiety, nervousness, depression, and even schizophrenia. Studies have suggested that niacinamide— as well as vitamins E and B6, and calcium pantothenate—may also be useful in the treatment of epilepsy, when used with anticonvulsants.

### Cancer

It appears from several studies that niacinamide is effective against more than one type of carcinogen. Thus, this nutrient may be useful in preventing several forms of cancer.

### RDIs AND CLASSIC DEFICIENCY SYMPTOMS

Severe niacin deficiency is a major factor in the development of pellagra, a disease characterized by "the three Ds": dermatitis, diarrhea, and dementia. To prevent these deficiency symptoms, the Reference Daily Intake for vitamin B3 is 20 milligrams for men and women.

Easily observable deficiencies of vitamin B3 generally occur only in alcoholics and other severely malnourished people. Niacin deficiency is also quite common in people who eat corn-based diets, because the niacin contained in the corn is unabsorbable. (An exception is corn that has been soaked in lime water, as is done in Mexico. This process releases the niacin.) Vitamin B3 requirements may be higher in people who have cancer; people who are taking the drug isoniazid, used to treat tuberculosis; women who are taking oral contraceptives; and people who have protein deficiencies.

*Food Sources:* Vitamin B$_3$ is found in beef, pork, fish, milk and cheese, whole wheat, potatoes, corn and corn products, eggs, broccoli, tomatoes, and carrots. However, some B$_3$ is often present in a form that is not absorbable. Since B$_3$ may be lost in cooking water, it is advisable to steam, bake, or stir-fry vegetables to spare as much of this vitamin as possible.

## SUPPLEMENTS

Both niacin and niacinamide are widely available as supplements. If you are treating circulatory problems or trying to lower your cholesterol and triglycerides, I recommend niacin rather than niacinamide.

Several types of niacin supplements are now on the market. They include immediate-release (IM) niacin; sustained- or time-release (SR) niacin; and inositol hexaniacinate (IHN), which contains niacin plus inositol. When using higher levels of IM niacin, individuals generally experience a "flushing" sensation, which often limits its use. Although SR niacin was designed to eliminate this sensation, it still produces flushing and gastrointestinal upset in some individuals. SR niacin is generally better tolerated, but at levels above 1,500 milligrams a day, elevated liver enzymes and liver toxicity have been reported. On the other hand, IHN, or "flush-free," niacin appears to be completely safe and without any flushing effect. Human studies using as much as 4,000 milligrams daily have shown IHN niacin to be free of side effects and adverse reactions. IHN has been shown to be beneficial for circulatory disorders, including Raynaud's disease and intermittent claudication.

## OPTIMUM DAILY INTAKE—ODI

For optimum general health, the basic Optimum Daily Intake for vitamin B$_3$ (10 to 25 percent of which should be niacin) is:

25–300 mg for men and women

Based on a thorough scientific review of vitamin B$_3$, and on my clinical experience, the following amounts of B$_3$ appear to be valuable for:

| Condition | Suggested Dosage |
|---|---|
| Anxiety, depression | 100–500 mg niacin or niacinamide (under professional advice) |

| | |
|---|---|
| Circulatory problems | 50–500 mg niacin |
| Emotional or physical stress | 100–500 mg niacin or niacinamide |
| High triglycerides and/or cholesterol | 250–500 mg niacin (up to 2,000 mg under professional advice) |

*Remember:* If you have a medical condition or psychiatric disorder, please consult with your physician before taking supplements.

## TOXICITY AND ADVERSE EFFECTS

There is no known toxicity of this vitamin in doses of 2 grams (2,000 milligrams) or less. In individuals with liver disorders, though, high-dose niacin therapy needs to be closely monitored by a physician, since it can cause elevations in liver function tests. Also consult with a professional if you have a history of ulcers, as high doses may also exacerbate a pre-existing gastric or duodenal ulcer.

In healthy people, the only adverse effect of niacin supplementation is a temporary flush, which makes you turn red and perhaps slightly itchy. However, by taking niacin after a meal, or by taking an aspirin an hour before you take the niacin, you can lessen or prevent the flush without losing the beneficial effects. Caution must be exercised when using time- or sustained-release (SR) niacin, since taking higher doses of sustained-release niacin, even under professional advice, yielded reports of liver toxicity. The newer "flush free" form, inositol hexaniacinate (IHN) appears to be much safer.

# Chapter 14

# VITAMIN B$_6$ (PYRIDOXINE)

itamin B$_6$, also known as pyridoxine, is one of the most essential, widely utilized vitamins in the body. As a coenzyme, B$_6$ participates in over sixty enzymatic reactions involved in the metabolism of amino acids (the building blocks of protein) and essential fatty acids. It is, therefore, needed for the proper growth and maintenance of almost all our body structures, and for almost all our body functions.

## FUNCTIONS AND USES

### The Nervous System

One of the many systems dependent on vitamin B$_6$ is the nervous system. For instance, vitamin B$_6$ is necessary for the production of serotonin and other neurotransmitters in the brain—substances that, when deficient, appear to be associated with depression. Although "megavitamin" therapy for psychiatric symptoms is controversial, many studies indicate an association between B$_6$ deficiency and emotional illness, including depression and schizophrenia. Many practitioners, including myself, feel that there is enough evidence to warrant its use as an alternative treatment when psychotropic drugs fail or result in toxicity. Others suggest that it be used with psychotropic drugs.

Research shows that B$_6$ may have a much greater effect on the nervous system than previously thought. For example, a number of studies report that patients with carpal tunnel syndrome—a neurological condition that leads to weakness and pain of the wrist and hand—respond positively to B$_6$ supplementation, especially when combined with vitamin B$_2$. In addition, infants fed formulas low in vitamin B$_6$ have suffered epileptic-like convulsions, weight loss, nervous irritability, and stomach disorders. These problems, as well as other forms of childhood epilepsy, have been found to respond to B$_6$ supplementation. Autistic children also have been shown to improve when given B$_6$ along with magnesium.

## Women's Health

B6 is also important for women who suffer from premenstrual syndrome (PMS), a condition that can include depression, irritability, fatigue, painful and swollen breasts, bloated abdomen, swollen fingers and ankles, headache, stomachache, and backache. Many studies have shown that B6 reduces or eliminates these symptoms for most women. The reason for this is unclear, but it may be that high estrogen levels after ovulation result in an increased need for B6 or a decreased ability to absorb it. In addition, B6 tends to act as a natural diuretic, promoting the formation and release of urine. This would also help reduce PMS symptoms. Certainly, I have seen remarkable results in my own patients with B6 supplementation, and many researchers suggest that B6 be tried before progesterone is considered.

A number of studies have shown that women who take oral contraceptives tend to have lower blood levels of this vitamin. This may be responsible for the lethargy, fatigue, and mental depression experienced by some women on oral contraceptives, since B$_6$ supplementation improves these symptoms.

B$_6$ is of special concern for both pregnant and lactating women, as studies have shown that the requirement for this nutrient increases at these times. Moreover, studies have found that pregnant women consume only 50 percent of the RDA during the last month of pregnancy, and that breastfeeding women consume only 60 percent of the RDA after delivery. These figures are of importance not only for the expectant mother, but for her infant, too. For instance, according to one study, B$_6$ supplementation can reduce or cure the nausea and vomiting of pregnancy. Another study found that Apgar scores— a measure of a newborn's health—were significantly better for infants of mothers who took an amount several times the RDA of B$_6$ than for those who took an amount close to the RDA. Adequate levels of B$_6$ are also vital in lactating women because of the previously mentioned association of B$_6$ deficiency with convulsions and irritability in some infants.

## Blood and Blood Vessels

Vitamin B$_6$ is also needed for healthy blood and blood vessels. It is required by the body to turn iron into hemoglobin, and to produce red blood cells and antibodies. A deficiency can therefore cause anemia and a depression of immune system responses. Studies also indicate that vitamin B$_6$ may help prevent arteriosclerosis (hardening of the arteries), and that low levels may increase the risk of heart attack.

## Other Uses

Asthmatics may benefit from B₆ supplementation, as may those with sickle cell anemia; diabetes; and Chinese restaurant syndrome, an adverse reaction to monosodium glutamate (MSG), the symptoms of which include facial pressure, tingling and burning of the skin, chest pain, headache, and heartburn. This nutrient has also been shown to be of use in the treatment of recurring kidney stones in adults, and in kidney failure in some infants. In addition, experiments with animals suggest that a diet deficient in B₆ may be involved in premature aging. Another experiment suggests that B₆ holds promise as a treatment for melanoma, a deadly form of cancer.

## RDIs AND CLASSIC DEFICIENCY SYMPTOMS

The most frequently diagnosed and well-recognized deficiency symptoms of vitamin B₆ occur in the skin and nervous system. The changes in the skin and mucous membranes are similar to those caused by other members of the B-complex group, and include seborrheic dermatitis, particularly around the nose, eyes, eyebrows, the skin behind the ears, and the mouth; acne; cheilosis and stomatitis, which are characterized by tiny sores and cracks in and around the mouth; and glossitis (inflamed tongue). B₆ deficiency is also associated with nervous system problems such as depression, confusion, dizziness, insomnia, irritability, nervousness, a pins and needles feeling in the hands and feet, and even brain wave abnormalities and convulsions.

While the list of benefits and uses of B₆ is a long one, it is difficult for men and women to obtain even their RDIs of 2 milligrams, and pregnant and lactating women to obtain their RDI of 2.5 milligrams from food. Certain members of the population, such as women, dieters, adolescent girls, alcoholics, and the elderly, have consistently been found to take in less than the RDA. For instance, one study of seventy-four female college students (excluding those taking oral contraceptives) determined that only one of them was getting the full RDA of B₆. In addition, many people may require more than the RDI. Among the situations that raise B₆ requirements are exposure to radiation; the use of certain medications, including oral contraceptives, isoniazid, penicillamine, and cycloserine; tobacco use; air pollutants; cardiac failure; and, of course, stress.

*Food Sources:* All foods contain small amounts of B₆. Those foods thought to contain the highest amounts of this nutrient include eggs, fish, spinach, carrots, peas, meat, chicken, fish (especially herring and salmon), brewer's yeast, walnuts, sunflower seeds, and wheat germ. Sources of moderate amounts of B₆ include brown rice and other whole grains, blackstrap molasses, avocados, cantaloupes, bananas, cabbage, and beans.

However, it has recently been discovered that data on the vitamin B$_6$ content of foods is unreliable, since the amount of B$_6$ in foods does not necessarily represent the amount that is bioavailable—active in the tissues after ingestion. This is true to some degree of all nutrients, but studies have shown that the bioavailability of the B$_6$ content of foods may in fact be quite limited. In addition, this content is affected by heat, oxygen, and light. In fact, up to 70 percent of the B$_6$ in foods may be lost during cooking, processing, and refining.

## SUPPLEMENTS

Vitamin B$_6$ is available as pyridoxine hydrochloride, the most commonly available form; and pyridoxine 5 phosphate, which may be better absorbed. These forms have been shown to be equally active in experimental animals, which probably means that they act similarly in humans also.

## OPTIMUM DAILY INTAKE—ODI

For optimum general health, the basic Optimum Daily Intake for vitamin B$_6$ is:

25–300 mg for men and women

Based on a thorough scientific review of vitamin B$_6$, and on my clinical experience, the following amounts of B$_6$ appear to be valuable for:

| Condition | Suggested Dosage |
| --- | --- |
| Anxiety, depression | 100–500 mg |
| Asthma | 50–300 mg |
| Carpal tunnel syndrome | 50–500 mg |
| Emotional or physical stress | 100–500 mg |
| Kidney stones (oxalate) | 100–300 mg |
| Oral contraceptive use | 50–300 mg |
| Premenstrual syndrome | 50–300 mg |
| Water retention | 100–300 mg |

*Remember:* If you have a medical condition or psychiatric symptoms, please consult with your physician before taking supplements. High doses of B$_6$ should not be used in people who are taking levodopa, a drug used in the treatment of Parkinson's disease.

## TOXICITY AND ADVERSE EFFECTS

B$_6$ is relatively nontoxic, but some problems with the nervous system have been reported. This occurs only with huge doses of 2,000 to 6,000 milligrams of $B_6$ daily, although there are isolated cases of toxicity with smaller doses. These side effects appear to be reversible when the dosage is discontinued. In addition, dependency has been induced in healthy adults who were given 200 milligrams daily for thirty-three days. This dependency results in a deficiency when supplementation is stopped abruptly.

# Chapter 15

# VITAMIN B$_{12}$ (COBALAMIN)

I n 1926, scientists determined that a certain form of anemia could be reversed or controlled by eating a half pound of raw or lightly cooked liver daily. By 1948, B$_{12}$, the nutrient that was responsible for eliminating the anemia, had been isolated. We now know that this B vitamin, also known as cobalamin, is a coenzyme needed by the body to form healthy blood, and to perform a variety of other functions, as well.

## FUNCTIONS AND USES

### The Blood

As already mentioned, the best-known function of vitamin B$_{12}$ is the role it plays in blood formation. Specifically, this nutrient is needed to form red blood cells in the marrow. Without an adequate amount of B$_{12}$, pernicious anemia results, with symptoms that include pallor and fatigue.

### The Nervous System

Vitamin B$_{12}$ is involved in the production of myelin, a fatty substance found in the sheath that covers our nerves. Therefore the association between B$_{12}$ deficiency and impaired nervous system function is well established. B$_{12}$ deficiency may play a part in many mild to severe physical and emotional symptoms such as confusion, moodiness, memory loss, peripheral neuritis, leg and finger incoordination, depression, and psychosis. These can occur even when there are no signs of changes in the blood to indicate either low levels of B$_{12}$ or anemia.

Recent studies have also uncovered a possible link between Alzheimer's-like dementia and low vitamin B$_{12}$ levels in the blood. Although it is not known whether there is a direct causal relationship between the two, it may be that prolonged low blood levels of B$_{12}$ produce the irreversible neurological changes seen in this disease.

## Cancer

Vitamin $B_{12}$ may also play a role in cancer prevention. When combined with ascorbic acid, this nutrient has been shown to inhibit the formation of cancer in laboratory mice. In addition, a study of smokers found low levels of both $B_{12}$ and folate, especially in those with precancerous changes. Vitamin supplementation decreased these abnormal cells.

## RDIs AND CLASSIC DEFICIENCY SYMPTOMS

The classic deficiency disease of $B_{12}$ is pernicious anemia, whose symptoms can include weight loss, weakness, pale skin, and psychological disturbances. This type of anemia is rather common and appears most frequently in alcoholics, the elderly, and strict vegetarians (non-lacto-ovo). It is imperative to use diagnostic tests to distinguish $B_{12}$ anemia from folic acid anemia. If folic acid is given to someone already deficient in $B_{12}$, severe $B_{12}$ deficiency will develop, as the body needs vitamin $B_{12}$ to utilize folic acid. If $B_{12}$ is given to someone already deficient in folic acid, severe folic acid deficiency will develop. To prevent overt deficiencies, the RDI for vitamin $B_{12}$ is 6 micrograms for men and women, and 8 micrograms for pregnant and lactating women.

Certain conditions can cause $B_{12}$ deficiency even when there is adequate dietary intake of the nutrient. When an inherited defect prevents the body from manufacturing sufficient quantities of a substance called intrinsic factor, normal absorption of the vitamin cannot take place. In addition, prolonged excess exposure to nitrous oxide ("laughing gas") may result in lowered blood levels of this vitamin. Although early studies suggested that vitamin C supplementation may also destroy $B_{12}$, subsequent studies using improved technology have shown that large doses of vitamin C do not have this effect. On the contrary, the absorption of the cyanocobalamin form of $B_{12}$ is slightly increased in the presence of vitamin C. Some medications, though, do interfere with absorption of this nutrient. (See the Drug-Nutrient Interaction Table on page 234.)

Although we have the ability to produce $B_{12}$ in the intestines, we are not sure how much of this can be absorbed by the body.

*Food Sources:* Generally, the amount of $B_{12}$ in foods is small. All sources are animal in origin: lamb and beef kidneys; and lamb, beef, calf, and pork livers are among the foods highest in $B_{12}$. Good sources include beef, herring, and mackerel. Egg yolk, milk, cheese, clams, sardines, salmon, crab meat, and oysters also have reasonable amounts.

Vitamin $B_{12}$ is not stable in the presence of heat, acid, or light, and is susceptible to oxidation, so care is required during the storage and cooking of foods.

## SUPPLEMENTS

Cyanocobalamin is the form of $B_{12}$ that is most widely used in oral supplements. Hydroxycobalamin is the form of $B_{12}$ used in injections, which are recommended in cases of $B_{12}$ malabsorption.

## OPTIMUM DAILY INTAKE—ODI

For optimum general health, the basic Optimum Daily Intake for vitamin $B_{12}$ is:

25–500 mcg for men and women

Based on a thorough scientific review of vitamin $B_{12}$ and on my clinical experience, the following amounts of $B_{12}$ appear to be valuable for:

| Condition | Suggested Dosage |
|---|---|
| Anxiety, depression | 100–500 mcg |
| $B_{12}$ anemia | 250–500 mcg |
| (injections by your physician may be necessary if you have malabsorption) | |
| Emotional or physical stress | 100–500 mcg |

*Remember:* If you have a medical condition or psychiatric symptoms, please consult with your physician before taking supplements.

## TOXICITY AND ADVERSE EFFECTS

Vitamin $B_{12}$ has no known toxicity.

# Chapter 16

---

# FOLIC ACID

F olic acid, also known as folate or folacin, was identified and named in the 1940s. This nutrient takes part in a variety of body processes, ranging from the synthesis of genetic material to the transmission of nerve signals.

## FUNCTIONS AND USES

### Cell Replication and Tissue Growth

In one of its most important roles, folic acid works closely with vitamin $B_{12}$ in the metabolism of amino acids and the synthesis of proteins, and in the production of genetic material (RNA and DNA). Thus, it is vital to healthy cell division and replication, and to tissue growth. A number of its therapeutic uses are related to this function.

### *Dysplasia*

Because of folic acid's role in cell division, a deficiency of this nutrient is associated with dysplasia, an abnormal growth of tissues. Researchers have had some success in using folic acid to treat various types of dysplasia, including the very common cervical dysplasia. Evidence suggests that in some women, the use of oral contraceptives causes a localized folate deficiency in the cells of the cervix, somehow making them more susceptible to cancer-causing viruses or chemicals. Because dysplasia is considered pre-cancerous, when the condition is severe, surgical removal of the suspicious cells is generally recommended. Fortunately, folate has helped stop or reverse cervical dysplasia in a number of women taking oral contraceptives. I have recommended folic acid to many patients whom physicians have referred to my office for this problem. When their physicians gave them follow-up exams, they were delighted to find a reversal of the dysplasia.

## Birth Defects

Because of the rapid cell multiplication that takes place during pregnancy, the mother's need for folate is great. Pregnancy may deplete the mother's supply of folic acid as the rapidly growing fetus makes increased demands on her body's nutrient stores. This may cause anemia in the mother, and birth defects in the child. In one study, one group of mothers whose children were born with harelips—one or more splits in the upper lip—were given folic acid prior to and during the first trimester of their next pregnancy, while another group remained unsupplemented. Only one of the supplemented mothers gave birth to another child with harelip; in the unsupplemented group, there were fifteen recurrences. Since oral contraceptives may also affect the level of folate in the blood throughout the body, any woman who discontinues use of the pill to become pregnant should make sure she has adequate folate stored in her body before she conceives.

The greatest attention received by folic acid is due to its ability to prevent defects of the neural tube, the structure in the embryo that gives rise to the brain, the spinal cord, and other parts of the central nervous system. In 1992, the U.S. Public Health Service released an advisory stating that "in order to reduce the frequency of neural tube defects and their resulting disability, all women of childbearing age in the United States who are capable of becoming pregnant should consume .4 milligrams (400 micrograms) of folic acid per day for the purpose of reducing their risk of having a pregnancy affected with spina bifida or other neural tube defects." The current RDI for pregnant and lactating women is twice that amount—800 micrograms. It should be noted, though, that the studies showing the most remarkable results did not use supplementation of folic acid only. In one study, for example, $B_{12}$ supplementation along with folic acid actually demonstrated superior results in preventing neural tube defects. In another study, multivitamins containing 800 micrograms of folic acid along with a multimineral supplement also demonstrated excellent results.

## The Nervous System

Folic acid derivatives are coenzymes for neurotransmitters—the chemicals that permit the sending of signals from nerve fiber to nerve fiber. Because of this important function, folic acid may cause certain nervous system-related disorders. Some studies have suggested that a folic acid deficiency can produce minor and major mental problems and mood changes, including depression, schizophrenia, and dementia. Since large doses of this vitamin have been reported as improving the condition of a certain congenital form of mental retardation, folate may also be connected with other forms of mental retardation and low IQ (intelligence quotient).

## The Immune System

Many aspects of the immune system are affected by a deficiency in folic acid, including the ability to recognize invading microbes, and the number and strength of our white blood cells. Thus, folic acid, when deficient, may render us less resistant to disease.

## The Blood

Like vitamin $B_{12}$, discussed in the previous chapter, folic acid is needed for the proper formation of red blood cells. Without adequate amounts of folic acid, a specific type of anemia results, characterized by oversized red blood cells.

## RDIs AND CLASSIC DEFICIENCY SYMPTOMS

The classic deficiency disease of folic acid is a type of anemia in which the red blood cells are improperly formed. The symptoms of this condition include irritability, weakness, sleeping difficulties, and pallor. Diagnostic tests *must* be used to distinguish folic acid anemia from $B_{12}$ anemia. If $B_{12}$ is given to someone already deficient in folic acid, severe folic acid deficiency will develop. If folic acid is given to someone already deficient in $B_{12}$, severe $B_{12}$ deficiency will develop. Classic folic acid deficiency symptoms most often occur in alcoholics and people with intestinal malabsorption usually due to the aging process, gastrointestinal surgery, or some other disease or condition of the digestive system. To prevent such overt deficiency, the RDI is 400 micrograms for men and women, and 800 micrograms for pregnant and lactating women.

Studies have shown that aspirin; nitrous oxide, an anesthetic gas; anticonvulsants; sulfasalazine, used for inflammatory bowel disease; and methotrexate, an anticancer drug, may interfere with folate absorption or utilization. In addition, there may be an increased need for this nutrient during illness, injury, and surgery, during which times the body repairs itself. It logically follows that folic acid requirements increase during any time of stress.

A word should be said about folinic acid, a synthetic derivative of folic acid that is used in very high doses to "rescue" cancer patients from methotrexate toxicity. It should not be confused with the vitamin folic acid. Folic acid does not interfere with the efficacy of methotrexate. Unfortunately, many patients are still advised not to take folic acid with this chemotherapy drug, thus putting them at risk for folic acid deficiency.

*Food Sources:* Folic acid is found in many types of foods. The best natural sources of folic acid are beef liver, lamb liver, pork liver, and chicken liver; deep green leafy vegetables, such as spinach, kale, and beet greens; and asparagus, broccoli, whole wheat, and brewer's yeast. However, it has been estimated that only 25 to 50 percent of the folic acid in food is biologically available. In addition, cooking and other types of processing can reduce folic content by 50 to 90 percent. For instance, 68 percent of the folic acid in whole wheat is removed when the grain is processed into white flour.

## SUPPLEMENTS

Folic acid is available without a prescription in amounts up to 0.8 milligrams (800 micrograms), either as an individual supplement or as part of a multivitamin formula. Stronger supplements are available only with a doctor's prescription.

## OPTIMUM DAILY INTAKE—ODI

For optimum general health, the basic Optimum Daily Intake of folic acid is:

### 400–1,200 mcg for men and women

Based on thorough scientific review of folic acid, and on my clinical experience, the following amounts of folic acid appear to be valuable for:

| Condition | Suggested Dosage |
|-----------|------------------|
| Anxiety, depression | 400–800 mcg |
| Cervical dysplasia | 800–5,000 mcg (5 mg) |
| Emotional or physical stress | 400–800 mcg |
| Folic acid anemia | 800–2,000 mcg (2 mg) |

*Remember:* If you have a medical condition, or any psychiatric symptoms, please consult with your physician before taking supplements.

## TOXICITY AND ADVERSE EFFECTS

There is no known toxicity of folic acid. However, women who are taking folic acid supplements, especially if they are current or former users of oral contraceptives, are at risk for lower plasma zinc concentrations. I recommend that these women take additional zinc to prevent lowered zinc levels. Also, make sure you are taking $B_{12}$ supplements along with your folic acid supplements. Before prescribing high therapeutic doses, I recommend a screening for both folic acid and $B_{12}$ anemia.

# Chapter 17

---

# PANTOTHENIC ACID

In 1933, pantothenic acid was recognized as a substance that stimulates growth. We now know that this nutrient is needed for a wide range of processes throughout the body.

## FUNCTIONS AND USES

Our bodies convert pantothenic acid to coenzyme A, which is used in a variety of biological processes involving the metabolism of fats, carbohydrates, and proteins, and the synthesis of hormones, bile, and hemoglobin. It is also needed for the production of sphingosine and acetylcholine, two very important substances involved in nerve transmission. Some of the ways in which this nutrient specifically affects function are discussed below.

### Emotional and Physical Stress

There are no documented cases of naturally occurring pantothenic acid deficiency. However, when deficiencies were artificially created in humans, headache, fatigue, insomnia, and nervous system-related symptoms such as anxiety and depression did occur. Some of these symptoms are no doubt due to the fact that pantothenic acid is used in nerve transmissions and in the production of hormones that control our reactions to emotional and physical stress and the fight or flight response. This is why this vitamin has long been considered an "anti-stress" vitamin. Interestingly, laboratory animals fed a pantothenic-rich diet show significant improvement in exercise tolerance. This may hold true for humans too. Some studies actually show that pantothenic acid helps delay the onset of fatigue, especially when combined with other members of the B complex. One study in particular showed that human subjects given 10 milligrams of pantothenic acid daily were significantly better able to withstand cold water stress. This may be connected with the nutrient's role in helping us resist stress in general.

There is some indication that pantothenic acid helps improve our ability to heal and withstand the stress of physical injury. For example, the surgical scars of supplemented laboratory animals healed better than did the scars of unsupplemented animals. In another study, a preparation that included pantothenic acid reduced the effects of ultraviolet radiation on animals. Another preparation containing a pantothenic-like substance was applied to human subjects with sports-related injuries. As a result, there was significant decrease in swelling and increase in joint mobility.

### The Immune System

Deficiencies in pantothenic acid have been shown to adversely affect the immune system in both humans and animals, indicating that the nutrient also has a role in our system of defense. It has been found that some people with rheumatoid arthritis—an autoimmune disorder—have significantly lower blood levels of pantothenic acid than do people without this disorder. The lower the levels of this nutrient, the more severe the symptoms appear to be. Studies have shown that when rheumatoid arthritis patients are given pantothenic acid, their symptoms of stiffness, disability, and pain are often alleviated. When the treatment is withdrawn, symptoms reappear. Similar results were achieved in patients with osteoarthritis.

Pantothenic acid has also proved effective in the treatment of chronic discoid lupus, another autoimmune disorder. In one study, the condition of thirty out of thirty-seven patients improved with massive doses of 6 to 10 grams per day, followed by lower maintenance levels of 2 to 4 grams.

### Cardiovascular Disease

Because of pantothenic acid's role in metabolizing fats, this nutrient has been used to lower blood cholesterol levels and treat related problems. In one study, supplementation of pantethine—a more active form of pantothenic acid—in amounts of 900 milligrams per day, brought about a statistically significant lowering of serum cholesterol levels and improved lipid metabolism in 1,045 hyperlipidemic patients, some of whom were diabetic (Types I and II). The authors concluded that pantethine should be considered for the treatment of high cholesterol and lipid abnormalities in patients with diabetes mellitus, and in other patients at high risk for such cardiovascular disorders.

### RDIs AND DEFICIENCY SYMPTOMS

The RDI for pantothenic acid has been established at 10 milligrams per day.

*Food Sources:* Pantothenic acid appears in a wide variety of foods. The best sources are eggs, potatoes, saltwater fish, pork, beef, milk, whole wheat, peas, beans, and fresh vegetables. Significant amounts of pantothenic acid are lost in foods when they are canned, cooked, frozen, or otherwise processed. For example, 50 percent of the pantothenic acid in grains is lost during the milling process.

## SUPPLEMENTS

Pantothenic acid is available in two forms: as calcium pantothenate, which is 92 percent pantothenic acid and 8 percent calcium; and as a more active metabolite known as pantethine, which is very unstable and extremely expensive.

## OPTIMUM DAILY INTAKE—ODI

For optimum general health, the basic Optimum Daily Intake for pantothenic acid is:

25–500 mg for men and women

Based on a thorough scientific review of pantothenic acid, and on my clinical experience, the following amounts of pantothenic acid appear to be valuable for:

| Condition | Suggested Dosage |
|---|---|
| Anxiety, depression | 100–500 mg |
| Emotional or physical stress | 100–500 mg |
| High cholesterol | 900 mg pantethine |
| Joint inflammation | 100–2,000 mg |
| Lupus | 6–10 g, gradually tapering to 2–4 g as maintenance |
| Osteo- and rheumatoid arthritis | 50–2,000 mg |

*Remember:* If you have a medical condition or psychiatric symptoms, please consult with your physician before taking supplements.

## TOXICITY AND ADVERSE EFFECTS

Pantothenic acid has no known toxicity. Nevertheless, doses of over 2,000 milligrams per day should be taken only under professional advice.

# Chapter 18

# BIOTIN

B iotin is an important coenzyme that is involved in a number of processes. It is not considered to be a true vitamin since it is made in our
bodies by intestinal bacteria.

## FUNCTIONS, USES, AND DEFICIENCIES

Like several of the other B vitamins, biotin is necessary for the metabolism of
carbohydrates, fats, and protein. Biotin deficiency symptoms include seborrheic dermatitis, which is most commonly seen in infants; and hair loss. When
due to a deficiency, these conditions do respond to supplementation. However, there has been no convincing evidence to support the widely touted use
of biotin as a cure for baldness. Biotin will work to restore hair only if there
is an underlying skin condition due to a deficiency in this nutrient.

Just as biotin deficiency can cause hair loss, it has also been known to result
in appetite loss, nausea, numbness, depression, and high blood cholesterol.
There is some evidence that biotin supplementation helps to prevent and treat
nervous system disorders seen in patients undergoing long-term hemodialysis. These patients' symptoms are similar to those of Alzheimer's patients,
and include disorientation, speech disorders, memory loss, restless legs,
tremors, and difficulty in walking.

Because biotin is both manufactured by the body and found in many foods,
only a few small groups of people have been found to be overtly biotin
deficient. These groups include infants who are born with a genetic defect;
bodybuilders and other people who eat large quantities of raw eggs, which
contain a substance that inhibits biotin absorption; and people who are
undergoing long-term therapy with antibiotics or sulfa drugs—substances
that may reduce the synthesis of biotin by intestinal bacteria. (For more
information about drug interactions, see the Drug-Nutrient Interaction Table
on page 234.)

## RDIs

The RDI for biotin has been established at 300 micrograms per day.

*Food Sources:* Foods high in biotin are chicken, lamb, pork, beef, veal, liver, brewer's yeast and other nutritional yeasts, soybeans, milk, cheese, saltwater fish, whole wheat flour, and rice bran. Biotin is stable during normal cooking and processing. Eggs, another excellent source of biotin, contain a substance that inhibits biotin absorption in the body. However, cooking destroys this substance.

## SUPPLEMENTS

Biotin is available as d-biotin, and is included in most B-complex and multivitamin supplements. Although it is also available as an individual supplement, I have never felt the need to supplement biotin individually.

## OPTIMUM DAILY INTAKE—ODI

For optimum general health, the Optimum Daily Intake for biotin is:

### 300 mcg for men and women

*Remember:* If you have a medical condition or psychiatric symptoms, please consult with your physician before taking supplements.

## TOXICITY AND ADVERSE EFFECTS

Biotin is considered to be nontoxic.

# Chapter 19

# CHOLINE, INOSITOL, AND PABA

Relatively little is known about these three nutrients. Members of the B-complex group, they are synthesized in the body, and therefore are not considered essential vitamins. However, they are involved in many important body processes.

## FUNCTIONS AND USES

Both choline and inositol seem to be involved in the body's use of fats and cholesterol, and have been shown to alleviate or prevent the accumulation of abnormal quantities of fat in the liver. Choline is used in the transport and metabolism of fats. Inositol is involved in the synthesis of phospholipids, which are essential to the digestion and absorption of fats, facilitate the uptake of fatty acids by the cells, and regulate the transport of material in and out of the cells.

Choline is also used by the body to make acetylcholine, a neurotransmitter that permits the sending of messages from nerve fiber to nerve fiber. Thus, an adequate supply of choline is critical for optimum nerve function. It has been demonstrated, for example, that a deficit of this nutrient may play a role in the development of certain neurologic disorders, such as Huntington's chorea, Parkinson's disease, and Alzheimer's disease. In doses of 500 to 3,000 milligrams per day, choline has resulted in a significant improvement in children who were seriously developmentally delayed.

Lecithin (phosphatidyl choline), a natural source of choline, is a structural component of cell membranes. It is used successfully to treat some cases of tardive dyskinesia, another neurological disorder. This condition, which results in facial twitches, is a common side effect of the heavy use of tranquilizers such as Thorazine. Lecithin has also been widely advocated in the treatment of high serum cholesterol. However, studies have generally failed to prove its effectiveness except at extremely high intakes of 12 to 35 grams per day.

PABA (para-aminobenzoic acid) appears necessary for the body's formation of folic acid, and for the metabolism of protein. Although it has proved to be effective in combating gray hair in animals, there is only anecdotal evidence that this nutrient has the same effect in human beings. Because of its ability to protect against sunburn when applied to the skin, PABA is a common ingredient in sunscreens. There is no evidence that oral doses of PABA have a similar effect.

## RDIs AND DEFICIENCIES

There have been no known cases of naturally occurring choline, inositol, or PABA deficiency, and RDIs for these nutrients have not been established.

*Food Sources:* Choline is found in legumes, organ and muscle meats, milk, and whole grain cereals, and is particularly high in egg yolk. Inositol is distributed in fruits, vegetables, whole grains, meats, and milk. PABA is found in brewer's yeast, liver, kidney, whole grains, and molasses.

## SUPPLEMENTS

Choline, inositol, and PABA are generally included in B-complex and multivitamin formulas, in amounts similar to those of the other B vitamins. They are also available as individual supplements.

Choline comes in three forms: choline bitartrate, choline dihydrogen citrate, and phosphatidyl choline (lecithin). I usually recommend lecithin, a natural substance high in this nutrient, since it is more absorbable and less irritating at higher levels than are the other two forms. Lecithin comes in several forms: capsules that contain oil, liquid, and granules.

Inositol is available in tablet and powder form. The tablets are preferable, as they are easier to take and cheaper than the powder. (It has been said that the price of the powder is high because it is allegedly purchased by those who intend to use it to cut cocaine. There is no evidence that inhalation of inositol confers any additional effects, or is of any therapeutic benefit.) PABA is included in nutritional supplements as para-aminobenzoic acid.

## OPTIMUM DAILY INTAKE—ODI

For optimum general health, the Optimum Daily Intake is:

Choline: 25–500 mg for men and women
Inositol: 25–500 mg for men and women
Lecithin: 12–35 g for men and women (therapeutic dose for lipid, neurologic, and psychiatric disorders)
PABA: 25–500 mg for men and women

There is not enough evidence at this time to warrant a high intake of these nutrients for most people, since large doses may prove harmful if taken over an extended period of time. However, if you are suffering from a neurologic, psychiatric, or lipid disorder, you may want to try taking large amounts of lecithin under the advice of a professional. Both I and other practicioners have had good results recommending lecithin to patients with mild cases of shingles—up to two capsules of 1,200 milligrams each three times a day.

## TOXICITY AND ADVERSE EFFECTS

There may be adverse effects if these nutrients are taken in high doses. Patients who have been treated with high oral doses of lecithin (choline) have complained of dizziness, nausea, diarrhea, depression, and a fishy odor on their breath and skin. Recent studies show that high doses of PABA (8 to 48 grams daily) are associated with side effects such as malaise, fever, liver disease, and lowered white blood cell counts.

*Chapter 20*

# VITAMIN C (ASCORBIC ACID)

A scorbic acid—or vitamin C, as it is commonly known—has spent a good deal of time in the limelight over the years. The nutrient first came to the public's attention through the work of Linus Pauling, who researched the vitamin's ability to help the body combat the common cold and other disorders. Later, vitamin C's role as an antioxidant received much attention. Despite media hype, though, most people don't realize just how many important functions are performed by this nutrient.

## FUNCTIONS AND USES

### Vitamin C's Antioxidant Powers

A good deal of vitamin C's usefulness seems to stem from its role as an antioxidant. In this role, vitamin C prevents the free-radical damage that contributes to aging and aging-related diseases, including cancer and cardiovascular disorders. In addition, ascorbic acid prevents other antioxidant vitamins, including A and E, from being oxidized, thus keeping them potent.

### The Immune System

Perhaps foremost among vitamin's C's many functions is the major role it plays in the immune system, where, according to growing evidence, it helps increase resistance to a range of diseases, including infections and cancer. Studies of both animals and humans have shown that excesses of vitamin C stimulate the production of lymphocytes, an important component of our immune system. Ascorbic acid also appears to be required by the thymus gland (one of the major glands involved in immunity), and increases the mobility of the phagocytes, the type of cell that "eats" bacteria, viral cells, and cancer cells, as well as other harmful foreign invaders.

Since vitamin C levels in the blood and body tissues decrease with age, it is not surprising that some elderly subjects who receive vitamin C supplements show enhanced immunity. A recent study demonstrated that men who consume 300 milligrams of vitamin C daily, through food and supplements, have a 40-percent lower death rate from heart disease and other causes than do those whose intake is less than 50 milligrams. Many laboratory studies have indicated that vitamin C inactivates a variety of viruses and bacteria in test tube conditions. Although the research regarding vitamin C and the prevention of colds is conflicting, many studies have shown that it can shorten the duration and lessen the intensity of the symptoms of upper respiratory infections. So while taking vitamin C may not lessen the number of colds you get, it may make them milder. Vitamin C has also been used to reduce the symptoms of asthma and allergies, particularly in cases of seasonal allergic rhinitis. Like many other practicioners, I have used vitamin C with my own patients with superb results.

### Emotional and Physical Stress

Another important role of vitamin C is the one it plays in our ability to handle all types of physical and mental stress. Vitamin C is needed by the adrenal glands to synthesize hormones, and the normally high levels of ascorbic acid in these glands are especially depleted during high-stress occurrences, such as surgery; any kind of illness, including infections and injuries; cigarette smoking; and the use of birth control pills. Research reveals that recovery from injury or surgery can be dramatically accelerated through the use of vitamin C supplementation. In a study in which subjects were given eight to fifty times the RDA (460 to 3,000 milligrams), recovery time was reduced by 50 to 70 percent. The higher the dosage, the shorter the recovery time.

### Cancer

The studies of vitamin C as a means of cancer treatment are, unfortunately, conflicting at this point. However, some research has indicated that the vitamin may be an effective form of cancer therapy.

In 1976, pioneering research conducted by Drs. Edwin Cameron and Linus Pauling studied one hundred terminally ill cancer patients, and concluded that the patients who received supplemental ascorbic acid lived an average of 4.2 times longer than did those who did not receive the supplement. Some supplemented patients lived 20 times longer.

A 1990 follow-up study conducted by Drs. Abram Hoffer and Linus Pauling looked at the effects of high-dose vitamin C therapy (12 grams a day) on cancer patients whose disease was progressing despite treatment with surgery, chemotherapy, and radiation. Patients were also given large daily doses of other nutrients, including 1.5 to 3 grams of niacin, 250 milligrams of vitamin $B_6$, other B vitamins, 800 international units of vitamin E, 30,000 international units of beta-carotene, and 200 to 500 milligrams of selenium. Included in the study were forty patients with cancer of the breast, ovary, uterus, or cervix, and sixty-one with other types of cancer; all of these patients received the nutritional regimen. A control group of thirty-one cancer patients did not receive the regimen. For those patients not receiving the supplements, the mean survival time was 5.7 months. Of those patients who did receive the supplements, 80 percent were considered to be good responders, with a mean survival time of 122 months for patients with cancer of the breast, ovary, uterus, and cervix; and 72 months for patients with other types of cancer. Even the 20 percent considered "poor responders" lived twice as long, on average, as did the unsupplemented cancer patients.

Laboratory research has borne out the results of these human studies. Such research has shown that ascorbic acid can inhibit the growth of leukemia cells and increase the cell-killing ability of various drugs and hormones. Since vitamin C appears to enhance chemotherapy in addition to boosting immunity, many practitioners, including myself, recommend vitamin C supplements to their patients who have cancer, usually in addition to conventional cancer therapy. Hospital protocol is supposed to recommend that 500 milligrams of vitamin C be given to cancer patients. Unfortunately, not all hospitals follow this protocol.

Even traditionalists such as the National Cancer Institute and the American Cancer Society feel that the evidence is strong enough to warrant a diet high in vitamin C as a possible *preventive* measure. Vitamin C's ability to enhance the immune system, discussed earlier, is just one way in which the nutrient contributes to cancer prevention, as is the vitamin's antioxidant function. Another protective mechanism involves nitrosamines and similar substances. Nitrosamines are proven carcinogens in animals and humans. Our bodies are exposed to nitrosamines in food and cigarette smoke. In addition, we ingest nitrites and nitrates, the precursors of nitrosamines, in food (vegetables and cured packaged meats such as bacon, sausage, hot dogs, and ham), water, polluted air, and cigarette smoke. Studies have shown that vitamin C blocks the process by which the body uses these substances to make nitrosamines, and should therefore also block the formation of the tumors that nitrosamines could generate. Studies have correlated a high intake of dietary vitamin C with a reduced risk of cancer of the stomach, colon, bladder, lung, esophagus, and cervix.

It is especially important that cigarette smokers take in adequate amounts of vitamin C. One study showed vitamin C to be anticarcinogenic in laboratory rodents who were exposed to benzopyrene, a very potent carcinogen found in cigarette smoke, including secondhand smoke. Another study found that smokers need a daily intake of nearly two and a half times the RDA to maintain the concentration of ascorbic acid found in nonsmokers.

In addition to the protective properties of orally administered vitamin C, various studies have shown that topical application of vitamin C may protect the skin from the free-radical damage associated with ultraviolet (UV) light. Many companies are now adding vitamin C and other antioxidants to their sunscreens and skin-care products. Animal studies have demonstrated a protective effect of vitamin C administration during radiation treatment for cancer. Both topical and oral vitamin C may prove to be protective during this treatment in humans, as well.

### Cardiovascular Disease

Vitamin C also acts in many ways to help prevent high blood pressure and atherosclerosis—the hardening of the arteries that can lead to heart attack and stroke. Both human and animal studies have linked increased levels of vitamin C with a reduction of serum cholesterol. It is thought that vitamin C may play a role in moving cholesterol from the arteries to the liver, where it is converted into bile acids and then, eventually, eliminated from the body along with fiber. Vitamin C may also help repair damaged arterial walls, and so prevent cholesterol deposits from forming. In addition, as an antioxidant, it reduces the oxidation of LDLs (low-density lipoproteins, the "bad" cholesterol), and thus helps prevent any damage from occurring in the cell wall in the first place.

In one clinical trial, patients with atherosclerosis given 1,000 milligrams of vitamin C daily, could walk farther without feeling pain or breathlessness than could unsupplemented patients. In another study, surgical patients given 1,000 milligrams of vitamin C daily, when contrasted with unsupplemented patients, had a 50-percent lower incidence of deep vein thrombosis—a blood clot that can cut off the blood supply to a major organ such as the heart, lung, or brain. Some studies have shown that an increase in vitamin C is associated with higher levels of high-density lipoproteins (HDLs). Often called "good" cholesterol, HDLs appear to protect the body from heart disease.

It has been discovered that elevated levels of lipoprotein(a), another fatty substance that can be measured in the blood, is a risk factor for stroke. Drs. Linus Pauling and Matt Rath have found that optimal vitamin C also prevents the deposition of lipoprotein(a) in the vascular wall.

### Other Uses

Vitamin C has other functions, as well. It is essential for the growth and repair of tissues in all parts of the body. It is needed for the formation of collagen, present in connective tissue, and for the formation of bone and cartilage. It is needed for the repair of fractured bones. When given before and after dental extraction, vitamin C causes the gum tissues to heal more rapidly. It is needed to convert folic acid, a B vitamin, into its active form. It increases our ability to absorb iron from nonanimal foods, such as raisins and spinach. It also plays a role in the storage of iron in the bone marrow, spleen, and liver, and improves the bioavailability of selenium.

## RDIs AND CLASSIC DEFICIENCY SYMPTOMS

The classic deficiency disease for vitamin C is scurvy. Early symptoms of scurvy are subtle and difficult to diagnose: listlessness, weakness, irritability, vague muscle and joint pains, and weight loss. Symptoms of advanced scurvy are bleeding gums, gingivitis, loosening of the teeth, and extreme weakness and fatigue. The RDI established to prevent these overt symptoms of scurvy is 60 milligrams for men and women.

Yet, many experts feel that the RDI is far too low, and that we are at high risk of not getting the amount of ascorbic acid we need. Unlike most other animals on this planet, we are incapable of producing vitamin C in our bodies. Neither can we store it for very long. Therefore, we must depend upon our food to supply us with what we need every day. Many researchers argue that *optimum* intake of vitamin C is the amount that would be synthesized by humans if we had the enzyme necessary to make vitamin C. Animals that produce their own vitamin C have high levels of ascorbic acid in their tissues. It has been shown that mammals synthesize the equivalent of 3,000 to 19,000 milligrams per day, when calculated for a human weighing 154 pounds. In humans, maximum body pools—the highest level of a substance that the tissues can absorb until they are saturated—have been estimated at 1,500 milligrams per day, but have been reevaluated by others at 5,000 milligrams of vitamin C for a 154-pound person. It is estimated that a daily dose of about 200 milligrams of vitamin C would maintain a body pool of this size in a healthy individual if he or she were totally devoid of stress of any kind. Even the government has begun to question the adequacy of the RDI for vitamin C. A 1996 study completed by Dr. Mark Levine and colleagues of the National Institutes of Health examined vitamin C requirements in healthy volunteers. The researchers concluded that the current recommendation of 60 milligrams should be increased to 200 milligrams per day.

As another means of calculating optimum daily intake, scientists have studied the handful of other animals that do not produce vitamin C: guinea pigs, primates, and certain fish. Their discovery has startling implications for human beings: Per body weight, primates and guinea pigs consume the equivalent of 2,000 milligrams of vitamin C per day. When under stress, they may ingest the equivalent of up to 7,000 to 10,000 milligrams of vitamin C per day. By law, animal chow for guinea pigs and monkeys must provide, respectively, the equivalent of 1,100 milligrams and 1,250 milligrams daily.

This data suggests that an optimum intake for humans may be 1,000 milligrams or more daily—an amount far higher than the RDI of 60 milligrams!

*Food Sources:* The foods that are highest in vitamin C include broccoli, Brussels sprouts, black currants, collards, guava, horseradish, kale, turnip greens, parsley, and sweet peppers. Also high on the list are cabbage, cauliflower, chives, kohlrabi, orange pulp, lemon pulp, mustard greens, beet greens, papaya, spinach, strawberries, and watercress. Sources of moderate amounts of ascorbic acid are asparagus, lima beans, Swiss chard, gooseberries, red currants, grapefruit, limes, loganberries, melons, okra, tangerines, potatoes, and turnips. (Notice that citrus fruits such as oranges and grapefruits do not have the highest ascorbic acid content; however, their skin is high in bioflavonoids, substances that increase the amount of vitamin C that is absorbed.)

Ascorbic acid is easily destroyed when exposed to oxygen, and this process is accelerated by light and heat. Vegetables begin to lose vitamin C as soon as they are cut. Freshly squeezed orange juice, which is not likely to be that high in vitamin C in the first place, quickly begins to lose its supply of this nutrient, too. As a result, there is almost no vitamin C to speak of in the juice sold in bottles and cartons. Since vitamin C is sensitive to heat and is lost when large quantities of water are used in cooking, vegetables should be eaten raw, lightly steamed, or cooked in a small amount of water to retain the greatest amount of this nutrient.

## SUPPLEMENTS

Vitamin C supplements are available both as ascorbic acid and as mineral ascorbates. You should be aware that the vitamin C in most supplements has been synthesized from natural, inexpensive substances such as starch, molasses, or sago palm. The "natural" vitamin C found in supplements is extracted from rose hips, which contain one percent ascorbic acid. Rose-hips vitamin C supplements actually contain mostly synthetic vitamin C, as a vitamin C supplement made entirely from rose hips would be enormous in size and very expensive. However, rose hips probably contain complementary substances that enhance the absorption of the vitamin, so that there may be some advantage to taking supplements which contain them. I do recommend that you buy ascorbic acid supplements which contain bioflavonoids (see Chapter 35), as these substances have been shown to increase vitamin C absorption.

In some supplements, ascorbic acid has been mixed with minerals to form mineral ascorbates. The most readily available mineral ascorbate is calcium ascorbate, which is sometimes mixed with other mineral ascorbates, such as magnesium ascorbate and sodium ascorbate. The advantage of calcium and other mineral ascorbates is that these are buffered forms of vitamin C—a desirable trait for some individuals, because they are nonacid and gentler to the stomach. People who have difficulty with oral doses of straight ascorbic acid can use these buffered products without getting acid stomach or diarrhea.

Vitamin C is widely available in the form of chewable tablets. Although convenient, high intakes of these tablets are not recommended for two reasons. First, they are usually loaded with sugar. Second, they may cause the pH of the saliva to fall so low that calcium is leached from tooth enamel.

Ascorbic acid is also available in the form of a powder that is to be dissolved in liquids. Although cheaper than tablets and capsules, the powder is less convenient to take. In addition, it, too, can damage tooth enamel, and so should be sipped through a straw if high dosages are taken frequently during the day.

## OPTIMUM DAILY INTAKE—ODI

For optimum general health, the basic Optimum Daily Intake for vitamin C is:

500–5,000 mg for men and women
(along with 500–5,000 mg bioflavonoids)

Based on a thorough scientific review of vitamin C, and on my clinical experience, the following amounts of vitamin C appear to be valuable for:

| Condition | Suggested Dosage |
|---|---|
| Allergies or asthma | 3,000–7,000 mg |
| Bleeding gums | 1,000–3,000 mg |
| Cancer prevention | 5,000–10,000 mg |
| Coronary heart disease prevention | 500–4,000 mg |
| Enhanced immunity | 1,000–5,000 mg |
| Exposure to cigarette smoke and polluted air | 1,000–5,000 mg |
| High levels of stress | 1,000–5,000 mg |
| Surgery, wounds, injuries | 5,000–10,000 mg |

Your Optimum Daily Intake may vary from day to day, depending on various factors. For example, you may want to raise your intake temporarily during times of stress, or when you have a cold or another type of infection. After such a period of time, remember to decrease your supplementation *gradually* until it is back to your normal ODI.

It is best to spread your total intake of vitamin C over the course of the day.

For example, if you take 3,000 milligrams total, take 1,000 milligrams at each meal. There are two advantages to this. First, because Vitamin C is rapidly excreted from the body, divided doses ensure a more constant level of blood and tissue saturation. Second, divided doses reduce the likelihood of any adverse effects, such as acid stomach or diarrhea.

Absorption varies widely from person to person. Studies have shown that one person may be able to absorb 3 grams of this vitamin without any excess spilling over into the urine. Other subjects are able to absorb only 100 milligrams at one time, and will excrete anything over that.

*Remember:* If you have a medical condition, please consult with your physician before taking supplements.

## TOXICITY AND ADVERSE EFFECTS

There is no proven toxicity for vitamin C. You may have heard that vitamin C causes kidney stones, but no studies show any relationship between vitamin C and the formation of kidney stones (calcium oxalate) in healthy people. Keep in mind, though, that vitamin C may actually interfere with the accuracy of certain commercial kits used by physicians to determine oxalate in the urine. A 1993 study suggests that kits using decarboxylase may be preferable. However, if you have a history of kidney problems of any kind, you should take vitamin C only under the guidance of a qualified professional. With alterations in kidney function, the mechanism that handles vitamin C excretion may not be working properly, so that caution may be warranted.

Early studies suggested that large doses of vitamin C destroy vitamin $B_{12}$ in the body. Subsequent studies using improved techniques have shown that vitamin C does not have this effect.

One common adverse effect of very high levels of vitamin C—5,000 milligrams a day and up—is intestinal gas and loose stools. This effect is benign and completely reversible. In fact, many practitioners, including myself, advise using this effect as a guide to finding your personal Optimum Daily Intake, particularly if you suffer from chronic fatigue, HIV infection, or AIDS. Many practitioners recommend that you start with lower daily doses of vitamin C (2 to 6 grams) and add 1 to 2 grams each week until bowel intolerance symptoms—gas, bloating, and/or diarrhea—appear. Then cut back on the dosage just until the symptoms are eliminated. Interestingly, it often appears that as someone gets better, their bowel tolerance decreases, and they need less vitamin C. I have noticed this occurring in myself. When I have a cold or the flu, I can take as much as 10 grams of vitamin C a day, with no bowel intolerance symptoms. But when I'm well, this amount does cause symptoms.

Some practitioners believe that if you take very high doses of vitamin C, and then suddenly stop supplementation, you may experience "rebound scurvy." A recent review study found that there is no basis for this belief. However, if you are concerned, you can easily prevent this by reducing your dosage slowly over a period of a few weeks.

Vitamin C is used by the liver to detoxify drugs and other chemicals, and appears to protect the body from the side effects that accompany many drugs. For instance, it has been shown to prevent acetaminophen (e.g., Tylenol) toxicity to the liver without hindering the drug's effectiveness. However, when taking other long-acting drugs, you may want to consult with a professional about taking high doses of ascorbic acid.

# Part Three

---

# THE MINERALS

# Chapter 21

# CALCIUM

Our bodies contain approximately 1,200 grams—about 2.5 pounds—of calcium, 99 percent of which is stored in our bones and teeth. The remaining 1 percent of calcium—10 to 12 grams, or about a third of an ounce—is distributed throughout the body in the bloodstream and the fluids surrounding our cells.

## FUNCTIONS AND USES

### Hypertension

Recent studies indicate that the high incidence of hypertension (high blood pressure) in the United States may be a result of low calcium intake combined with high sodium intake. In one study, forty-eight hypertensive men were treated with 1,000 milligrams of calcium for eight weeks. Twenty-one of them (44 percent) achieved a therapeutically meaningful reduction in their blood pressure. In many cases, the result was similar or superior to that achieved with blood pressure medication.

In another study, women with high blood pressure were given either 1,500 milligrams of calcium *or* hypertensive medication for four years. The calcium-supplemented group achieved a significant drop in their systolic blood pressure. The unsupplemented group experienced a *rise* in their blood pressure, *even though they were taking hypertensive medication.*

Studies have also revealed a worldwide correlation between pregnancy-related hypertension and low calcium intake. In countries characterized by an average calcium intake of 1,000 milligrams per day or more, pregnancy-related hypertension occurs in fewer than 1 out of 200 pregnancies. In societies in which calcium intake is under 500 milligrams per day, the incidence is ten to twenty times higher.

Calcium supplementation is free of the unpleasant side effects so frequently encountered with antihypertensive drug treatment, including impotence, fatigue, exercise intolerance, weight gain, dizziness, and impaired concentration. As the studies indicate, calcium therapy can be an effective medication-free means of treating high blood pressure. Hypertensives who are salt-sensitive seem to benefit most.

## Colon Cancer

There is also some evidence that calcium helps prevent colon cancer. Epidemiological studies have shown that colon cancer incidence is lower in people who receive more sunlight exposure and consume more dairy foods. Several studies suggest that people who eat a typical high-fat diet may be protected from colon cancer by consuming 1,200 to 1,500 milligrams of calcium daily. The authors found that within two to three months after supplementation was begun, tests of the subjects' colon linings showed that the number of fast-growing cells associated with cancer had significantly decreased. In a Dutch study of over 2,500 people, those with a low intake of calcium had a higher risk of being diagnosed with colorectal cancer, and a higher death rate from this form of cancer, as well. It should be noted that one source of dietary calcium—yogurt—provides the body with *two* forms of protection. In addition to the calcium, yogurt contains "friendly" bacteria (acidophilus) that inhibit the effects of known colonic carcinogens.

## The Bones

Most of the attention paid to calcium is due to its role in maintaining strong, healthy bones. As we have seen, although most of the calcium in the body is found in the bones, calcium performs various vital functions throughout the body. Thus, our bones are designed to provide more than a rigid framework for our bodies. They also function as a kind of bank from which the body can draw the calcium it needs for other purposes. This is an ongoing dynamic process during which bone—which, despite its seeming permanence, is a live tissue—is constantly being broken down and re-formed. In the process, about 600 to 700 milligrams of calcium are exchanged in the bone of normal adults every day. Normally, if there is sufficient calcium being absorbed from the diet, the blood and bone calcium levels stay in balance and fluctuate only slightly. However, from the body's point of view, it is more important to maintain enough calcium in the blood to keep the heart beating regularly than it is to keep the bones strong and hard. So if the diet is deficient in calcium, the body will always choose to maintain a certain level of calcium in the blood by drawing it out of the bone. This is accomplished through a complex system involving hormones, especially the parathyroid hormone, and vitamin D. Even if there is adequate calcium in the diet, a lack of vitamin D will seriously impair the body's ability to make use of the mineral.

The survival mechanism just discussed can cause some problems if a calcium-deficient diet is consumed over a long period of time. Eventually, there is so much calcium lost from the bone that osteoporosis—loss of bone mass, or thinning of the bone—occurs. The bones become porous, brittle, and so weak that a person may easily suffer a fracture from such normal activities as sneezing, bending over, or receiving a hug. The vertebrae of the spinal column may compress or fracture, causing pain, disability, loss of height, and a hunched-over appearance. If calcium is lost from the bones of the jaw, periodontal disease may result. Hip fracture is also a common sign of osteoporosis, and is a major source of disability among the older population. Indeed, osteoporosis is occurring in epidemic proportions in an estimated 15 to 20 million Americans. Women over the age of fifty (postmenopausal) are especially at risk, but many younger people and older men are affected as well. Osteomalacia, or softening of the bone, is another common problem that is caused by inadequate calcium intake.

The growing consensus is that osteoporosis is not a disease that comes on suddenly in middle or old age. Many studies have correlated a long-term low-calcium diet, perhaps beginning at the age of thirty or earlier, with the development of osteoporosis and periodontal disease. In children, the deficiency symptom of poor calcium intake is rickets, a condition in which the bones grow too weak to support the weight of the child, with deformity being the highly visible result. There is some recent evidence that a suboptimum calcium intake in childhood may help set the stage for bone loss in later life, even when there are no obvious problems during childhood.

Because the body gives top priority to the maintenance of normal calcium levels in the blood, blood tests are an ineffective means of determining calcium levels in either the bone or the diet. The blood may be perfectly normal, while the bone level is poor. The clinical signs of calcium depletion from the bone are insidious, and so are not usually apparent until the symptoms of osteoporosis begin to appear. Even x-rays are incapable of picking up bone loss until 30 to 40 percent of the bone has disappeared. Once osteoporosis is diagnosed, it can usually be slowed or halted with appropriate therapy, but it can be difficult to reverse. For this reason, I feel that the best course of action is prevention. That is why I recommend that calcium supplementation be started as early as possible, and preferably by age twenty.

## Other Functions

In addition to the functions just discussed, calcium is used to activate the enzymes involved in fat and protein digestion and in the production of energy. It is involved in blood clotting and the transmission of nerve impulses. Calcium also regulates the contraction and relaxation of the muscles, including the heart. And it aids in the absorption of many nutrients, especially vitamin B$_{12}$.

## RDIs, DEFICIENCIES, AND FACTORS
## THAT INFLUENCE ABSORPTION

Although calcium intake is clearly a major factor in the development of the diseases of calcium deficiency—osteoporosis, osteomalacia, and rickets—it is not the only factor. There are many other circumstances that influence the absorption and utilization of the calcium you consume. These include other elements of the diet, exercise, and any medication taken.

Some studies have linked diets high in protein and fat—especially when the fat and protein come from foods of animal origin—with the loss of calcium from the bone. However, it is difficult to isolate other factors such as vitamin D, calcium, and phosphorus intake in these studies. Therefore, the results have been conflicting.

One important dietary element is phosphorus intake. Most researchers advise that the ratio of calcium to phosphorus should be at least 1 to 1. In other words, you should take in at least as much calcium as you do phosphorus. If phosphorus intake is much higher, it may impair the absorption of calcium, as well as increase the amount drawn out of the bone. So if your diet contains many phosphorus-rich foods such as meats, soft drinks, and food additives, your phosphorus intake may be too high to maintain a good calcium balance.

A 1985 study suggests that an adequate amount of *all* the micronutrients can make a significant difference in the body's proper and efficient metabolism of calcium. One group of women was given a calcium and vitamin D supplement, and experienced an improvement in bone density. The other group received a balanced supplement of calcium, vitamin D, and 100 percent of the RDA for over fifteen other vitamins and minerals. This group experienced a *two to three times greater increase in bone density*. A growing body of evidence seems to indicate that several trace minerals, including zinc, manganese, copper, boron, and essential fatty acids, as well as vitamin D and the B vitamins, all play a role in preventing, halting, and reversing osteoporosis.

The RDI for calcium has been established at 1,000 milligrams for everyone over the age of four, except for pregnant or lactating women, for whom the RDI is 1,300 milligrams. However, research has shown that a large percentage of people develop osteoporosis even when their intake is at this level. This suggests that 1,000 milligrams may not be enough, especially during the early time in your life when you are developing peak bone mass and, for women, after menopause. In fact, the American Medical Association and many research scientists recommend at least 1,500 milligrams for postmenopausal women.

Interestingly enough, recent research has discovered that our ancient human ancestors who lived during the Paleolithic Age ingested approximately 1,600 milligrams of calcium per day. Evolutionary theory suggests that we are genetically "programmed" to require a similar amount. The richest food source is milk and dairy products. Over three glasses of milk or the equivalent is needed to attain the RDI of 1,000 milligrams, but many people do not include anywhere near this amount in their diet. While the lactose in milk may increase calcium absorption, we are not sure whether lactose-intolerant people—who have trouble digesting milk—experience an impairment in calcium absorption. They are likely, however, to avoid milk products, and so are at particularly high risk of calcium deficiency.

One study found that two thirds of the women in America between the ages of eighteen and thirty—the period during which peak bone mass is developing—ingest less than the RDI. After the age of thirty-six, three fourths have calcium intakes less than the RDI. Fully one fourth of all U.S. women ingest less than 300 milligrams on any given day. Further exacerbating the situation is that absorption of whatever calcium is in the diet begins to decrease during the ages of forty to fifty, and in some cases, perhaps as early as thirty. After menopause, estrogen levels decrease, an event that has also been implicated in bone loss. Estrogen therapy, which may have some disturbing side effects, is often prescribed in an attempt to prevent bone loss in postmenopausal women. In fact, estrogen therapy slows bone loss, at best. Many practitioners prefer calcium therapy over estrogen therapy, as calcium, when taken with other nutrients, appears to *increase* bone density.

I also advise my patients to get regular physical exercise, because studies have shown that physical exercise may improve calcium absorption and utilization, and may therefore play a crucial role in the prevention and treatment of osteoporosis. Aerobic exercise and weight training have been shown to increase bone mass in athletes, in the elderly, and in people recovering from a decrease in bone mass that occurs during a decrease in physical activity. Loss of bone mass is most pronounced in people undergoing full bed rest, who lose 200 to 300 milligrams of calcium per day. A diet that is adequate for a healthy adult may not provide enough calcium to offset prior illness-related losses. Increasing the calcium intake alone during the illness will not offset these losses, either. However, resumed physical activity combined with adequate calcium intake will restore normal bone mass.

As mentioned earlier, another factor that can affect calcium absorption is any medication being taken. Among the many medications that can affect the absorption and utilization of calcium are antibiotics, oral contraceptives, anticonvulsants, and laxatives. (For details, see the Drug-Nutrient Interaction

Table on page 234.) When such medications are taken, calcium intake should be increased.

*Food Sources:* Dairy foods such as milk, cheese, and yogurt are outstanding sources of calcium. If you do not consume such foods, it is extremely difficult to achieve a satisfactory intake of dietary calcium. In addition to its being a superb source of calcium, milk contains lactose, a substance that may increase the absorption of calcium in our bodies. Other foods that can make a substantial contribution include canned salmon and sardines (including the bones), and green leafy vegetables such as collard greens, turnip greens, and mustard greens. Clams, oysters, and shrimp are also good sources of calcium, followed by kale, broccoli, soybeans, and soybean products such as tofu.

It has been estimated that we actually absorb as litle as 20 to 40 percent of the calcium in our food. Part of the problem may be oxalic acid, a substance found in spinach, Swiss chard, beet greens, cocoa, and rhubarb. This substance may bind with calcium to prevent its absorption in the colon. Phytic acid, or phytates—substances found in the outer layers of cereal grains—may also interfere with calcium absorption. However, the evidence is inconclusive, and many scientists discount it. In addition, the inhibitory effect of such substances appears to occur only when calcium intake is low, and oxalic acid or phytate intake is quite high. In addition, the fermentation of yeast, as found in leavened bread, destroys much of the phytate in the flour. In fact, when vegetarians were studied, it was found that they have less incidence of osteoporosis than nonvegetarians. Since vegetarians as a group eat a diet high in phytates, it seems unlikely that calcium absorption is significantly affected by this substance.

## SUPPLEMENTS

Calcium supplements are available as tablets, as flavored chewable squares, and in liquid form. The supplements generally combine pure, or "elemental," calcium with other chemicals, or "salts." The forms most commonly available are calcium aspartate, calcium carbonate, calcium citrate, calcium gluconate, and calcium lactate. When buying calcium supplements, remember to consider the amount of *elemental* calcium, not the amount of calcium salts. Of the three forms, calcium carbonate contains the greatest amount of elemental calcium: 40 percent. Many people prefer this form because the higher calcium content allows them to take fewer pills to obtain their Optimum Daily Intake. However, the other forms may have specific therapeutic value. Another factor to consider is absorbability. I generally recommend calcium carbonate and calcium lactate, since they appear to be very absorbable. Calcium citrate, which is also quite absorbable, may be a particularly good choice for the elderly. Often, elderly individuals have low levels of hydrochloric acid in their stomachs, and so do best with calcium citrate, which requires little hydrochloric acid for absorption.

I advise you to take your calcium supplements along with magnesium and vitamin D, as these three nutrients work together to enhance one another's absorption and utilization in the body. Also, if calcium supplements are taken without magnesium, it may result in a magnesium deficiency—a deficiency that has been implicated in osteoporosis. The calcium-to-magnesium ratio should be approximately 2 to 1. Fortunately, there are now many supplements that contain calcium carbonate or calcium lactate and magnesium in the proper proportions. There are also supplements that combine calcium with vitamin D.

Dolomite is a supplement that contains both calcium and magnesium. However, because this product contains these minerals in their least absorbable form, I do not recommend its use. Bone meal, another source of calcium, is highly absorbable. However, this form contains substantial amounts of phosphorus, and most people get quite enough—and often too much—phosphorus from their diets.

Many antacids are being promoted as calcium supplements since these products contain calcium carbonate. However, some of these also contain aluminum, a toxic mineral that can interfere with calcium absorption and have many deleterious effects on the body. One study showed that these adverse effects include high levels of calcium excreted in the urine, bone resorption (loss of minerals from the bone), impaired fluoride absorption, and phosphorus depletion, all of which may ironically contribute to bone disease. If you choose to use antacids as your source of calcium, be sure to read the label to check that aluminum is not an ingredient.

## OPTIMUM DAILY INTAKE—ODI

For optimum general health, the basic Optimum Daily Intake for calcium is:

1,000–1,500 mg for men and women

Based on a thorough scientific review of calcium, and on my clinical experience, the following amounts of calcium appear to be valuable for:

| Condition | Suggested Dosage |
|---|---|
| Broken bones and fractures | 1,000–2,000 mg |
| High blood pressure | 1,000–1,500 mg |
| Osteoporosis | 1,200–2,000 mg |

Calcium should be taken with magnesium in a ratio of 2 to 1, and with vitamin D to aid in absorption. Since the body is unable to absorb 1,000 milligrams all at once, divide your total ODI into halves or thirds and take them two or three times a day.

*Remember:* If you have a medical condition, please consult with your physician before taking supplements.

## TOXICITY AND ADVERSE EFFECTS

Calcium has no known toxic effects. A panel of the Food and Drug Administration (FDA) concluded that calcium intakes of 1,000 to 2,500 milligrams daily do not result in hypercalcemia—high levels of calcium in the blood. Although hypercalcemia may be seen in certain medical conditions and in cases of vitamin D overdose, a high intake of calcium is not in itself a causative factor. The development of kidney stones in connection with high calcium intake is rare. One study demonstrated that calcium citrate does not cause kidney stones.

Some people report a feeling of relaxation and drowsiness after taking calcium supplements. This has never been documented in a scientific study. However, if you experience this particular effect, you can do what I suggest to my patients: Take advantage of the drowsiness by scheduling your calcium supplements in the evening before retiring.

# Chapter 22

# PHOSPHORUS

hosphorus is the second most abundant mineral in the body, after calcium. There are approximately 600 to 700 grams of this mineral—1.25 to 1.5 pounds—in the average-size person, which represents about 1 percent of total body weight. As is the case with calcium, most of the body's phosphorus (80 to 90 percent) is found in the bones and teeth. The rest is distributed throughout the body in the cells, and in the blood and other fluids. The ratio of calcium to phosphorus in the bone is about 2 to 1. However, in the soft tissues, the proportion of phosphorus is much higher.

## FUNCTIONS AND USES

First and foremost, phosphorus strengthens bones and teeth. But this mineral also plays a part in almost every important chemical reaction in the body. Most of its actions have to do with the utilization of fats, protein, and carbohydrates. One function is to combine with fats in the blood to make phospholipids, which, in turn, become the part of the cell that regulates the transport of materials in and out of the cell walls. Phosphorus is also involved in the transport of fats in the circulatory system.

Phosphorus is involved in energy metabolism, storage, and regulation. It also plays a role in such cellular processes as muscle contraction, the transfer of nerve impulses, hormone secretion, and protein synthesis. Additionally, it is a component of the nucleic acids—RNA and DNA—which control heredity and the replication of cells. Moreover, many of the B vitamins are effective only when combined with this mineral in the body. Finally, phosphorus plays an important part in our buffer system, which maintains the proper acid-base balance (pH) within the body.

## RDIs AND DEFICIENCY SYMPTOMS

Considering the many ways in which phosphorus is used within the body, it is fortunate that most people have no trouble getting more than the Reference

Daily Intake of 1,000 milligrams for men and women, and 1,300 milligrams for pregnant and lactating women. Although there is some evidence that phytates—substances found in whole grains—interfere with the absorption of essential minerals, there is doubt as to whether this occurs on a large enough scale to be of practical importance. Although long-term phytate consumption has not been specifically investigated, vegetarians, who consume a high-fiber diet rich in phytates, have not been found to be deficient in phosphorus. The long-term use of aluminum-containing antacids, however, may deplete the body of phosphorus to such a degree that deficiency is a real possibility. Symptoms of phosphorus deficiency include weakness, loss of appetite, loss of bone mass, and loss of calcium.

The actual absorption, storage, and excretion of phosphorus is dependent on mechanisms involving vitamin D and parathyroid hormone. Like calcium, phosphorus exists in a complex give-and-take relationship between the bones, the blood, and the soft tissues of the body. It is continuously being deposited and released from the bone "bank" as blood levels fluctuate in response to dietary intake and excretion. In addition, phosphorus levels and calcium levels influence each other. It has been suggested that phosphorus and calcium intake should be approximately equal—in a ratio of 1 to 1—even though the ratio in bone is 2 to 1. However, excess phosphorus consumption is common, with an average daily intake of 1,500 to 1,600 milligrams. This means that in most diets, phosphorus intake exceeds calcium intake. A convincing body of evidence suggests that this overly high phosphorus intake, coupled with long-term low calcium intake and high protein intake, is a major dietary factor in the demineralization that leads to osteoporosis. For instance, in a study of female athletes, those who drank carbonated beverages—which are rich in phosphorus— had more than twice as many fractures as did those who did not include high-phosphorus beverages in their diet. (See Chapter 21 for more information on calcium and osteoporosis.)

*Food Sources:* Phosphorus is found in nearly all foods, but is especially high in carbonated soft drinks, milk and other dairy products, meat, and fish. Nuts, beans, and grains are also high in phosphorus.

### SUPPLEMENTS

Rather than adding phosphorus supplements to their diet, most people appear to require a *reduction* of phosphorus. Foods that are particularly high in phosphorus include meat and carbonated beverages. Traditionally, a calcium-to-phosphorus ratio of 1 to 1 is recommended. However, as a general rule, a higher percentage of phosphorus (70 percent) than calcium (40 percent) is absorbed from the diet. In addition, the calcium-to-phosphorus ratio in the bone is 2 to 1. Bearing this in mind, you may want to manipulate the ratio slightly in favor of calcium to maintain a more favorable balance in the body.

## OPTIMUM DAILY INTAKE—ODI

For optimum general health, the Optimum Daily Intake for most people can usually be met through dietary sources. Possible exceptions may include the elderly, menopausal women, and individuals on restricted diets. For this population, the ODIs are:

200–400 mg for men and women

*Remember:* If you have a medical condition, please consult with your physician before taking supplements.

## TOXICITY AND ADVERSE EFFECTS

Too much phosphorus may lead to an increase in the excretion of calcium, and, consequently, to osteoporosis.

# Chapter 23

# MAGNESIUM

Your body contains between 20 and 28 grams of magnesium. Half of this amount is found in the bones. The remainder activates hundreds of enzymes throughout the body, and is critical for proper cell function.

## FUNCTIONS AND USES

### Bones and Teeth

Like calcium and phosphorus, magnesium is required for strong, healthy bones and teeth. This mineral plays an important part in bone growth, and helps prevent tooth decay by holding calcium in tooth enamel. Understandably, poor magnesium intake has been implicated in disorders such as osteoporosis.

### Muscles

One of magnesium's most important roles is that of helping the muscles to relax. When calcium flows into muscle tissue cells, the muscle contracts. When calcium leaves and magnesium replaces it, the muscle relaxes. These functions are no doubt related to the association of magnesium deficiency with the occurrence of muscle spasms, tremors, and convulsions. Many professionals now successfully use magnesium malate supplements—a combination of magnesium and malic acid—in the treatment of fibromyalgia, a disorder characterized by many tender knots in the muscles; and in the treatment of chronic fatigue, which may also involve muscle aches and pains.

### Psychiatric Disorders

Low magnesium appears to be associated with psychiatric problems. In a study of 165 boys, it was found that those with symptoms of depression, schizophrenia, and sleep disturbances had lower levels of magnesium in the blood than did boys without these disorders. In another study, it was found that the average magnesium levels of autistic children were also well below average. In fact, there is some evidence that autistic children may improve when given large doses of magnesium along with vitamin B$_6$.

In adults, insufficient magnesium may be accompanied by a loss of sensation in the extremities and, if severe, tremors, convulsions, muscle contractions, confusion, delirium, and behavioral disturbances. One study found that psychiatric patients who had attempted suicide had lower magnesium levels than did nonsuicidal psychiatric patients and healthy individuals.

### Cardiovascular Disease

Magnesium—along with sodium, potassium, and calcium—appears to affect the muscle tone of the blood vessels, which may explain why magnesium supplementation has been shown to help control cardiovascular disease. For example, research indicates that magnesium supplementation is effective in lowering some types of high blood pressure in individuals with low magnesium levels. In addition, research has shown that people suffering from angina, which can be caused by a spasm of the blood vessel leading to the heart, are benefited by magnesium supplementation. People with high blood pressure often experience spasms in the blood vessels of the retina, which can eventually affect vision. In studies, these people, who tend to have low levels of magnesium, have experienced a regression of this disease when taking magnesium supplements. Diabetes is another disease that can damage the blood vessels of the retina, possibly leading to severe vision problems and even blindness. Again, there is evidence that low levels of magnesium may be an additional risk factor in the development and progression of this complication.

### Other Functions

Magnesium has many functions other than those just discussed. For instance, magnesium plays an important role in maintaining the function of the nerves. It also stabilizes the enzymes that produce cellular energy, and thus is involved in energy regulation and metabolism. It also plays a role in proper insulin production. Finally, this nutrient may prove useful in preventing certain complications of pregnancy, such as prematurity and intrauterine growth retardation.

### RDIs AND DEFICIENCIES

Since magnesium is widely distributed in foods, severe deficiencies are most often found in those whose food intake is low or imbalanced, such as alcoholics and diabetics. However, many other groups of people may be at risk. It has been estimated that as much as 60 percent of the United States population is at risk for magnesium deficiency. For instance, people using a number of drugs, including antibiotics and diuretics, may have depleted magnesium.

Oral contraceptives, too, have been found to lower blood magnesium. Since low magnesium levels result in blood clots, this may help explain why there is a higher incidence of thrombosis among women on the pill. (For more information on the effect of drugs on magnesium levels, see the Drug-Nutrient Interaction Table on page 234.) In addition, magnesium may be too low in people with malabsorption syndromes or gastrointestinal disorders such as Crohn's disease. We are also beginning to recognize that bulimics are at risk because of their prolonged diarrhea and/or vomiting. Stress has also been implicated in depleted magnesium levels, which may account for the typical "Type A" personality's increased risk for cardiovascular disease. One study suggested that stress may also be in part responsible for the lowered magnesium levels in women with premenstrual tension.

The RDI for magnesium is 400 milligrams for men and women, and 450 milligrams for pregnant and lactating women.

*Food Sources:* Magnesium is widely distributed in foods. Those foods with the highest magnesium content include milk and other dairy products, meat, seafood, nuts, blackstrap molasses, soybeans, seeds, and wheat germ. Whole grains such as oatmeal, cornmeal, and rice are also good sources.

Bear in mind, however, that the magnesium content of food varies considerably with the magnesium content of the soil in which the food is grown. In addition, much of the magnesium in food is lost during processing. For example, milling removes 59 percent of the magnesium from whole wheat. Cooking foods in water also causes this mineral to leach out.

## SUPPLEMENTS

The potency of magnesium supplements is determined by the amount of elemental magnesium. I recommend taking magnesium supplements as either magnesium carbonate or magnesium oxide, as these forms have the greatest potency. Magnesium oxide contains the greatest percentage of magnesium—60 percent—while magnesium carbonate is 40 percent magnesium. Other forms of magnesium, such as chelated magnesium, which is bound to amino acids; magnesium citrate; magnesium malate; and magnesium aspartate, are also available. Many practitioners prefer these forms in specific therapeutic regimens. Although they provide less magnesium per tablet or capsule than do magnesium oxide and magnesium carbonate, these forms do contain compounds that appear to have their own beneficial effects. Citrate, for example, is important for energy production. In addition, the magnesium in these supplements may be more bioavailable than that in the higher-magnesium products.

Magnesium works together with other nutrients, such as calcium and vitamin D. As explained in Chapter 21, calcium and magnesium supplements should be taken together. The consensus is that the calcium-to-magnesium ratio should be about 2 to 1, which is what I usually recommend. There are supplements that contain both calcium and magnesium in this ratio. Some researchers have had success using a ratio that is closer to 1 to 1. However, studies supporting this ratio are lacking at this time. Many people compromise by taking calcium and magnesium in a ratio of 2 to 1.5

## OPTIMUM DAILY INTAKE—ODI

For optimum health, the basic Optimum Daily Intake for magnesium is:

### 500–750 mg for men and women

Based on a thorough scientific review of magnesium, and on my clinical experience, the following amounts of magnesium appear to be valuable for:

| Condition | Suggested Dosage |
|---|---|
| Angina | 500–1,000 mg |
| Fibromyalgia and chronic fatigue | 6–12 tablets of magnesium malate* |
| High blood pressure | 500–750 mg |
| Oral contraceptive use | 500–750 mg |
| Osteoporosis | 500–1,000 mg |

*Six tablets supply approximately 300 mg magnesium and 1,200 mg malic acid.

*Remember:* If you have a medical condition, please consult your physician before taking supplements.

## TOXICITY AND ADVERSE EFFECTS

Magnesium toxicity is rare, except in individuals with kidney failure. In healthy individuals, large amounts of magnesium salts—3,000 to 5,000 milligrams daily—have a cathartic effect, and magnesium-containing products are often used as over-the-counter laxatives. These products, which include Epsom salts (magnesium sulfate), milk of magnesia (magnesium hydroxide), and magnesium citrate, work by drawing fluid into the intestines, and thereby stimulating contractions. Toxicity symptoms have been noted in subjects treated with 9,000 milligrams of this mineral.

# Chapter 24

# ZINC

Our bodies contain approximately 2 to 3 grams of zinc, which is distributed throughout the body. Zinc is an essential component of over twenty enzymes associated with many different metabolic processes. The highest concentrations of zinc are found in the eyes, liver, bones, prostate, semen, and hair.

## FUNCTIONS AND USES

### Growth and Reproduction

Perhaps the most critical role zinc plays is in the synthesis of the nucleic acids RNA and DNA, which are essential for cell division, cell repair, and cell growth. Thus, zinc is needed for reproduction, and for growth and development. Several studies have linked low zinc levels with complications during pregnancy, and with miscarriage and birth defects.

Studies have also found large percentages of children to be deficient in zinc. These children showed symptoms of suboptimal growth, in addition to a loss of taste acuity and poor appetite. When their zinc intake was increased, the symptoms improved. Animal studies and human studies of children and adults suggest that lethargy, passivity, and apathy are symptoms of marginal zinc deficiency, since these behavioral problems improve with zinc supplementation.

### The Eye

One of the highest concentrations of zinc in the human body is found in the eye, especially the iris and retina. Although the exact mechanisms of its functions are largely unknown, zinc seems to be involved in the activation of vitamin A, and thus is a factor in night vision. In addition, there is a growing body of evidence which indicates that poor zinc intake is related to such eye conditions as impaired color discrimination; cataract formation; and optic neuritis, the inflammation of the optic nerve.

## Physical and Mental Stress

There is some evidence that zinc levels fall after physical and mental stress. For instance, strenuous exercise has been shown to lead to significant losses of zinc, probably due to the increase in glucose metabolism, which requires zinc. It has also been discovered that zinc is depleted during upper respiratory infection accompanied by fever. In addition, severe burn victims have only two thirds the normal amount of zinc in their blood. Diabetics tend to have less zinc in their tissues, which may be related to many of their complications.

Studies have shown that zinc supplements may have therapeutic value in cases of physical stress. When hospital patients who were marginally deficient in zinc were given extra zinc, it helped restore the rate of healing to normal. Zinc may therefore be of benefit to people who have undergone surgery, or have sustained broken bones or wounds. Some physicians prescribe zinc to stimulate the healing process.

## Taste and Smell

Zinc is especially important in body systems that undergo a rapid turnover of cells. This includes the gastrointestinal system, and particularly the taste buds—a fact that may explain why a change in the ability to taste foods is often an early sign of zinc deficiency. This symptom may be accompanied by similar changes in the ability to smell. Foods may either have no taste or smell at all, or taste or smell unpleasant. All these factors contribute to a loss of appetite, but may be so insidious that they go unnoticed.

Many of my elderly patients report a heightened sense of taste after a few weeks of zinc supplementation. They often find this development quite remarkable, since prior to supplementation, they may not have recognized the loss of taste sensitivity. The elderly may benefit from zinc supplementation in another way, too, as zinc appears to play a role in increasing bone density in postmenopausal women.

## The Immune System

Zinc may exert a protective influence by boosting the immune system. Many studies have shown that a zinc deficiency can impair a large variety of immune functions and defense mechanisms in animals, and some studies have shown similar effects in humans. These effects—which include abnormalities and eventual shrinking of the spleen, thymus, and lymph nodes; and impaired production of antibodies—have been found to be correctable with zinc supplementation.

Low zinc levels, often accompanied by high copper levels, have been reported in people with many types of cancer. In a 1981 study, it was found that people with a certain type of lung cancer survived for a significantly longer period of time when they had high levels of zinc in their blood. It's not surprising that low levels of zinc are also found in people with AIDS (acquired immune deficiency syndrome). Since the beneficial effects of zinc on immunity are so well documented, and the therapy is nontoxic and inexpensive, some researchers suggest further studies involving immune deficiency diseases. Many of my patients who get frequent colds and sore throats have shown a marked decrease in these outbreaks with zinc supplementation.

## Other Protective Functions

Aside from its support of the immune system, zinc may protect the body in a variety of other ways. For instance, zinc has been shown to protect the liver from damage due to poisoning from the common cleaning solvent carbon tetrachloride. Zinc is also known to prevent the absorption of lead and cadmium, which we may be exposed to through our drinking water, car and bus exhaust fumes, and many other environmental factors. Through its influence on cell membrane stability, zinc may even help protect us from substances known to contribute to cancer, heart disease, and a variety of other disorders. Zinc is an essential component of superoxide dismutase (SOD), an antioxidant made by the body to combat free radicals.

## Anorexia Nervosa

Many studies suggest that there is a relationship between zinc depletion and anorexia nervosa. Researchers theorize that inadequate levels of zinc might somehow help trigger the development of this disease, which further depletes zinc levels, which further worsens disease symptoms, and so on, in a vicious cycle. My anorexia patients, as well as those of other practitioners, have improved with zinc supplementation, indicating that zinc may be helpful both in the treatment and in the prevention of this serious disease.

## Hormone Levels

Zinc has been shown to inhibit the production of prolactin, a pituitary hormone, and so is used therapeutically in men and women with abnormally high prolactin levels. Elevated prolactin levels can lead to distressing effects such as secretion of breast milk, enlarged breasts, and sexual dysfunction.

## The Prostate Gland

The prostate gland has one of the highest concentrations of zinc in the body. In general, low levels of zinc in the prostate appear to be associated with diseases of the gland. Zinc supplementation has been shown to reduce the size of the prostate and symptoms of benign prostatic hypertrophy (BPH) in the majority of patients. Zinc also inhibits the binding of androgens to receptors in the prostate gland, an action that may play a role in the prevention of prostate cancer and other diseases of the prostate gland.

## RDIs AND DEFICIENCY SYMPTOMS

Despite the fact that zinc is so necessary, there are no true storage depots for this mineral. Although relatively large amounts are found in the bone, along with other minerals, it does not appear that this zinc is readily available to the body. Instead, the body is dependent upon a continual external supply, as the relatively small body pool of biologically available zinc appears to be used rather rapidly. Therefore, deficiency signs tend to appear quite soon after depletion. It is now recognized that subclinical zinc deficiency may manifest itself as impaired ability to heal, impaired acuity of taste and smell, loss of appetite, and impaired night vision. Prolonged zinc deficiency may result in failure to grow, mental disturbances, lethargy, skin changes, and susceptibility to frequent infections. Testicular function may also be adversely affected. This is probably the origin of the oyster's reputation as an aphrodisiac, as oysters have a high zinc content.

The RDI for zinc is 15 milligrams for all men and women. In spite of its importance and seemingly wide availability in food, evidence indicates that many people do not get enough zinc from their diets. Marginally low intakes are common in large areas of the country because the soil is deficient in this mineral. (In fact, at one time, many farm animals were found to be deficient in this mineral, and they now receive zinc-enriched feed.) A 1979 study detected an average intake of 8.6 milligrams per day for humans, or just over half the RDI. In another survey, the zinc intake of elderly people was on the average less than half the RDI, indicating that this group is particularly at risk. It is worthwhile noting that the people in this survey suffered from the loss of taste sensitivity so common in this age group. In another study of the elderly, it was found that senile purpura—purple spots under the skin caused by bleeding—may also be due to a zinc deficiency. Indeed, zinc is used, both orally and topically, in the treatment of many skin conditions, including folliculitis (inflammation of the hair follicles); acrodermatitis enteropathica (a severe genetic skin disorder); acne vulgaris (common adolescent acne); alopecia areata (a usually temporary form of hair loss); and leg ulcers.

Certain individuals are unable to absorb zinc, or absorb the mineral only poorly, and thus are at risk for zinc deficiency. These include babies with the hereditary disease acrodermatitis enteropathica, mentioned above; as well as people with malabsorption syndromes such as Crohn's disease, celiac disease, and short bowel syndrome. Also at risk are people with chronic kidney disease, sickle cell anemia, cystic fibrosis, pancreatic insufficiency, and other chronically debilitating disorders. These individuals may have subtle signs of zinc deficiency, including loss of appetite, impaired night vision, and depressed immune and mental functions. In one study, patients with highly active Crohn's disease had only 60 percent of the normal blood level of zinc.

Several drugs have been found to interfere with zinc absorption and metabolism. These include such commonly used substances as alcohol, diuretics, and oral contraceptives.

The dip of zinc levels associated with the use of oral contraceptives is probably the result of the drugs' hormone content, as zinc levels are also lower during pregnancy. In addition, the use of oral contraceptives has been found to reduce folic acid levels in some women, and so often leads to folic acid supplementation. Unfortunately, in large doses, folic acid has been found to lower zinc concentrations in the blood, which may make these women particularly prone to zinc deficiency.

Research on the use of diuretics for hypertension suggests that some unexplained side effects of the drugs may be the result of zinc depletion, rather than the drugs themselves. Impotency, for example, appears to be connected to low zinc levels. The association of diuretic therapy with zinc deficiency may have important implications for patients who suffer heart attacks, as the deficiency may retard the healing of the injured heart.

The water you drink may also affect zinc levels. Excessive copper intake, commonly resulting from copper pipes, worsens an already existing zinc deficiency. In addition, there is some evidence that the calcium bicarbonate found in hard tap water may interfere with zinc absorption and utilization.

*Food Sources:* Although some zinc is found in nearly all foods, the mineral is especially plentiful in meats, poultry (particularly dark meat), fish and other seafood (oysters are notably high), liver, eggs, legumes such as peanuts, and whole grains. Approximately 73 percent of the zinc is removed from whole grains during the milling process that produces white flour. The flour is then "enriched," a process that replaces several vitamins and iron, but not zinc.

The biological availability of zinc in different foods varies. It is estimated that as little as 40 percent of dietary zinc is actually absorbed. Some studies have suggested that the zinc in meats and seafood is better absorbed than is the zinc in grains. Zinc deficiency is known to occur in populations whose zinc intake is far in excess of the RDI, but is derived solely from grain sources. This has led to the concern that vegetarians may need a higher intake of zinc. However, when vegetarians were recently studied, it was found that they had adequate zinc levels. It may be that the soybean products popular in vegetarian cuisine help supply the extra zinc and enhance its absorption.

## SUPPLEMENTS

Zinc is available as individual supplements, and as part of many multivitamin and multimineral formulas. In supplements, pure or "elemental" zinc is combined with other compounds. Of these, I feel that zinc gluconate and zinc citrate, which are sometimes referred to as chelated zinc, are the best choices for most people, as they are relatively inexpensive and well tolerated. Zinc sulfate is the least expensive, but can be very irritating to the stomach. Many practitioners use other forms of zinc, such as zinc picolinate and zinc orotate, because they believe they are the most absorbable forms. Unfortunately, there is no convincing data to support these claims.

Since zinc supplements combine elemental or pure zinc with another compound, when buying supplements you must consider the amount of elemental zinc, which is commonly listed on the product label. For example, 80 milligrams of zinc gluconate usually contain 10 milligrams of elemental zinc, and 220 milligrams of zinc sulfate supply 50 milligrams of elemental zinc.

### OPTIMUM DAILY INTAKE—ODI

For optimum general health, the basic Optimum Daily Intake for zinc is:

### 22.5–50 mg for men and women

Based on a thorough scientific review of zinc, and on my clinical experience, the following amounts of zinc appear to be valuable for:

| Condition | Suggested Dosage |
|---|---|
| Decreased sense of taste and smell | 30–50 mg |
| Enhanced immunity | 30–50 mg |
| Enhanced wound healing | 30–50 mg |
| Poor night vision | 30–50 mg |
| Prostatitis | 30–50 mg (up to 100 mg under professional advice) |

*Remember:* If you have a medical condition, please consult with your physician before taking supplements.

### TOXICITY AND ADVERSE EFFECTS

The symptoms of zinc toxicity are gastrointestinal irritation and vomiting. Zinc is actually recognized as an emetic—a substance that induces vomiting.

However, this form of toxicity occurs only when 2,000 milligrams or more have been ingested. Studies have shown that even when up to ten times the RDA of 15 milligrams is given for prolonged periods of time, there are no adverse reactions.

There is some evidence that an excessive intake of zinc—more than 50 milligrams per day taken for an extended period of time—may lower copper levels and aggravate a marginal copper deficiency. This may, in fact, be a beneficial, rather than an adverse, effect for some people. Although copper is an essential nutrient, there are people with copper levels that are far too high for optimum health. In fact, high-level zinc supplementation has been used therapeutically to treat Wilson's disease, a potentially fatal disorder characterized by excessive copper accumulation in tissues. Nevertheless, researchers recommend that patients on long-term zinc supplementation of more than 50 milligrams a day have their copper levels, lipids, and immune function monitored.

Short-term experiments suggest that 150 milligrams of zinc twice a day decrease levels of high-density lipoproteins (HDLs, or "good" cholesterol), and raise levels of low-density lipoproteins (LDLs, or "bad" cholesterol) and/or serum cholesterol, causing a less desirable ratio. However, studies are needed to assess long-term effects. The results of another study, using 50 milligrams of zinc per day, showed the opposite effect: HDL cholesterol increased and overall cholesterol decreased. In addition, diastolic blood pressure decreased. At one time, my HDLs were 46 and my total cholesterol was 225. After three years of taking 100 milligrams of zinc daily, my HDLs are 98 and my cholesterol is 185. My HDL levels certainly have not suffered from the excess zinc. Of course, I take a *balance* of other supplements along with zinc, and also do aerobic exercise four times a week.

# Chapter 25

# IRON

Every cell in the body contains and requires iron, a mineral that is needed for all body functions. Thus, iron stores are carefully guarded by the body and, when depleted, cause diverse symptoms.

## FUNCTIONS AND USES

### Oxygen Transport and Storage

Approximately 75 percent of the body's iron is found in our red blood cells in the form of hemoglobin, a protein-iron compound responsible for carrying oxygen from our lungs to all of the parts of our body. About 5 percent of our iron is found in a substance called myoglobin. This protein, a form of hemoglobin that is found in the muscles, carries and stores oxygen for the muscles. The iron helps hemoglobin and myoglobin to carry and hold the oxygen, and then release it for use by every cell in the body.

### Energy Production

Iron is present in a variety of enzymes—catalysts that help chemical changes take place throughout the body. Many of the iron-containing enzymes are involved in the production of energy.

### The Immune System

Iron is also of key importance in maintaining many of the functions of our immune system. While either too much or too little of the mineral may create problems, most problems are due to a deficiency.

## RDIs AND DEFICIENCY SYMPTOMS

The major deficiency disease for iron is hypochromic microcytic anemia, often called iron deficiency anemia. In this form of anemia, the red blood cells are smaller than normal and pale in color due to low amounts of hemoglobin.

Because of the low hemoglobin content of the blood, the tissues of the body become oxygen-starved, leading to symptoms such as listlessness, fatigue, irritability, difficulty swallowing, paleness, heart palpitations during exertion, and a general lack of well-being.

However, because the symptoms of anemia appear only after all the body's stores of iron have been depleted, the usual tests for anemia are an unsatisfactory means of detecting iron depletion. Moreover, numerous studies have shown that even in the absence of anemia, iron deficiency may have a detrimental effect on learning ability, endurance, and general well-being. For example, when chronically fatigued women were studied, the researchers concluded that some of these women might have been suffering from iron deficiency, even though their hemoglobin was in the accepted range. Apparently, their normal range for hemoglobin was higher than average. In other studies, women who were clearly iron deficient and women who had low-normal hemoglobin levels were found to have a low tolerance for cold, which improved when they received iron supplements. Runners who are iron deficient, but nonanemic, have been found to have less endurance. When college students were studied, it was found that low iron may play a part in faulty attention span. Another study indicated that iron supplementation of iron-deficient children improves their ability to learn. Finally, both infants with anemia and infants with signs of iron deficiency, but no anemia, have shown significant improvement in mental development scores when supplemented with iron.

Because iron plays a role in immune system function, other deficiency symptoms include increased susceptibility to infection, reduced white blood cell counts, and impaired antibody production. Other widely diverse signs of possible iron deficiency are becoming increasingly recognized. Angular cheilosis, an inflammation of the corners of the mouth, has most frequently been seen in vitamin B deficiencies. However, according to one report, iron deficiency was present in a much higher percentage of sufferers. Animal experiments suggest that iron deficiency may contribute to high levels of fat in the blood and liver. In addition, new data indicates that a craving for salt may be a sign of iron deficiency.

Of all the nutrient allowances, the allowance for iron is the most difficult to obtain from dietary sources. This is why iron deficiency is the most common single nutrient deficiency in the world. Vast numbers of individuals become deficient in iron at some time in their lives, and large segments of the population are chronically deficient.

While iron deficiency is far from uncommon in men, children, and the elderly, the highest risk category is menstruating women. Healthy men have an iron reserve of 1,000 milligrams, and lose an average of 1 milligram of iron per day. In menstruating women, the iron reserve is not more than 200 to 400 milligrams. These women lose an average of 1.5 milligrams per day, and sometimes as much as 2.4 milligrams per day. In a study of female college students, only six of the seventy-four women studied—about 12 percent— were getting the RDA for iron. Other surveys have shown that 10 to 30 percent of women have iron deficits. The RDI for iron is 18 milligrams for all men and women. Yet women and girls have lower caloric requirements, and consequently *cannot* meet their needs even when they follow a diet of carefully selected foods.

Pregnant women are at particularly high risk for low iron, with deficiencies as high as 60 percent. I usually recommend supplements for these women because their needs cannot met by the average diet. Often, they had a marginal iron intake before becoming pregnant. Therefore, their iron stores are below optimum, putting them and their babies at risk.

Some researchers have expressed concern that vegetarian women may be at an even higher risk for low iron intake than are nonvegetarians. Based on an actual analysis of their diet, the average intake is 11 to 14 milligrams per day for lacto-ovo vegetarian women. Although this is below the RDI, nonvegetarian women appear to have similarly low intakes.

Even when iron intake is sufficient, various factors can affect iron absorption. Low stomach acid, removal of part of the stomach, and malabsorption syndromes have all been shown to reduce iron absorption. In addition, calcium phosphate salts, tannic acid in tea, and antacids tend to interfere with absorption. Phytates, a substance found in whole grains, may interfere with iron absorption, too. However, the evidence for this is inconclusive.

*Food Sources:* Foods that are highest in iron are meat (especially liver), poultry, and fish. Other substantial sources are eggs, breads and cereals (either whole grain or iron-enriched), leafy vegetables, potatoes and other vegetables, fruit, and milk.

The absorbability of iron from foods varies widely. The "organic" iron found in red meats is the most absorbable (10 to 30 percent). Plants contain "inorganic" iron, only 2 to 10 percent of which is absorbed by our digestive tracts. In addition, large quantities of iron are lost from food that is cooked in water. However, when you cook acidic foods in cast-iron cookware, iron from the cookware leaches out into the foods, increasing its iron content considerably. In addition, vitamin C enhances the absorbability of iron in nonanimal foods and prevents it from being converted into its unstable form, which may cause oxidative stress and cell damage from free radicals.

## SUPPLEMENTS

Iron is available as an individual supplement and as a part of many vitamin-mineral formulas. The most common form is iron sulfate, which is very inexpensive, but can be irritating to the digestive tract. I recommend iron glycinate, iron fumarate, and iron gluconate, since they are less irritating to the digestive tract and less likely to cause constipation. As when buying other minerals, look for the "elemental" content when choosing an iron supplement.

## OPTIMUM DAILY INTAKE—ODI

For optimum general health, the basic Optimum Daily Intake for iron is:

15–25 mg for men
18–30 mg for women

Based on a thorough scientific review of iron, and on my clinical experience, the following amounts of iron appear to be valuable for:

| Condition | Suggested Dosage |
|---|---|
| Chronic fatigue | 15–20 mg |
| Iron deficiency anemia | 20–30 mg |
| Poor attention span | 15–20 mg |

*Remember:* If you have a medical condition, please consult your physician before taking supplements.

Anemia due to iron deficiency will respond fairly rapidly to supplementation. Nevertheless, supplements should be continued for several months to fully replenish the body's stores. You should be aware that anemia may also be due to a vitamin $B_{12}$ or folic acid deficiency. (See Chapters 15 and 16 for details.) Other possible causes of anemia are internal bleeding, the adverse effects of certain drugs, and the presence of toxins in the body. There is also a condition called "sports anemia." Not a true anemia, this problem is due to abnormal destruction of red blood cells through mechanical injury, rather than inadequate iron intake. Thus, routine iron supplementation is not justified. Be sure to consult with your doctor if you show signs of anemia.

## TOXICITY AND ADVERSE EFFECTS

The toxicity of iron is low, and harmful effects of daily intakes of up to 75 milligrams per day are unlikely in healthy individuals. The body has a highly effective mechanism that prevents an overload of iron from entering it and causing toxicity. The amount of iron the body absorbs is carefully regulated by the intestines according to the body's needs. The greater the need, the higher the rate of absorption. Growing children, pregnant women, and anemic individuals have higher rates of absorption. When a deficiency occurs, the rate of absorption increases to two to three times higher than normal. (Unfortunately, this response does not appear to be sufficient to prevent anemia in iron-deficient subjects who are only mildly anemic and whose iron intake is marginal.)

There have been conflicting scientific reports concerning iron and the risk of coronary heart disease. Some studies have shown that high iron levels in the blood appear to increase the risk of heart disease, while other studies have failed to confirm these findings. Some studies have demonstrated that high levels of serum ferritin (a complex in which iron is stored in the tissues) or of total iron binding capacity (TIBC) appear to increase the risk of heart disease, while other studies have failed to confirm these findings, as well. What does all this mean?

We know that antioxidants are our natural defense against free radical oxidative stress, and that iron is a very powerful pro-oxidant—an initiator of oxidative stress. (For more information about oxidative stress, see Chapter 3.) The discrepancies in the study findings may be the result of the *balance* of antioxidants and iron. Even though iron is essential to the functioning of our bodies, too much iron combined with poor antioxidant defense, due to poor intake of antioxidants, would put anyone at high risk for increased oxidative stress, which is believed to be a culprit in heart disease. Since we can easily measure iron, TIBC, and ferritin levels in our blood, these levels should routinely be screened during physical exams. If high levels are present, a reduction of iron intake should be discussed with your physician.

In some cases, a dangerous condition known as hemochromatosis can cause the excessive absorption of iron. This results in a build-up of excess iron in the tissues of many organs, possibly leading to damage to the liver, heart, pancreas, and other organs. In genetic hemochromatosis, there is inappropriately high absorption of dietary iron from birth. Acquired hemochromatosis may occur as a result of transfusions, medical conditions, or excessive long-term iron intake. This condition, too, can easily be detected through blood tests. If the tests confirm the condition, steps should be taken to avoid iron in food and supplements, and to avoid foods cooked in cast iron cookware or stored in metal cans.

# Chapter 26

# COPPER

The body contains about 100 to 150 milligrams of copper. It is stored in the liver, brain, heart, and kidneys, and is found in the hair.

## FUNCTIONS AND USES

Copper helps your body absorb and use iron to synthesize hemoglobin. It also plays a role in maintaining the integrity of myelin, the fatty substance that is a constituent of the covering of some nerves. Copper is needed for taste sensitivity; the maturation of collagen, a component of connective tissue, bone, cartilage, and skin; the formation of elastin, a protein that forms certain tissues; and bone development. It is also an important part of a number of enzymes required for energy production; the oxidation of fatty acids; and the formation of melanin, a skin pigment. Copper is also involved in the metabolism of ascorbic acid. And copper plays a role in the immune system. It is, in fact, an essential component of superoxide dismutase (SOD), an antioxidant made by the body to combat free radicals. Experimentally induced copper *deficiencies* or *excesses* have each been reported to increase the severity of a wide variety of infections in laboratory animals.

Drugs containing copper complexes have been shown to be effective in combating many inflammatory diseases, including rheumatoid arthritis, osteoarthritis, ankylosing spondylitis, rheumatic fever, and sciatica. Copper-containing drugs are also used in the treatment of ulcers, convulsions, chorea, cancer, and diabetes. It is thought that the drugs' positive effects are due to the copper complexes' ability to facilitate or promote tissue repair processes that use copper-dependent enzymes.

While human copper deficiency is not a common problem, abnormally high blood copper levels are often seen in people with viral infections, rheumatoid arthritis, rheumatic fever, lupus erythematosus, myocardial infarction, leukemia, and certain cancers, although the causes for the increased levels of copper are unexplained. It may be that excess copper plays a role in the development and progression of these diseases, or it may be that the body is circulating more copper in an attempt to deal with the diseases. When experimental animals were given oral contraceptives, their blood copper levels were significantly elevated. Copper is best measured in a blood component known as ceruloplasmin—the copper-protein compound in which 95 percent of the body's circulating copper is found. This measurement can be made as part of any routine blood test.

## RDIs AND DEFICIENCY SYMPTOMS

The RDI for copper is 2 milligrams for all men and women. Copper is so widely available in foods and through the use of copper cooking utensils that, as previously mentioned, deficiency of this mineral is thought to be rare in humans. Many believe that even a diet that is poor in other nutrients is likely to furnish sufficient copper. However, recent research suggests that the typical American diet may not contain the amount of copper it was originally thought to contain (see "Food Sources," below). In addition, there are some groups who are at particular risk of suboptimal copper intake.

Much of our understanding of copper deficiency is the result of symptoms of deficiency in animals. In animal studies and human reports, deficiency symptoms have included anemia, skeletal defects, degeneration of the nervous system, defects in the pigmentation and structure of the hair, reproductive problems, and abnormalities in the cardiovascular system. Mild copper deficiency in animals has also resulted in elevated serum cholesterol, especially when the zinc intake was high. Copper supplements have been shown to lower total cholesterol and raise HDL cholesterol (the "good" kind) in experimental animals and humans who have copper deficiency. Copper supplementation, along with supplementation of calcium and other minerals, has also been shown to increase bone density in postmenopausal women.

In humans, deficiency may occur in severely malnourished individuals, in which case the symptoms are anemia, impaired immunity, and bone disease. Similar symptoms have also been detected in premature infants fed a diet of only cow's milk, which is low in copper. In addition, people who suffer from sprue or celiac disease may have difficulty absorbing copper. And there is evidence that an excess of zinc may interfere with copper absorption, increasing the requirements for copper. Pregnant women may also be at risk for copper deficiency. In a study that looked at twenty-four healthy women during their pregnancy, the intake of dietary copper was far below normal, and even when supplements brought daily intake up to 2.7 milligrams, this was marginal in meeting the women's needs. This may be a cause for concern, as research has demonstrated that a copper deficiency in pregnant animals may cause birth defects in offspring.

*Food Sources:* Copper is widely distributed in foods, with liver, shellfish, meats, nuts, legumes, whole grain cereals, and raisins being the richest sources. Early data indicated that the average dietary intake of copper was 2 to 5 milligrams. However, more recent surveys indicate a much lower intake, often substantially below 1 milligram per day. We don't know whether this discrepancy is due to an actual decline in copper intake or differences in measuring intakes. Another factor to consider is that only 25 percent of the copper ingested is absorbed, and that many people eat highly processed, demineralized foods. Drinking water may contribute to your total daily copper intake, but this varies with the type of piping used and the hardness of the water.

## SUPPLEMENTS

Copper is available as an individual supplement, and is often included in multivitamin-mineral formulas, as well. The most common available forms of this supplement are copper gluconate and copper sulfate. Copper citrate is also available. I generally recommend copper gluconate, as it is gentler to the digestive tract. However, when taken in amounts as small as 2 milligrams, any of the forms may be well tolerated.

## OPTIMUM DAILY INTAKE—ODI

For optimum general health, the Optimum Daily Intake for copper is:

### 0.5–2 mg for men and women

There is not enough data to permit me to make recommendations for specific conditions and concerns at this time. I recommend using the zinc-to-copper ratio to determine the amount of copper that should be consumed. For most individuals, this ratio can range from 10 to 1, to 15 to 1. For example, if you ingest 30 milligrams of zinc and 2 milligrams of copper a day, your zinc-to-copper ratio would be 15 to 1.

*Remember:* If you have a medical condition, please consult with your physician before taking supplements. If you suffer from Wilson's disease, please do not take a copper supplement (see "Toxicity and Adverse Effects," below).

## TOXICITY AND ADVERSE EFFECTS

In Wilson's disease, a rare hereditary disorder, copper accumulates in the liver and is then released and absorbed by other parts of the body, causing toxicity.

The symptoms of this condition include hepatitis, degeneration of the lens of the eye, kidney malfunction, and neurological disorders. Acute excessive doses of copper produce nausea, vomiting, abdominal pains, diarrhea, headache, dizziness, and a metallic taste in the mouth. If untreated, this can lead to death.

# Chapter 27

# MANGANESE

Manganese is less abundant in the body than any of the minerals discussed in previous chapters. The human body contains between only 10 and 20 milligrams of this mineral.

Most of the information now available on manganese is the result of animal experiments. When this is combined with human data, it appears that despite the relatively small amount of this mineral found in the body, manganese has many important uses.

## FUNCTIONS AND USES

### Metabolism

Perhaps the best-known role of manganese is its involvement in various enzyme systems. Manganese works with dozens of different enzymes that facilitate processes throughout the body, including protein, fat, and carbohydrate metabolism.

### Growth, Development, and Repair

Manganese is required for normal growth and development, and for the repair of bones and connective tissue. Studies have associated low manganese levels in human infants with birth defects ranging from cleft palate to bone deformities. Manganese also appears to help maintain bone density in postmenopausal women.

### The Nervous System

Another important role of manganese involves the proper functioning of the nerves. For instance, animals fed manganese-deficient diets show an increased susceptibility to convulsions. According to a study involving young human patients, insufficient manganese may also exacerbate a tendency to have epileptic seizures.

## The Immune System

Experiments have yielded evidence suggesting that manganese deficiencies may also affect the immune system. Antibody response and the activity of macrophages, granulocytes, and phagocytes—cells that protect the body from bacteria and other foreign invaders—are all stimulated by manganese. In addition, manganese is a component of the enzyme superoxide dismutase (SOD), a powerful free radical scavenger that prevents the cellular damage associated with the aging process and with cancer.

## Glucose Tolerance

Experiments indicate that manganese deficiency may also play a role in glucose tolerance. In one animal study, when glucose was given to manganese-deficient rats, their insulin output was 76 to 63 percent that of manganese-sufficient rats. It has also been reported that oral manganese supplements significantly lowered blood glucose levels in a patient who was unresponsive to insulin. This data has exciting implications for people with blood sugar problems.

## RDIs and DEFICIENCIES

The RDI for manganese is 2 milligrams for all men and women. This amount is roughly what you would consume if you were eating the typical American diet of highly refined foods. However, researchers have noted that diets high in refined carbohydrates may not supply adequate manganese. There is an especially high risk of deficiency when manganese requirements are increased, as during pregnancy or times of rapid growth.

In view of the fact that manganese is poorly absorbed and is severely lacking in refined foods, many practitioners, including myself, feel that the recommendation of 2 to 5 milligrams per day is much too low.

*Food Sources:* Good sources of manganese include nuts and seeds (especially hazelnuts and pecans), avocados, seaweed, and whole grains such as oatmeal, buckwheat, and whole wheat. Other fruits and vegetables contain moderate amounts of this mineral. Refined grains are a poor source of manganese, as milling removes 73 percent of the manganese content, and the enrichment process does not put it back.

In general, the manganese in food is poorly absorbed in the intestines. In experimental conditions, it has been shown that phytates—present in whole grains—may interfere with manganese absorption. However, it is probable that this effect occurs to a significant degree only when extremely high amounts of fiber are eaten.

## SUPPLEMENTS

Manganese is available in individual supplements and in some multivitamin-mineral formulas. The most common available forms of this supplement are manganese gluconate, manganese sulfate, and manganese citrate. I generally recommend the gluconate form, as it is gentler to the digestive tract.

## OPTIMUM DAILY INTAKE—ODI

For optimum general health, the basic Optimum Daily Intake for manganese is:

### 15–30 mg for men and women

Based on a thorough scientific review of manganese, and on my clinical experience, the following amounts of manganese appear to be valuable for:

| Condition | Suggested Dosage |
| --- | --- |
| Cancer prevention | 15–30 mg |
| Impaired glucose tolerance | 20–30 mg |
| Osteo- and rheumatoid arthritis | 15–30 mg |
| Osteoporosis | 15–30 mg |

*Remember:* If you have a medical condition, please consult with your physician before taking supplements.

## TOXICITY AND ADVERSE EFFECTS

The toxicity for manganese is low when it is ingested in the form of either manganese-rich foods or supplements. Toxicity can occur, however, when manganese is inhaled, as in the case of certain miners who are exposed to high concentrations of manganese oxide in the air. In these situations, even small doses can cause psychiatric abnormalities and nerve disorders. Manganese toxicity may also occur as a result of manganese-contaminated well water.

# Chapter 28

# CHROMIUM

As adults, our bodies contain approximately 6 grams of chromium. The highest concentrations of this mineral are found in the hair, spleen, kidneys, and testes. The heart, pancreas, lungs, and brain also contain this trace mineral, but in lower concentrations.

## FUNCTIONS AND USES

Chromium's primary role in the body is to activate enzymes involved in the metabolism of glucose and the synthesis of proteins. Its chief functions in the body and therapeutic uses are related to this activity.

### Glucose Metabolism Disorders

Commonly known as blood sugar, glucose is the fuel that our cells "burn" for energy. The hormone insulin regulates the amount of glucose in our blood by "escorting" glucose into our cells so that it can be stored for later use. This prevents our blood sugar from rising too high, as occurs in diabetes, or from falling too low, as occurs in hypoglycemia. Because chromium is the major mineral involved in insulin production, it should come as no surprise that a lack of this mineral interferes with the maintenance of healthy blood sugar levels. There is strong and growing evidence that many disorders of glucose metabolism—namely, diabetes and hypoglycemia—may, in fact, be chromium-deficiency states.

In experiments, chromium supplementation has actually been found to improve glucose tolerance in some diabetics and in people with impaired glucose tolerance. In one study, for example, ten elderly individuals were given chromium supplementation. For four of the subjects—the "chromium responders"—all abnormal features of the glucose-tolerance test (GTT) disappeared in a short time. These subjects previously had mild abnormalities on their GTT, while the nonresponders had more severe abnormalities. This suggests that the nonresponders might have been so severely deficient in chromium that it would have taken longer for them to show any improvement. In general, when I have recommended chromium supplements to insulin- and noninsulin-dependent diabetics, along with a diet and exercise program, their physicians were able to reduce their insulin injections or stop their oral medications. Chromium supplementation also improves the insulin resistance associated with diabetes. It is beneficial for hypoglycemics, as well.

### Cardiovascular Disorders

Chromium depletion has also been implicated in hypercholesterolemia (high cholesterol in the blood), again because of its role in insulin production and glucose regulation. Glucose is the primary source of energy for the body, so if chromium depletion results in ineffective insulin levels and seriously impaired glucose metabolism, the body must rely on lipid (fat) metabolism for energy. This is a less-than-satisfactory situation, because some of the by-products of lipid metabolism are made into cholesterol. Many researchers believe that the accelerated atherosclerosis seen in diabetics may be the result of this process. In fact, studies have shown that chromium deficiency tends to decrease the liver's uptake of cholesterol and fatty acids, which could favor the accumulation of lipids in the arteries. In laboratory experiments, rats fed a chromium-deficient, high-sugar diet showed a dramatically increased accumulation of cholesterol in the arteries. On the other hand, when rats fed a high-sugar diet were supplemented with chromium, the nutrient significantly lowered their serum cholesterol levels and resulted in less accumulation of lipids in the arteries. Epidemiological evidence has borne out the results of these laboratory experiments. In several Eastern nations in which low serum cholesterol levels are common, high chromium concentrations have been found in the tissues. Moreover, studies have shown that chromium supplements increase high-density lipoproteins (HDLs, or "good" cholesterol), and lower low-density lipoproteins (LDLs, or "bad" cholesterol), in addition to lowering overall cholesterol.

### Body Fat Reduction

A preliminary study by Dr. Gary Evans indicated that chromium picolinate was effective in increasing lean body mass (muscle) and reducing the percentage of body fat in male athletes. There were also reports that lean body mass was increased in females on a weight training program. A weight reduction program appeared successful with chromium picolinate, L-carnitine, and fiber. However, much of this work is preliminary and has not yet been duplicated by other researchers.

## RDIs AND DEFICIENCY SYMPTOMS

The established RDI for chromium is 120 micrograms. According to long-term studies in human subjects, 200 to 290 micrograms are required daily to maintain a balance or near-balance of chromium. However, the estimated chromium intake for the average American is 50 to 100 micrograms per day. This amount is lower than the amount consumed in Italy, Egypt, South America, and India. Even a diet that is considered to be adequate in other respects may be marginal in chromium, and chromium deficiency is believed to be relatively common in the United States, with 80 percent of the population affected, according to some estimates. This is no doubt due at least in part to the refining of grains, which removes over three quarters of the chromium. (As explained in Chapter 27, refining also removes 73 percent of the manganese. It is interesting to note that a lack of both of these minerals has been implicated in diabetes.)

It is believed that athletes may be at particular risk for marginal chromium deficiency. Strenuous running places considerable stress on the body and increases the energy requirements by seven- to twentyfold. This results in changes in hormones and other substances that function in glucose metabolism.

*Food Sources:* Brewer's yeast, beer, meat (especially liver), cheese, and whole grain cereals and breads are good sources of chromium. Leafy vegetables contain chromium, but in a form that is poorly absorbed. White rice and white bread—both refined products—are poor sources of this mineral. The milling of grains removes up to 83 percent of the chromium, none of which is replaced during the enrichment process.

## SUPPLEMENTS

Chromium is available as an individual supplement and as a component of some multivitamin-mineral formulas. It is produced in several forms, including chromium chloride, GTF (glucose tolerance factor) chromium, chromium polynicotinate, chromium dinicotinate, and chromium picolinate. In GTF chromium, the mineral is generally combined with niacin, cysteine, glycine, and glutamic acid.

There appears to be some disagreement as to the true form of GTF chromium. Chromium polynicotinate is considered by some to be the true form that was discovered by Dr. Walter Mertz in 1959. Several studies have demonstrated that this form has excellent glucose-lowering properties, as well as antioxidant activity in the liver and kidneys. However, *all* forms of chromium have been shown to improve glucose tolerance, blood lipids, and insulin resistance.

In my clinical practice, I have found that individuals respond differently to the various types of chromium. Therefore, if you don't achieve the desired results with one chromium supplement, you should try another form.

## OPTIMUM DAILY INTAKE—ODI

For optimum general health, the basic Optimum Daily Intake for chromium is:

### 200–600 mcg for men and women

Based on a thorough scientific review of chromium, and on my clinical experience, the following amounts of GTF chromium appear to be valuable for:

| Condition | Suggested Dosage |
|-----------|------------------|
| Diabetes | 400–600 mcg |
| High cholesterol, high LDLs, and low HDLs | 400–600 mcg |
| Hypoglycemia | 200–600 mcg |
| Impaired glucose tolerance | 400–600 mcg |

*Remember:* If you have a medical condition, please consult with your physician before taking supplements, especially if you have diabetes.

## TOXICITY AND ADVERSE EFFECTS

There is no known toxicity for chromium, except in the cases of chromium mining and industrial exposure, which cause chromium dust to be inhaled.

# Chapter 29

# SELENIUM

S elenium is present in all the tissues of the body, but is concentrated most highly in the kidneys, liver, spleen, pancreas, and testes. People do not consume enough selenium both because of the type of diet they eat, and because of the low selenium content of the soil in which their food is grown. The selenium content of soil varies widely, with many areas showing serious depletion. In fact, there have been several reports of selenium deficiencies in livestock raised on selenium-depleted soil.

## FUNCTIONS AND USES

### Cancer

Selenium's best-known and perhaps most important biological function relates to its role as an antioxidant and anticancer mineral. As we have seen in other chapters, free radicals damage our cells, possibly leading to the development of cancer and other degenerative diseases. Selenium is an activating component of the enzyme glutathione peroxidase, which protects our cells from this damage.

Many animal studies have proven that selenium deficiency increases the incidence and rate of growth of cancers in animals that are either exposed to a variety of potent carcinogens or receive transplanted tumors. Companion studies have shown that high selenium intake protects against these cancers. For example, in one study in which rats were exposed to a potent carcinogen, only 15 percent of those who were also given selenium developed liver cancer, as compared with 90 percent of the unsupplemented rats. In another study, the occurrence of cancer was 10 percent in the supplemented group versus 80 percent in the control group. In yet another animal study, selenium supplementation reduced colon cancer incidence by more than 50 percent. In another study, selenium protected against UV-induced skin damage and cancer, retarding the onset and number of skin lesions, and reducing inflammation, blistering, and pigmentation.

In humans, there is ample epidemiological evidence that high selenium is correlated with a lower incidence of many types of cancer. For instance, researchers have found that cancer risk is significantly lower in people living in areas with selenium-rich soil, in people with a high-selenium food supply, and in people with higher blood levels of selenium, when compared with people with lower intakes and blood levels. Selenium intakes in the people studied were close to 750 micrograms per day, with no toxic side effects noted. In a survey that spanned twenty-seven countries, including the United States, it was found that the cancer death rate was lower in those people whose typical diets were high in selenium. This and other cancer studies indicate that selenium is especially protective against cancer of the breast, colon, and lung. Data also suggests protection against tumors of the ovaries, cervix, rectum, bladder, esophagus, pancreas, skin, liver, and prostate, as well as against leukemia.

Since 1969, it has been known that the blood levels of cancer patients are low in selenium. In general, cancer patients with lower-than-average selenium levels have a greater number of primary tumors, more recurrences, more distant metastases (tumors that have spread to distant parts of the body), and a shortened survival time. In a study of 12,000 people conducted in Finland, the risk of fatal cancer in people with the lowest levels of serum selenium was nearly six times higher than that in people with the highest selenium concentrations.

Like other nutrients, of course, selenium cannot do its work alone. In several studies, it has been shown that selenium and vitamin E—and perhaps vitamin A, too—have a synergistic effect. For example, in one study, male smokers who died of cancer had lower levels of serum selenium, vitamin A, and vitamin E, when compared with healthy control subjects. It is well known that vitamin E enhances the antioxidant effect of selenium. In addition, it has been found that supplementation with selenium alone and with selenium plus vitamin E in excess of the RDAs stimulates the immune system in experimental animals. This effect is particularly pronounced when the diet is high in polyunsaturated fats—a factor that has been linked to a higher incidence of certain cancers.

These studies show promise for the prevention and possible treatment of cancer with selenium supplementation. When combined with other supplements, the anticancer effect may be even greater. The National Cancer Institute is conducting ongoing "chemopreventive" trials of several individual nutrients, including selenium, vitamin E, and vitamin A. However, often these trials are limited to 200 micrograms of selenium per day, which may be too low a dose to assess the potential protective effect of this mineral. Larger doses of selenium have been shown to be protective in animals, and safe in humans. In addition, we are not sure of the extent to which selenium supplementation influences the later stages of cancer development. If its influence is strongest in the early stage, it will be very difficult for these trials to prove the connection between low selenium and cancer because of the long latency period for most cancers. (For example, it may take up to fourteen years for a single breast cancer cell to multiply and produce a tumor large enough to be detected by currently available diagnostic methods.) Finally, evidence of the synergism of nutrients has led many researchers to emphasize the need to consider several nutrients in any given diet and cancer study, instead of focusing on just one nutrient per study.

## Cardiovascular Disease

In humans, a link has been found between selenium and heart disease. People found to have overt selenium deficiencies—alcoholics with cirrhosis of the liver, and people receiving long-term intravenous feeding—have also been found to suffer from heart problems that respond to selenium supplementation. In eastern Finland, which has one of the highest mortality rates from heart disease in the world, it was found that low selenium in the blood was associated with up to a six- or sevenfold increase in the risk of death from heart disease. In addition, children in certain areas of China in which the selenium content of the soil is low are known to develop a heart disease called Keshan's disease. Their heart problems, too, respond to selenium supplementation.

## Other Functions

There is some evidence that selenium may also prove effective in the treatment or prevention of several other disorders. A study using 400 micrograms of selenium and approximately 25 international units of vitamin E markedly improved skin conditions such as acne and seborrheic dermatitis in the test subjects. A Danish study examined patients with rheumatoid arthritis and found that they had lower levels of selenium. Those with the lowest levels had the more severe form of this disease. Moreover, a recent study conducted in Japan suggests that selenium and vitamin E may enhance the responsiveness of arthritis patients to conventional treatment. A fascinating study conducted in Scandinavia showed a correlation between low selenium levels and the incidence and severity of muscular dystrophy; one patient who was treated with selenium supplements showed considerable improvement after one year. Finnish researchers have also conducted a study on elderly patients, who were given large doses of selenium and vitamin E for one year. After two months, researchers found an obvious improvement in their patients' mental well-being, including less fatigue, depression, and anxiety, and more mental alertness, motivation, and self-care. Finally, selenium has been shown to protect against the toxic effects of mercury, arsenic, and copper.

## RDIs AND DEFICIENCY SYMPTOMS

Selenium deficiency symptoms may include muscular weakness and discomfort. Recent studies have shown that people with celiac disease—an inborn inability to digest gluten—are at high risk for low selenium, along with other nutrients, either because their low-gluten diets are also low in selenium, or because of their absorption problems. Down's syndrome patients have also been found to have low levels of selenium and other antioxidants.

In one study, refinery workers were found to have low selenium levels in spite of their dietary intake of 217 micrograms per day, which is more than three times higher than the RDI. This study indicates that because of the workers' exposure to free radicals on the job, their bodies were utilizing large amounts of selenium to produce the protective enzyme glutathione peroxidase. This suggests that exposure to toxic environmental chemicals increases the requirement for this mineral.

The RDI for selenium is 70 micrograms for all men and women.

*Food Sources:* There are no accurate available measurements of the selenium content of foods. However, it appears that the richest sources of selenium are seafoods, meats, and organ meats—if the animals of origin ate a diet high in selenium. Whole grains can be good sources, but, similarly, this depends on the selenium content of the soil in which they were grown. Fruits and vegetables generally contain very low amounts of selenium.

The refining process strips foods of much of their selenium content. In one study, it was found that a highly refined diet contains 61 percent less selenium than does a diet rich in unrefined foods. Cooking also reduces the content significantly, especially if the cooking water is discarded. Vitamin C seems to enhance the absorption of selenium.

## SUPPLEMENTS

Selenium is most often available as an individual supplement, although some multivitamin-mineral formulas are beginning to include this mineral. I recommend selenium in the form of selenomethionine, which is extracted from selenium-rich yeast or ocean plants. This form is the least toxic and appears to be the most absorbable.

## OPTIMUM DAILY INTAKE—ODI

For optimum general health, the basic Optimum Daily Intake for selenium is:

> 100–400 mcg for men and women living in low-selenium areas
> (this includes coastal areas and glaciated areas)
> 50–200 mcg for men and women living in high-selenium areas

Based on a thorough scientific review of selenium, and on my clinical experience, the following amounts of selenium appear to be valuable for:

| Condition | Suggested Dosage |
|---|---|
| Arthritis | 50–400 mcg |
| Cancer prevention | 200–400 mcg |
| Heart disease | 100–300 mcg |
| Mercury accumulation | 50–200 mcg |

*Remember:* If you have a medical condition, please consult with your physician before taking supplements.

## TOXICITY AND ADVERSE EFFECTS

Animal poisoning due to high-selenium soil is well known. The evidence so far seems to indicate that for toxicity to occur in humans, the intake must be very high indeed. Various studies have shown that long-term intakes of up to 500 to 750 micrograms per day have produced no signs of toxicity in humans. Data extrapolated from animal studies suggests that toxicity does not occur in humans ingesting less than 1,000 to 2,000 micrograms per day. The Food and Nutrition Board has stated that overt selenium toxicity may occur in humans ingesting 2,400 to 3,000 micrograms daily. (But for some reason, the board still claims that the maximum intake of selenium should not exceed 200 micrograms.) Toxicity symptoms, which include a garlic odor in breath, urine, and sweat, have been reported among people living in high-selenium areas and among certain workers exposed to selenium. Some data, when combined with selenium's known teratogenic effect in animals, suggest that extremely high levels of selenium may also cause birth defects in humans.

# Chapter 30

# IODINE

Our bodies contain 20 to 30 milligrams of iodine. Approximately three quarters of this is found in the thyroid gland, while the remainder is distributed throughout the body, mostly in the fluid that bathes our cells.

## FUNCTIONS AND USES

### The Thyroid Gland

As indicated by its high concentration in the thyroid gland, iodine is important for the proper functioning of that gland. Specifically, it is a necessary constituent of the thyroid hormones, which are used to regulate physical and mental growth, the functioning of the nervous system and muscles, circulatory activity, and the metabolism of all nutrients.

### Other Uses

Recent data indicates that iodine may have functions in other parts of the body, as well. For example, the results of a study of iodine-deficient children in China suggest that hearing loss may be an iodine-deficiency disorder. In addition, iodine supplements are used in the event of a nuclear accident to prevent the absorption of radioactive iodine by the thyroid gland, protecting against thyroid damage and, possibly, thyroid cancer.

## RDIs AND CLASSIC DEFICIENCY SYMPTOMS

The classic iodine deficiency disease is goiter, a condition in which the thyroid gland becomes enormously enlarged in an effort to compensate for insufficient hormone production. If the thyroid cannot overcome this insufficiency, symptoms of listlessness, lassitude, and sluggishness appear. Goiter may also appear in people who ingest large amounts of goitrogens—substances that decrease the production of a thyroid hormone by preventing the utilization of iodine. Goitrogenic foods include rutabagas, strawberries, peaches, peanuts, soybeans, spinach, radishes, cabbage, turnips, mustard, and cassava root. Cooking usually inactivates goitrogens.

The RDI for iodine is 150 micrograms for all men and women. The estimated intake in the United States is between 64 and 677 micrograms per day—a wide range because of widely varying soil conditions, fertilizer use, and food processing. Areas in the United States in which iodine deficiency is most common are called "goiter belts," and include the Midwest, the Pacific Northwest, and the Great Lakes region. Switzerland, Central America, the mountainous regions of South America, New Zealand, and the Himalayas also suffer a high incidence of goiter owing to low-iodine soil. Simple goiter is found most often in women, especially during adolescence, pregnancy, and menopause.

Since the introduction of iodized table salt, the incidence of goiter has fallen dramatically. In the United States, it remains to be seen whether the recent efforts to reduce salt consumption will have any effect on goiter incidence.

*Food Sources:* The richest and most consistent food sources of iodine are seafoods, including fish, shellfish, and plants. Seaweed is extremely high in iodine, with as much as 50,000 micrograms in a 3-ounce serving. Most land vegetables are rather low in iodine, unless they are grown near the seacoast or in soils enriched with iodine-containing fertilizers.

The iodine content of meat, dairy products, and eggs depends upon the iodine content of the animals' diet. Livestock destined for consumption may be encouraged to lick salt blocks that contain iodine so that their meat will be higher in this mineral.

For many individuals, the most important dietary source of iodine is iodized salt, 1 gram of which supplies about 76 micrograms of iodine.

## SUPPLEMENTS

Many individuals are supplemented with iodine through the use of iodized table salt. However, if you do not wish to increase your consumption of salt, iodine is also available in tablets as "sea kelp," and in concentrated liquid drops and tablets. The topical antiseptic known as tincture of iodine is not to be used orally because it is poisonous if ingested.

## OPTIMUM DAILY INTAKE—ODI

For optimum general health, the Optimum Daily Intake for iodine is:

150–300 mcg for men and women living in low-iodine areas
and consuming low-iodine diets
0–150 mcg for men and women routinely consuming iodized salt
and/or seaweed products

Keep in mind that individuals who consume iodized salt or seaweed may not require iodine supplementation. However, they can safely consume the lower-range amounts usually found in multinutrient supplements.

*Remember:* If you have a medical condition, please consult your physician before taking supplements. If you are allergic to iodine, you may need to avoid this mineral.

## TOXICITY AND ADVERSE EFFECTS

An intake of up to 1,000 micrograms of iodine per day is considered safe. Toxicity symptoms include rash, headache, difficulty in breathing, and a metallic taste in the mouth. Very high doses—20,000 micrograms per day—can paradoxically cause a form of goiter called "iodide goiter." This has been seen in certain groups of Japanese who consume great quantities of seaweed daily.

# Chapter 31

# POTASSIUM

Our cells contain more potassium than any other mineral. A total of approximately 250 grams of this nutrient can be found in the adult body.

## FUNCTIONS AND USES

### Cardiovascular Disease

A growing body of evidence indicates that low levels of potassium are associated with high blood pressure, and therefore deserve more attention. This association may be especially strong when the sodium-to-potassium ratio is high. Some researchers feel that in some cases, low potassium may play a more significant role in hypertension than high sodium does. In several studies, for instance, potassium supplementation significantly lowered blood pressure without sodium restriction. As some researchers have pointed out, diets restricted in calories, sodium, and cholesterol are often recommended to people with cardiovascular disease. It is unfortunate that such diets also tend to reduce nutrients such as calcium and potassium, which may be essential for maintaining normal blood pressure.

Potassium may prove to be of value to the cardiovascular system in other ways, as well. In one animal study, rats were given stroke-inducing diets. The group that was supplemented with potassium suffered a 2-percent rate of fatal strokes, as compared with the 83-percent rate of the unsupplemented group. In another animal study, potassium supplementation was able to protect against the kidney damage resulting from hypertension. In both studies, these remarkable effects occurred even when potassium did not reduce blood pressure.

### Other Uses

Potassium is essential for maintaining the fluid balance in our cells, and is required for the enzymatic reactions taking place within them. Potassium is used to convert glucose into glycogen for storage and later release. It is also used for nerve transmission, muscle contraction, hormone secretion, and other functions.

## RDIs AND DEFICIENCY SYMPTOMS

Potassium deficiency symptoms include nausea; vomiting, which can lead to further potassium losses; listlessness; feelings of apprehension; muscle weakness, muscle spasms, and cramps; tachycardia (rapid heartbeat); and, in extreme cases, heart failure.

There is no Reference Daily Intake for potassium, but it has been estimated that the average American diet contains from 2 to 6 grams per day. Potassium deficiency can result from severe malnutrition, alcoholism, anorexia nervosa, vomiting, or diarrhea, or from illnesses that seriously interfere with appetite. Potassium may also be depleted following severe tissue injury due to surgery or burns, and during prolonged fevers. The excessive use of steroids, laxatives, and some diuretics also encourages potassium loss. If a person already has heart disease, low potassium can worsen the picture. Thus, patients with hypertension who are taking diuretics under a doctor's care are often given potassium supplements to counteract the effect.

In the body, potassium must exist in balance with sodium. Although sodium may be an important dietary determinant of blood pressure, variations in the potassium-to-sodium ratio in the diet affect blood pressure under certain circumstances. So when considering potassium levels, we must consider sodium levels as well, and watch out for high-sodium foods, including canned goods, luncheon meats, sausages, and frozen foods.

*Food Sources:* Potassium is found in a wide range of foods. Dairy products (except for cheese, because potassium is lost in the whey), meats, poultry, and fish are all good sources. Legumes, fruits, vegetables, and whole grains are also respectable sources. People who are taking diuretics for the treatment of high blood pressure are frequently advised to eat fruits such as bananas, oranges, and tomatoes for their potassium content. However, the amount of potassium in these foods is minimal compared with the amount excreted in urine as a result of diuretic use. It would take an enormous number of bananas per day to provide the recommended amount of potassium for a patient taking diuretics. Many physicians often prescribe high-dose potassium supplements for these patients.

Bear in mind, too, that potassium is lost through cooking, although the amount of potassium lost varies according to the cooking method used. A boiled potato may have lost up to 50 percent of its original potassium content. A steamed potato, only 3 to 6 percent. Some researchers have suggested adding modest amounts of salt substitute containing potassium chloride to boiling water, as this prevents the potassium from leaching out during cooking.

## SUPPLEMENTS

Potassium is available in tablet and liquid form. Levels above the ODI should be taken only under the advice of a professional.

## OPTIMUM DAILY INTAKE—ODI

Since potassium is so widely available in fresh foods, most people do not require a potassium supplement. Rather, most people should be advised to reduce sodium intake so that a sodium-to-potassium ratio of 1 to 1 is achieved. If, however, you wish to take a supplement, the Optimum Daily Intake of potassium is:

99–300 mg for men and women

Your physician may suggest higher levels of potassium if you are taking certain diuretics, or if you are trying to lower your blood pressure. Keep in mind, though, that high amounts of this nutrient should be taken only under professional guidance.

*Remember:* If you have a medical condition, please consult with your physician before taking supplements.

## TOXICITY AND ADVERSE EFFECTS

Potassium toxicity is seen when daily intakes exceed 18 grams, an amount that is unlikely to be ingested through food. Toxicity usually occurs only through the uneducated use of supplements, or when an individual has kidney failure. Excess potassium may cause muscle fatigue, irregular heartbeat, and possibly heart failure.

# Chapter 32

# BORON

We have known about the existence of boron, a trace mineral, for a long time. Only recently, however, were the health benefits of this nutrient discovered.

## FUNCTIONS AND USES

### The Bones

Based on the limited data we have so far, it appears that boron has a remarkable effect on the prevention of bone loss and demineralization. In a study conducted by researchers at the United States Department of Agriculture, boron was given to postmenopausal women, who are at high risk of developing osteoporosis. The results of this study suggest that boron works very much like estrogen to prevent the loss of minerals from the bone. As a result of this and other studies, boron is considered to be an essential mineral and a useful adjunct, along with calcium and vitamin D, in the maintenance of bone health and the prevention of osteoporosis. Future studies may demonstrate boron as a safer alternative to estrogen-replacement therapy. (See Chapter 21 for a more detailed discussion of osteoporosis.)

### The Immune System and Inflammation

Animal research suggests that boron enhances the utilization of vitamin $D_3$, and modulates immune and inflammatory processes. Thus, boron may be useful in the treatment and/or prevention of osteoarthritis. In one study, subjects with osteoarthritis were given 6 milligrams of boron daily, or a placebo. A significant improvement was obtained in 50 percent of the subjects receiving the boron supplement, compared with an improvement in only 10 percent of those receiving the placebo. Other data has shown that people with arthritis have lower boron concentrations in their bones and synovial fluid than do people who do not have arthritis.

## RDIs AND DEFICIENCY SYMPTOMS

There is no established RDI for boron, and no deficiency symptoms have been identified.

*Food Sources:* Fruits and vegetables are the best sources of boron; meat and fish are poor sources. A diet containing a variety of foods, including fruits and vegetables, supplies 1.5 to 3 milligrams of boron per day.

## SUPPLEMENTS

Boron is available as an individual supplement and in combination with other minerals, such as calcium and magnesium.

## OPTIMUM DAILY INTAKE—ODI

There is no Optimum Daily Intake for boron. However, 3 milligrams per day were used in the Department of Agriculture study. In general, 3 to 6 milligrams are being used by clinicians in the treatment of postmenopausal women at high risk of osteoporosis.

*Remember:* If you have a medical condition, please consult with your physician before taking supplements.

## TOXICITY AND ADVERSE EFFECTS

There are no reported adverse effects with doses of 3 to 6 milligrams of boron per day.

# Part Four

---

# BEYOND VITAMINS
# AND MINERALS

# Chapter 33

# COENZYME Q$_{10}$

oenzyme Q$_{10}$ is also known as ubiquinone, because it is ubiquitous—it exists everywhere in the body. Although coenzyme Q$_{10}$ (or CoQ) behaves like a vitamin in that it serves as a catalyst in certain reactions, it isn't considered a true vitamin because it is synthesized in the cells.

## FUNCTIONS AND USES

### Energy Production

Coenzyme Q$_{10}$ acts as a catalyst in the chain of chemical reactions that create adenosine triphosphate (ATP), a compound that yields the energy needed by cells to function. Due to CoQ's role in energy production, it stands to reason that a low concentration of this substance is detrimental to health in general. Not surprisingly, CoQ is most abundant in organs that require a large supply of energy, especially the heart and liver, and in the immune system.

### CoQ's Antioxidant Powers

Like a number of other vitamins, CoQ is an antioxidant. Similar in structure to vitamin E, another antioxidant, CoQ has been shown to scavenge harmful free radicals, and thus may help prevent cell damage in a variety of conditions. (For more information on antioxidants, see page 29.)

### Cardiovascular Disease

Most of the research on CoQ involves the heart, since this nutrient is most concentrated in that organ. The research concerning CoQ's effects in patients with heart disease is quite remarkable. For example, a number of clinical trials suggest that CoQ supplements benefit people with angina, with no adverse effects. Some studies show that CoQ supplementation increases the time in which people with angina are able to exercise. In another study, CoQ was found to be an effective drug therapy in the actual treatment of angina. Data from many human studies indicates that this nutrient may protect the heart from damage due to heart attack. Numerous studies also suggest that CoQ reduces the amount of tissue damage that occurs during open heart surgery and, possibly, heart transplantation.

In Japan, considerable research has been conducted on the beneficial effects of CoQ supplementation for patients with congestive heart failure. This prompted the Japanese government to approve CoQ in the treatment of this condition. Several large-scale studies have demonstrated that CoQ is extremely effective at improving the symptoms associated with congestive heart disease, preventing a worsening of serious complications, reducing hospital admissions, and improving the overall quality of life. CoQ therapy has been given both alone and with conventional medicine, and no side effects have been noted in studies utilizing as much as 100 to 300 milligrams each day. One study was able to improve symptoms in patients who had not been helped by standard diuretic and digitalis therapy.

The results of human and animal studies suggest that CoQ also decreases irregular heartbeat (arrhythmia) even in those patients receiving psychotropic drugs, of which arrhythmia is a common side effect. CoQ may also help in the treatment of mitral valve prolapse and the resulting chronic fatigue by reducing myocardial thickness, a thickening of the heart muscle that may affect heartbeat regularity.

In addition to helping people with established heart disease, CoQ may also prevent disease by reducing some of the risk factors associated with heart problems. For example, human studies have demonstrated that CoQ significantly protects low-density lipoproteins (LDLs, or "bad" cholesterol) from oxidation and lowers elevated serum cholesterol. At the same time, it raises high-density lipoproteins (HDLs)—the "good" cholesterol that helps protect against heart disease. (For more information on HDLs and LDLs, see the inset Understanding Cholesterol on page 32.) Studies also suggest that CoQ may lower high blood pressure. In several studies, including a controlled study of twenty hypertensive patients, 100 milligrams of CoQ taken daily lowered both systolic and diastolic blood pressure. (For an explanation of systolic and diastolic blood pressure, see the inset Understanding Blood Pressure on page 189.)

### Cancer

Certain cancer patients may benefit from CoQ supplementation, since animal studies have indicated that CoQ protects heart tissue from Adriamycin (doxorubicin hydrochloride), a cancer chemotherapy drug that is highly toxic to the heart. Several researchers have reported similar effects in humans. Yet this nutrient is rarely recommended to patients undergoing treatment with this common medication.

# Understanding Blood Pressure

*Blood pressure is a measurement of the force exerted by the blood on the wall of your blood vessels. It is measured at two points in the heart's pumping rhythm. Systolic pressure is measured at the point at which the heart muscle is contracting—in other words, when the heart is beating. Diastolic pressure is measured when the heart relaxes between beats. The combined pressure is expressed as a fraction, with the systolic pressure given first. For example, in a normal reading of 120/80, 120 represents the systolic pressure, and 80 represents the diastolic pressure. Individuals with blood pressure readings of 140/90 are usually considered borderline hypertensive, while those with even higher systolic and diastolic readings are considered hypertensive. Runners, athletes, and other people who engage in regular aerobic exercise generally have lower-than-average blood pressure readings, showing that less force is needed to move the blood through the body. As a result, the heart doesn't have to work as hard. This is why regular aerobic exercise is associated with a lower risk of all types of heart disease and is therapeutic for hypertension.*

*An estimated 40 million Americans have high blood pressure. Because the heart must work harder to pump the blood through the circulatory system of a hypertensive person, this condition can lead to kidney failure, heart failure, or stroke. At times, high blood pressure is the result of an underlying condition, such as arteriosclerosis (hardening of the arteries) or atherosclerosis (a buildup of fatty plaque on blood vessel walls). Often, high blood pressure is associated with disorders such as obesity, diabetes, and hyperthyroidism. In addition, the chance of developing hypertension is increased by a number of lifestyle-related risk factors, including cigarette smoking, stress, excessive use of stimulants like coffee and tea, use of certain medications, and high sodium intake. Those with a family history of hypertension are most likely to suffer from this condition.*

CoQ may also have anticancer properties of its own. In 1993, one of the researchers who used CoQ with Adriamycin reported that ten patients survived for five to fifteen years with high-dose CoQ therapy. In 1994, a Danish researcher reported on thirty-two breast cancer patients who were treated with high-dose CoQ therapy. These patients had been treated with conventional therapy, but were at high risk for recurrence. After twenty-four months on CoQ supplements, all were still alive, when at least six deaths would have been expected. Six of the women showed a partial remission of the tumor. In two women, the tumors had disappeared entirely.

## Chronic Fatigue and Immune Dysfunction

Research has revealed that patients with chronic fatigue syndrome (CFIDS) and immune dysfunction may also benefit from CoQ supplementation. One study showed that many patients with this problem have lower levels of CoQ compared with healthy subjects. Supplementation with CoQ dramatically improved many of the symptoms associated with CFIDS, including headache, sleep disturbances, postexercise fatigue, exercise tolerance, and chronic fatigue.

## Other Uses

Coenzyme $Q_{10}$ appears to have other uses as well. There have been extensive reports of CoQ's effectiveness in treating many forms of muscular dystrophy and myopathy, both of which cause the weakening and wasting of skeletal muscles. The cardiac disease commonly associated with these conditions, and that may be associated with the weakened muscles, may also be improved with CoQ. This is the only known substance that safely offers improved quality of life for people with these conditions. Finally, some reports suggest that CoQ may benefit people with periodontal disease, diabetes, and deafness. This may be linked to the fact that levels of CoQ tend to decrease with age—a fact which may indicate that higher levels of the nutrient can help prevent or relieve age-related disorders.

## RDIs AND DEFICIENCY SYMPTOMS

There is no established RDI for coenzyme $Q_{10}$, and no deficiency symptoms have been identified.

*Food Sources:* Coenzyme $Q_{10}$ is most abundant in beef hearts, chicken hearts, and other hearts. Sardines, peanuts, and spinach are other good sources. Many plants contain a form of CoQ, but it may not act the same way in the body as does the form found in animal foods. Very little is known about CoQ in foods, as all studies have used supplements.

## SUPPLEMENTS

Coenzyme $Q_{10}$ is generally available in 10-, 30-, 50-, and 100-milligram capsules.

## OPTIMUM DAILY INTAKE—ODI

There is no Optimum Daily Intake for coenzyme $Q_{10}$. Generally, 50 to 300 milligrams have been used in clinical trials, and appear to be safe and effective. Some trials have used as much as 600 milligrams, but this higher dose should be used only under the guidance of a professional.

## TOXICITY AND ADVERSE EFFECTS

Even in high doses, CoQ results in few adverse effects. There have been some reports of gastrointestinal upset, loss of appetite, nausea, and diarrhea.

# Chapter 34

# ESSENTIAL FATTY ACIDS

Although a low-fat diet is generally healthier than one that is higher in fat, our bodies require a certain amount of fat for proper growth and functioning. Those fats that are necessary for good health and cannot be manufactured by the body are called essential fatty acids (EFAs). They are termed *essential* because, like vitamins and minerals, they must be provided by the diet. This chapter focuses on the two groups of essential fatty acids that have received the most attention: omega-3 and omega-6 fatty acids.

The omega-3 family includes alpha-linolenic acid, eicosapentaenoic acid (EPA), and docosahexaenoic acid (DHA). In certain plants, omega-3 fatty acids are found in the form of alpha-linolenic acid. In the body, this fatty acid is converted to EPA, which is then converted to DHA. The oils of certain fish contain preformed EPA and DHA, which are the active and most desirable forms of the omega-3 family. Ultimately, DHA is converted to a group of anti-inflammatory prostaglandins—hormonelike substances used throughout the body. It is this final conversion to prostaglandins that is responsible for omega-3's therapeutic effects.

The omega-6 family includes cis-linoleic acid, linoleic acid, and gamma-linolenic acid (GLA). Cis-linoleic acid is found in certain plants and vegetable oils. Linoleic acid is found in most plants and vegetable oils. In the body, some cis-linoleic acid is converted to GLA, the most therapeutic form of the omega-6 family. Preformed GLA can also be found in certain plants, with evening primrose, black currant, and borage oils being the most commonly used sources. The body ultimately converts GLA to another group of anti-inflammatory prostaglandins. Again, it is this final conversion that is responsible for omega-6's therapeutic effects. However, it should be noted that cis-linoleic acid and linoleic acid can also be converted to *pro*-inflammatory prostaglandins.

A balance of essential fatty acids is needed for good health. Unfortunately, the average American diet does not provide a balance. Instead, because it is so high in certain vegetable oils, it provides an excess of linoleic acid, which is generally metabolized into pro-inflammatory substances, and an insufficient amount of those fatty acids that are needed to make anti-inflammatory substances. Depending on your particular needs, you may want to add omega-3 EFAs, omega-6 EFAs, or both EFAs to your supplementation program.

## FUNCTIONS AND USES

As already explained, chief among the roles of the EFAs is the part they play in the body's manufacture of prostaglandins—hormonelike substances that are produced and used by all cells. Once manufactured, the prostaglandins regulate all of our body functions, including those of the cardiovascular, reproductive, immune, and nervous systems. In addition, fatty acids serve as structural parts of cell membranes, and therefore help protect the cells from invading toxins, bacteria, viruses, carcinogens, and allergens. It's easy to understand why research has linked fatty acid imbalances to a variety of chronic diseases, including heart disease, cancer, arthritis, allergies, and various immunological disorders.

### Cardiovascular Disease

Interest in fatty acids began when researchers observed that in spite of a diet incredibly rich in fat, the Greenland Eskimos had a very low rate of heart disease, as well as a low incidence of cancer and diabetes. Intrigued by this apparent paradox, researchers studied the Eskimo diet and discovered that it was high in EPA and DHA—omega-3 fatty acids found in the cold-water fish and marine mammals that form the bulk of the Eskimo diet. Subsequent studies in Japan, Sweden, and the Netherlands confirmed that the higher the consumption of omega-3-rich fish, the lower the incidence of heart disease.

Many studies have shown that EPA protects against heart disease. Platelets—the blood cells that enable our blood to clot and aggregate—can adhere to artery walls, contributing to atherosclerosis, or hardening of the arteries. By preventing this adhesion, EPA acts as a natural "blood thinner," and thus helps prevent atherosclerosis. Studies with GLA have yielded results similar to those achieved with EPA. Also, studies on evening primrose oil—a rich source of GLA—as well as studies on fish oil, have demonstrated positive results in improving lipid abnormalities in certain diabetic patients, provided they received vitamin E supplementation, as well.

It is interesting to note that because aspirin thins the blood, it has been widely touted as a heart-attack preventive. Yet several studies have suggested that fish oil—whether consumed in fish or in fish-oil supplements—is superior to aspirin in preventing heart disease, and is not associated with the ulcers, gastrointestinal bleeding, anemia, and other side effects that occur with aspirin use. In studies that used both aspirin and fish oil, the combination was more effective than aspirin alone. These factors, along with the fact that EPA appears to lower high levels of triglycerides, a risk factor in heart disease, makes fish oil a better, safer option in preventing cardiovascular disorders in people at high risk.

EFAs also appear to be effective in the treatment of existing heart disease. There is evidence that fish oil lowers blood pressure, and can reduce chest pain during exercise in people with angina. Because of its blood-thinning abilities, EPA may also be of use after bypass surgery and as an adjunct to angioplasty. In addition, GLA has been shown to reduce stress-induced hypertension in animals, and to help relieve the pain of angina in humans.

### The Immune System and Inflammation

Both EPA and GLA appear to have positive effects on immune function and inflammation. By blocking the pro-inflammatory prostaglandins, EPA tends to improve symptoms of asthma, atopic dermatitis, rheumatoid arthritis, Raynaud's disease, systemic lupus erythematosus, psoriatic arthritis, psoriasis, and gout. In a recent study using high levels of GLA (1.4 grams) from borage seed oil, patients with rheumatoid arthritis experienced a significant improvement of symptoms. In several studies, GLA relieved the symptoms of eczema and atopic dermatitis and reduced the amount of skin area that was affected. Studies using GLA have also shown clinical benefits in patients with autoimmune disorders such as lupus and multiple sclerosis. Since GLA's anti-inflammatory mechanism is slightly different from that of EPA, it appears to complement EPA's anti-inflammatory activities.

### Cancer

Numerous test tube and animal studies have shown that EPA and GLA may prevent or inhibit the growth of cancer, particularly breast cancer. It appears that GLA "normalizes" cancer cells without harming healthy cells, suggesting the possibility of an effective yet nontoxic treatment. EPA has shown promise in preventing bowel cancer. Human studies have shown that EPA helps prevent metastasis—the spread of cancer.

### PMS and Dysmenorrhea

In several studies, evening primrose oil, high in GLA, has reduced symptoms of premenstrual syndrome (PMS), including depression and irritability. Researchers believe that a deficiency of GLA causes an abnormal sensitivity to the hormone prolactin, which leads to symptoms of PMS. There are also reports that GLA may be an effective treatment for fibrocystic breasts.

Supplementation with essential fatty acids also appears to be beneficial in cases of dysmenorrhea—painful menstrual periods. In a study of adolescent girls, the group that received supplements of EPA, DHA, and vitamin E experienced a marked reduction of menstrual pain after two months of supplementation. The supplements apparently prevented a buildup of the pro-inflammatory prostaglandins in the cell membranes of the uterus—a buildup that produces symptoms such as cramps, nausea, vomiting, bloating, and headaches.

## Other Uses

GLA may also prove to be an important component of weight-loss programs. Preliminary data suggests that this nutrient enhances weight loss by stimulating fat metabolism, and thus burning extra calories. Animal studies suggest that both EPA and GLA may slow the progress of the kidney disease glomerulonephritis, and may help patients avoid dialysis. Finally, there is evidence that these essential fatty acids may be useful in the treatment of certain disorders of the central nervous system. There are reports that both EPA and GLA affect schizophrenia. Furthermore, EPA may help in cases of manic-depressive illness, and GLA in cases of hyperactivity in children.

## RDIs AND DEFICIENCY SYMPTOMS

There are no established RDIs for the essential fatty acids, and no deficiency symptoms have been identified.

## WHICH FATTY ACIDS SHOULD YOU TAKE?

The properties of omega-3 and omega-6 fatty acids overlap to a great degree. Both enhance the body's own anti-inflammatory process, acting like cortisone, but without the undesirable side effects. Both have cardioprotective and anticancer properties. So you might be left wondering: Which one should I take? The truth of the matter is that essential fatty acid supplementation is often a case of trial and error. As a general rule of thumb, I tend to use EPA when there is a family tendency of high cholesterol (170 or above), high triglycerides, heart arrhythmias, or other heart disease. For those with low cholesterol, I generally use GLA. For hormonal problems, I usually try GLA first. However, keep in mind that researchers and clinicians have observed individual responses to the different fatty acids, so you must be willing to experiment. Try one type of supplement for one month, and then switch to the other. Compare the results and stick with whichever one is most effective. If the results are not clear-cut, you may have to use both to achieve the balance that is right for you. In fact, some practitioners suggest giving EPA/DHA and GLA supplements together, and studies have shown that EPA and GLA used together yield the best results for some purposes, such as decreasing the inflammation of rheumatoid arthritis.

## OMEGA-3 FATTY ACIDS (EPA AND DHA)

*Food Sources:* Animals—primarily cold-water fish and seafood such as her-ring, salmon, tuna, cod, mackerel, and shrimp—generally have the highest levels of EPA. Flaxseeds and flaxseed oils are the richest sources of alpha-li-nolenic acid, which can be converted to EPA and DHA in the body. However, many factors can inactivate this process, including smoking, environmental toxins, aging, excessive saturated fat intake, alcohol, and certain medications. Fish oil, rich in the already active forms of EPA and DHA, is the more dependable source of this essential nutrient.

### Supplements

It is essential that EPA and DHA supplements include vitamin E to prevent rancidity, and that supplements be taken with additional vitamin E supplements to prevent oxidation in the body. In fact, some of the conflicting results of studies using fish oil may be due to the fact that in some cases, the supplements used did not contain any vitamin E to protect them. Study results have been superior when EPA has been consumed with a vitamin E supplement.

Per capsule, fish oil supplements generally contain between 180 and 400 milligrams of EPA *plus* 120 to 300 milligrams of DHA. Although cod liver oil contains EPA and DHA, large doses should be avoided, because the oil contains high amounts of vitamins A and D, which, if ingested in very high amounts, could be toxic.

### Optimum Daily Intake—ODI

There is no Optimum Daily Intake for omega-3 fatty acids. Population studies have generally shown that eating cold-water fish as little as two or three times a week—the equivalent of about one ounce per day—could have beneficial effects, especially regarding heart disease preven-tion. For people who prefer not to rely on fish as a source of EPA and DHA, I generally recommend four to six fish oil capsules. Most studies used eighteen or more fish oil capsules without controlling dietary fat intake. You can achieve the same clinical benefits by eating a low-fat diet and using lower amounts (four to six capsules). Because of this nutrient's blood-thinning effect, higher amounts should be taken only under professional supervision, especially if you are also taking blood-thinning medication.

*Remember:* If you have a medical condition, and particularly if you are on blood-thinning medication, please consult your physician before taking sup-plements.

### Toxicity and Adverse Effects

There are no known toxic effects of EPA, DHA, or alpha-linolenic acid. Blood-clotting times do decrease with supplementation, but are still within normal range. Some of my patients have complained that high-potency EPA supplements are difficult to digest and leave a fishy odor and taste.

## OMEGA-6 FATTY ACIDS (GLA)

*Food Sources:* With the exception of human milk, most foods contain very little active GLA. Plants from which we extract vegetable oils generally have the highest levels of omega-6 fatty acids, with corn oil and canola oil being the most commonly used. However, oils from these plants contain mostly linoleic acid and small amounts of cis-linoleic acid, which must first be converted in our bodies to the more active, potent gamma-linolenic acid before they can be further converted to prostaglandins. This conversion—like the conversion of alpha-linolenic acid to EPA and then DHA—may be inhibited by many factors, including aging; stress; alcohol; and diets high in saturated fat, trans-fatty acids (found in margarine), cholesterol, and sugar. Other vegetable oils (see below) are more potent sources of GLA, but these are not generally used as food.

### Supplements

Both in scientific studies and in clinical practice, capsules of evening primrose oil have been the mainstay of GLA supplementation. The problem is that each evening primrose oil capsule contains only 45 milligrams of GLA along with over 100 milligrams of linoleic acid—the essential fatty acid that has inflammatory effects. However, other, richer sources of GLA have been discovered, including borage oil and black currant oil. These oils supply more GLA—240 to 300 milligrams per capsule—while containing less linoleic acid—50 milligrams per capsule. Since most of us already have an overabundance of linoleic acid in our diet, I prefer to use GLA from borage and black current oils to correct the imbalance and obtain the desired therapeutic effect.

### Optimum Daily Intake—ODI

There is no Optimum Daily Intake for omega-6 fatty acids. For people at risk for the conditions mentioned earlier, I generally recommend 70 to 240 milligrams of GLA as a preventive measure. This is approximately two to six evening primrose oil capsules per day, or one GLA capsule from borage or black currant oil. Higher amounts should be taken only under professional supervision to avoid upsetting the fatty acid balance in your body.

*Remember:* If you have a medical condition, please consult with your physician before taking supplements.

## Toxicity and Adverse Effects

There are no known toxic or adverse effects for GLA.

# Chapter 35

# FLAVONOIDS

A flavonoid is one of a group of crystalline compounds found in plants. Flavonoids were discovered by the Nobel Prize-winning scientist Szent-Gyorgy in 1936. He later named this class of plant compounds vitamin P.

Since 1936, scientists have isolated more than 4,000 flavonoids. Yet even this large number may represent only a small fraction of all the flavonoids that exist in nature. These substances are responsible for the deep colors of berries, and are also found in the skins of citrus fruits, and in other fruits, vegetables, nuts, seeds, grains, legumes, tea, coffee, cacao, and wine. In addition, most medicinal herbs owe their therapeutic qualities to flavonoid compounds.

It should be noted that you will often hear flavonoids referred to as "bioflavonoids." While the term "flavonoid" is the more scientific of the two terms, "bioflavonoid" is often used to describe biologically active flavonoids. In addition, when purchasing vitamins that contain flavonoids, you will find that the term "bioflavonoid" is the one that is most frequently used. Be aware, though, that the terms are generally used interchangeably.

## FUNCTIONS AND USES

Hundreds of studies on flavonoids have demonstrated the substances' wide range of abilities. They possess antiviral, anticarcinogenic, anti-inflammatory, antihistamine, and antioxidant activities, and may therefore be useful in preventing and/or treating a wide variety of conditions.

Recently, flavonoids have received a lot of attention because of their impressive antioxidant properties. (For more information about antioxidants, see page 29.) Several of these compounds appear to be even more effective than the more familiar antioxidants—vitamins C and E, for instance—in their effects, such as that of protecting low-density lipoproteins (LDLs) from oxidation. They may also lower cholesterol levels, offering further protection against cardiovascular disease. And it appears that if we are eating lots of fruits, vegetables, grains, and legumes, the consumption of flavonoids would far exceed the consumption of other antioxidants, such as vitamin C. In fact, flavonoid consumption is estimated to be between 200 and 1,000 milligrams a day.

Of the thousands of these oddly-named compounds that exist, the flavonoids that have been the most studied are quercetin, rutin, naringin, hesperidin, genistein, baicalin, Pycnogenol (a product that combines several substances), catechin, and bioflavonoid complex. Many studies—in particular, those of Dr. Chithan Kandaswami and Dr. Elliot Middleton—have demonstrated the effectiveness of a variety of flavonoids in the prevention and treatment of various cancers. These studies, which have included cancers resistant to chemotherapy, have involved both cell lines (cultures of cells grown in petri dishes) and living organisms.

The flavonoids known as proanthocyanidins are, in particular, getting a good deal of attention. Most of the research on proanthocyanidins has used Pycnogenol—a product containing proanthocyanidins and related plant flavonoids from the bark of the French Maritime Pine tree—rather than grape seed extract, which also contains this type of flavonoid. Much of this research has focused on the ability of these substances to act as antioxidants, and on their beneficial effects on many types of circulation problems. Human trials have shown that these flavonoids can prevent peripheral hemorrhage, swelling of the legs due to water retention, diabetic retinopathy, and high blood pressure. Researchers have also reported success in using these substances to treat varicose veins, leg cramps, and other problems arising from insufficient blood flow.

There has been considerable research performed on the antiviral activity of flavonoids, especially with viruses associated with polio, influenza, hepatitis types A and B, herpes simplex 1, human T-cell leukemia virus type I, and HIV (human immunodeficiency virus). In *in vitro* (test tube) conditions, for instance, baicalin and quercetin have been shown to inhibit the replication of the HIV virus by 100 percent.

It is interesting to note that many medicinal plants used for centuries contain high levels of flavonoid compounds. Examples can be found in the popular Japanese herbal medicine known as *Sho-saiko-to,* which is used to treat chronic liver disease. When investigators examined the ability of these herbs to inhibit the growth of cancer cells, they discovered that the combination of herbs was better at inhibiting the cancer growth than was each of the herbs when acting individually. This clearly demonstrates the synergistic effect of flavonoids.

Flavonoids that behave as *phytoestrogens* do not increase estrogen levels, as this name might imply. Instead, they encourage a better balance of "good" to "bad" estrogen by binding to sites for bad estrogen, and helping our bodies metabolize the bad estrogen. An excess of the bad estrogen (estradiol) is implicated in breast cancer, prostate cancer, menopausal symptoms, premenstrual symptoms, endometriosis, fibrocystic breast disease, and possibly other hormonally related disorders. Flavonoids help the body convert estradiol to estriol, the safe and protective form of estrogen. In fact, estriol is the preferred form of estrogen used in Europe in hormone-replacement therapy. Rich sources of the phytoestrogens are found in soybean products, and may be one reason for the lower incidence of estrogen-dependent disorders found in Eastern countries whose cuisines include soybean foods. There are even reports of flavonoids being used successfully in the treatment of osteoporosis as a safe alternative to estrogen-replacement therapy.

Considering the hundreds of studies that have been performed on flavonoids, and the fact that many of the effects have been outstanding when compared with those of drug-intervention studies, it is puzzling that these substances are not used more frequently as a treatment option for HIV/AIDS, arthritis, hepatitis, and cardiovascular disease, as well as the host of other degenerative diseases that have responded in test tube, animal, and some human experiments.

## RDIs AND DEFICIENCY SYMPTOMS

There are no established RDIs for flavonoids, and no deficiency symptoms have been identified.

*Food Sources:* Flavonoids are found in fruits, vegetables, nuts, seeds, grains, and legumes (particularly soybeans and soy products), and in beverages such as tea, coffee, and wine. It is possible to obtain the basic ODI for flavonoids by eating a diet rich in these foods.

## SUPPLEMENTS

Supplements of many—but not all—of the various flavonoids are available individually and in combination. Those that are easiest to find include bioflavonoid complex, curcumin, hesperidin, Pycnogenol, quercetin, and rutin. Note that all flavonoids should be taken with vitamin C, as they increase vitamin C absorption and are themselves powerful antioxidants.

## OPTIMUM DAILY INTAKE—ODI

For optimum general health, the basic Optimum Daily Intake for flavonoids—alone or in combination—is:

250–1,000 mg for men and women
(to be taken with an equivalent amount of vitamin C)

For specific conditions, the following flavonoids have been found to be helpful for:

| Condition | Supplements | Suggested Dosage |
|---|---|---|
| Allergies, arthritis, asthma, and inflammation | Curcumin | 500–1,500 mg |
| Bruising and circulatory disorders, including phlebitis and varicose veins | Pycnogenol or proanthocyanidins | 50–100 mg |
| Bruising and circulatory disorders, including varicose veins | Bioflavonoid complex containing rutin and hesperidin | 1,000–5,000 mg |
| Cancer prevention (especially breast and prostate) and hormone imbalance | Genistein | 4,000–6,000 |
| Viral infections, including HIV; inflammations due to arthritis and injury; and allergies | Quercetin | 500–1,500 mg |

*Remember:* If you have a medical condition, please consult your physician before taking supplements.

## TOXICITY AND ADVERSE EFFECTS

There are no known toxicities or adverse effects for flavonoids.

# Chapter 36

# GARLIC

G arlic is a plant food used all over the world. In many ancient and modern cultures, garlic has been considered a potent medicinal herb, effective in combating heart disease, infections, and cancer. Recent studies support these traditional uses for garlic, making its medicinal properties better recognized and accepted in the United States. However, because garlic contains many active ingredients—including potassium, phosphorus, vitamins B and C, diallyl disulfide, amino acids, germanium, and selenium—researchers are not sure which ingredient does what at this point, or if garlic's components are working alone or in combination.

## FUNCTIONS AND USES

### Cardiovascular Disease

Studies have shown that garlic protects against heart disease—and, in some cases, treats existing cardiovascular problems—in a number of ways. For instance, garlic prevents platelets, the blood cells needed for clotting, from sticking to one another and to artery walls. By preventing excess clotting, garlic may protect against strokes and coronary thrombosis (blood clots within a coronary artery). It may also deter the development of atherosclerosis by reducing the chance that blood clots will adhere to artery walls. Perhaps it is no coincidence that in countries such as Italy and Spain, where garlic is an important part of the cuisine, arterial disease is much less common than it is in the United States.

In addition, there's strong evidence that garlic protects the body from heart disease by changing the proportions of the various fats in the blood. In numerous animal and human studies, components of garlic have been shown to lower blood levels of the harmful fats—cholesterol, triglycerides, low-density lipoproteins (LDLs), and very-low-density lipoproteins (VLDLs)—and raise levels of the beneficial high-density lipoproteins (HDLs). Studies have also demonstrated the antioxidant benefits of garlic, which include the protection of LDLs from oxidation, a function that prevents LDLs from sticking to artery walls. A recent "meta-analysis"—a review of previous studies—that appeared in the *Journal of the American Medical Association*—concluded that garlic significantly lowers cholesterol. In one study conducted by researchers at Loma Linda University, subjects were given either garlic or a placebo for six months. At the end of the study, 73 percent of the garlic group showed a 12- to 31-percent drop in cholesterol levels. Interestingly, these researchers reported that about half of those in the garlic group who regularly ate meat showed no significant improvement; in several, cholesterol actually rose. It appears that it is the individual on a vegetarian or high-carbohydrate diet who benefits most from garlic supplementation.

Many medical authorities feel that garlic can also reduce high blood pressure, perhaps by acting as a vasodilator—an agent that causes a widening of the blood vessels. Practitioners in several countries, including Japan and Austria, recognize the value of garlic in the treatment of this condition.

### Infection and Immunity

Garlic's efficacy as a treatment for infection was noted long ago in ancient Egypt, Greece, and Rome. Garlic eaters seemed to have more resistance to disease and fewer deaths in times of plague. During both World Wars, garlic was used to treat troops suffering from typhus, dysentery, and battle wounds. In the former Soviet Union, garlic is still known as "Russian penicillin."

It has been discovered that garlic does contain substances, such as sulphur-containing compounds, that act against bacteria. In addition, garlic has proven effective against viruses, fungi, and parasites. Both in human studies and in the laboratory, garlic has been effective, for example, against *Candida albicans*, a fungus responsible for many common infections; *Cryptococcal meningitis*, a fungal infection of the brain; and two groups of bacteria, *Streptococcus* and *Staphylococcus*.

### Cancer

Animal and human studies suggest that garlic may prove to be a potent weapon against cancer. A National Cancer Institute study found that people whose diets are rich in garlic and its relatives, such as onions, have a lower incidence of stomach cancer than do people who consume less garlic. Other researchers have found that garlic inhibits the growth of bladder cancer in mice, both by acting on cancer cells directly and by enhancing the effectiveness of immune cells. In one study in which animals were exposed to a carcinogen that induces breast cancer, raw garlic powder and garlic extract reduced the incidence of breast cancer by 40 to 64 percent. Add to this the fact that garlic does not have the adverse side effects of other forms of cancer therapy, and it's clear that this food could have implications for a safe, side effect-free treatment for not just stomach, bladder, and breast cancers, but other forms of cancer, as well. This therapy might be particularly useful as an adjunct to conventional cancer treatment.

## Liver Disorders

Garlic also appears to defend the body from certain toxins. In laboratory and animal studies, garlic extract was able to protect the cells in the liver from the damaging effects of potent chemicals like carbon tetrachloride. The researchers pointed out that each day, we come in contact with a variety of harmful chemicals and microorganisms, and that, as a result, the incidence of liver disorders seems to be rising. In the ongoing search for substances that prevent or cure liver conditions, perhaps garlic will provide at least part of the answer.

## New Recommendations

Garlic's properties are so extraordinary and so wide ranging that in 1990, a special World Congress was held in Washington, D.C., during which over fifty leading garlic researchers representing fifteen countries presented their most recent research, and discussed the significance of their findings with two hundred participating physicians and scientists. These experts concluded that garlic in various forms—from cooked garlic, garlic oil, and raw garlic juice, to aged garlic extract, such as Kyolic—can provide great health benefits, including the reduction of cardiovascular and cancer risks in people exposed to the stresses of modern industrialized life, such as the modern processed diet. Increased garlic intake may also help reduce the free-radical damage often associated with pollution and nuclear radiation. Interestingly, the researchers agreed that to provide health benefits, garlic products do not have to contain allicin—one of garlic's active ingredients—nor do they have to have a garlic odor.

Based on the data then available, the researchers urged the public to increase its consumption of garlic and/or garlic products, suggesting a daily intake of at least one gram. Research presented at subsequent conferences, such as Designer Foods III, held in Washington, D.C., in 1993, supported these initial conclusions and recommendations.

*Food Sources:* The consumption of fresh garlic is the least costly means of benefiting from this nutrient. Many studies either used fresh raw garlic, or examined diets that were rich in garlic and related vegetables, such as onions, leeks, and green onions. Although cooking seems to reduce garlic's effectiveness, most people prefer cooked garlic over raw, and eating cooked garlic is certainly preferable to eating no garlic at all. If, however, you want to avoid garlic's taste and odor, you can choose supplements, instead.

## SUPPLEMENTS

Garlic preparations are available as liquid extracts, oil-filled capsules, and tablets. The supplements generally contain 100 to 300 milligrams in each pill. Many of these forms are deodorized or specially coated. Fortunately, deodorized garlic seems to be just as effective as the fresh aromatic form. Many studies—such as those showing garlic's effectiveness in reducing cholesterol and protecting the liver—used Kyolic, an odor-modified garlic extract, or Kwai, a nonodor-modified product. In Germany, Kwai is actually prescribed as a treatment for high cholesterol.

## OPTIMUM DAILY INTAKE—ODI

There is no Optimum Daily Intake for garlic, but I generally recommend 200 to 1,200 milligrams per day—about 1 to 4 ounces of fresh garlic, or two to six capsules, depending upon the potency.

## TOXICITY AND ADVERSE EFFECTS

There doesn't appear to be any adverse effect from supplementation with six capsules per day. In some people, fats in the blood may initially rise during garlic supplementation, and then begin to drop. No adverse effects have been noted as a result of this transient rise, even among heart disease patients. Higher doses could cause a sudden drop in blood pressure, and so should be taken under professional supervision only. Some people may experience skin eruptions with higher doses, but this side effect subsides when supplementation is reduced or stopped.

# Chapter 37

# GLUTATHIONE AND N-ACETYLCYSTEINE (NAC)

Most people are accustomed to thinking of antioxidants as vitamins and minerals. But there are many other natural substances that function in this way. Glutathione, a powerful antioxidant enzyme produced in our bodies, is one such substance. N-acetylcysteine (NAC), an amino acid required by our bodies to produce glutathione, appears to possess particular antioxidant properties, as well.

## FUNCTIONS AND USES

As antioxidants, these two related substances are intimately involved in the detoxification process, and are important members of our defenses against environmental toxins and carcinogens. They also protect our cells from oxidative stress—damage that may occur from a variety of environmental insults. Because such damage plays a role in degenerative diseases and in the weakening of the immune system, it should come as no surprise that it is the degenerative diseases—cancer, cardiovascular disease, and arthritis, for instance—and viral infections that respond to glutathione and NAC supplementation. In general, the studies of NAC have focused on its use in the treatment of viral infections, while the studies of glutathione have concerned the treatment of cancer. However, there is considerable overlap in the function and use of these two antioxidants, and it is reasonable to assume that both work for many conditions.

### Infection and Immunity

As already mentioned, most studies of NAC have focused on its potential use as an antiviral agent, specifically in the treatment of HIV (human immunodeficiency virus) infection and AIDS (acquired immune deficiency syndrome). Studies have shown that NAC reduces the replication of HIV. Moreover, when NAC is given along with vitamin C and glutathione, the results have been more striking than when any of these substances is given alone. Other studies have suggested that NAC and glutathione may work together to extend the latency period of HIV, delaying the onset of opportunistic infections. Researchers have also suggested that glutathione supplementation, along with NAC, inhibits expression of HIV—meaning that although a person may test positive for HIV, he or she may otherwise show no evidence of the infection. These findings may offer a promising new means of interfering with the progression of this disease.

Several researchers have indicated that NAC and glutathione are both natural nontoxic anti-HIV agents, and that they may inhibit the replication of other viruses, as well. Reports at the Ninth International Conference on AIDS in Berlin suggested that NAC can actually prevent apoptosis, a process that programs cell death. This may have important implications, as in HIV infection, apoptosis is a permanent and chronic situation.

In both animal and human studies, both NAC and glutathione have been shown to help protect against damage to the immune system. Indeed, deficiencies of these antioxidants may result in depletion of many types of immune cells, including macrophages, phagocytes, and T-cells. Supplementation, on the other hand, has been shown to improve immune function. In addition, supplementation with glutathione has been shown to increase the activity of neutrophils, another type of immune cell.

## Cancer

In preliminary animal and cell culture studies, glutathione has shown promise as a natural cancer preventive and therapeutic agent. Studies on glutathione have suggested that it may be particularly useful in some cancer patients receiving chemotherapy. For example, in one study, intravenous glutathione was shown to protect against kidney damage induced by the medication cisplatin. Interestingly, the survival rates of ovarian cancer patients receiving both glutathione and cisplatin in the early, middle, and late stages of the disease, were extraordinarily high compared with the rates of those receiving cisplatin alone. Based on these results, the authors of the study concluded that this combination represents a promising approach to optimizing the clinical use of cisplatin in the treatment of ovarian cancer. In another study, high doses of glutathione appeared to improve survival in women with liver cancer. In animals, it prevented chemotherapy-induced hair loss when administered intravenously or applied topically.

## Detoxification

Numerous studies have demonstrated NAC's ability to protect against toxic substances. It has a long history of both oral and intravenous use as an antidote for acetaminophen (Tylenol) toxicity, which can result in liver necrosis (cell death). NAC has also been shown to be an antidote for carbon tetrachloride exposure, protecting against both liver and kidney damage. Workers at risk for exposure to this toxic and carcinogenic chemical include air transportation workers, automobile mechanics, dry cleaning workers, grain workers, hazardous waste workers, museum workers, pesticide applicators, pharmaceutical manufacturers, steel mill and blast furnace workers, telephone and telegraph equipment and manufacturing workers, and tin waste-recovery workers. Possibly as the result of environmental toxins in general, several studies have shown that sperm counts and motility have dropped by half all over the world. Glutathione may help reverse this trend, as infertile men who received glutathione injections have experienced a significant increase in the motility of their sperm, and a significant reduction in atypical sperm.

## Aging

As antioxidants, both glutathione and NAC show great promise as a means of protecting against many of the disorders associated with aging. Indeed, studies of large segments of the elderly population have shown low glutathione levels. Already-completed research show that glutathione and NAC may help stave off the ravages of aging in the eye, the heart, and the nervous system. Specifically, glutathione is known to defend the eye against degeneration by protecting the lens and the macula, a part of the retina, against oxidative stress. Thus, glutathione—as well as NAC, because it replenishes glutathione—may be useful in the prevention of both cataracts, the clouding of the lens of the eye, and macular degeneration, a condition that can eventually lead to blindness.

## Cardiovascular Disease

NAC appears to also be useful in the prevention and treatment of cardiovascular disorders. First, NAC has been shown to lower levels of lipoprotein(a). This is a significant finding, because high levels of lipoprotein(a) have been correlated with an increased risk of cardiovascular disease. In addition, antioxidants—including the enzyme glutathione peroxidase, of which glutathione is a component; NAC; and superoxide dismutase (SOD)—seem to reduce the oxidative stress that contributes to the surgical complications associated with cardiopulmonary bypass procedures.

## Pulmonary Disease

Mucomyst, an inhalant form of NAC, has long been used to manage bronchitis, asthma, and other lung disorders. NAC treats these diseases by breaking up mucus. In addition, NAC can help reduce the high levels of oxidative stress that these disorders can cause in the lung tissues.

## Parkinson's Disease

Studies have revealed that the brains of Parkinson's sufferers have reduced levels of glutathione. This deficiency may result in increased oxidative stress, which may then damage the mitochondria—the tiny powerhouses that produce energy in our cells. By preserving glutathione levels in patients with Parkinson's, we may be able to prevent, slow, or stop the progression of this disease.

## RDIs AND DEFICIENCY SYMPTOMS

There are no established RDIs for glutathione and NAC, and no deficiency symptoms have been identified.

*Food Sources:* Fresh whole fruits; vegetables; and just-cooked animal foods, including beef, chicken, and fish, appear to be the best sources of glutathione. Dairy foods and grains are poor sources of this substance, and processing and preservation, except for freezing, generally cause significant losses of glutathione in foods.

N-acetylcysteine is made from cysteine, an amino acid found in high-protein foods. Thus, the best sources of this substance are eggs, dairy products, fish, poultry, and meat.

## SUPPLEMENTS

Separate supplements are available as glutathione and N-acetylcysteine. Cysteine, the precursor of NAC, is also available in supplement form, but the NAC form appears to be more active. Although perfectly safe, NAC and glutathione are quite expensive. Therefore, most professionals reserve their use for individuals whose health is severely compromised.

## OPTIMUM DAILY INTAKE—ODI

There is no Optimum Daily Intake for either glutathione or N-acetylcysteine. However, researchers and practitioners generally use 1 to 3 grams of NAC, and 500 to 1,500 milligrams of glutathione per day.

*Remember:* If you have a medical condition, please consult with your physician before taking supplements.

## TOXICITY AND ADVERSE EFFECTS

There is no known toxicity for either glutathione or NAC when administered orally, although some gastrointestinal effects may occur at high doses. Although shown to be safe, intravenous and inhalant use should be supervised by a physician.

# Chapter 38

# L-CARNITINE

Although often called an amino acid because of its chemical makeup, L-carnitine is actually a vitamin-like nutrient, related in structure to the B vitamins. L-carnitine is the biologically active form of carnitine, and can be synthesized by the human body in the liver and kidneys. It can also be obtained, already formed, from animal foods.

## FUNCTIONS AND USES

### Energy Production

L-carnitine's most important function is the transport of fatty acids into the muscles, where they can be burned for energy. Because fatty acids are a major fuel source for working muscles, carnitine deficiency can reduce the amount of energy available to the body.

L-carnitine levels in muscles are increased by physical training. Moreover, supplementation appears to build stamina and endurance, and may therefore enhance exercise performance—particularly in people with low levels of this nutrient. Supplementation appears to be most beneficial in well-conditioned individuals and athletes, whom it helps resist fatigue. Carnitine is also often prescribed for individuals who suffer from muscle fatigue due to conditions such as fibromyalgia and chronic fatigue syndrome.

### Cardiovascular Disease

Just as L-carnitine plays an essential role in transporting fatty acids into other muscles for energy, it is needed to transport these substances into the heart, the most important muscle in the body. Understandably, much of the research concerning L-carnitine has focused on its use in the treatment of heart disease.

Approximately 60 percent of the energy for the heart muscle is supplied by fatty acids. Thus, myocardial (heart muscle) L-carnitine deficiency has been found to be associated with myopathic heart disease, aging, diabetes, diphtheria, and chronic heart failure. L-carnitine supplementation has been shown to help lessen the impairment of heart muscle function associated with these conditions.

L-carnitine supplementation appears to benefit the heart in other ways, as well. Human studies have also shown that carnitine supplementation improves exercise tolerance and heartbeat regularity in patients with angina pectoris; significantly reduces the extent of cardiac necrosis (cell death) in patients hospitalized for heart attack; decreases the incidence of heart failure and reduces the need for pacemaker transplants in patients with heart disorders; and reduces the number of deaths due to myocarditis (inflammation of heart muscle tissue). In addition, carnitine has been used successfully to treat hypertriglyceridemia (elevated blood triglycerides), a risk factor for heart disease. It also increases levels of high-density lipoproteins (HDLs), which have been associated with a reduced risk of heart disease.

### The Nervous System

L-Carnitine may also be important for healthy brain function, since it appears to influence the metabolism of several neurotransmitters—chemicals that facilitate the sending of signals from one nerve fiber to another. In a study involving people with Alzheimer's disease, the progression of the disease was significantly reduced in those receiving 2 grams per day of acetyl-L-carnitine—a particular form of carnitine—orally for one year.

### Detoxification

L-carnitine also seems to have some antioxidant properties, as well as the ability to help detoxify certain drugs. For example, it appears to protect the heart muscle from the damage caused by Adriamycin (doxorubicin hydrochloride), a drug used in cancer treatment.

### RDIs AND DEFICIENCIES

Vegetarians are at particular risk for low carnitine levels for two reasons. First, L-carnitine can be obtained only from animal foods. Second, certain nutrients—vitamin C, niacin, vitamin B6, iron, and the amino acid L-lysine—are essential for the synthesis of carnitine. Because cereal grains such as corn, wheat, and rice—mainstays of many vegetarian diets—are low in L-lysine, a vegetarian's ability to synthesize carnitine may be compromised. The cooking or toasting of these grains destroys L-lysine entirely.

L-carnitine loss has been documented in patients receiving dialysis. This loss has been related to the complications these patients often face, such as high blood lipids, cardiomyopathy (any disease of the heart muscle), muscle loss, and muscle cramps. Treatment with oral L-carnitine has been shown to replace lost carnitine and improve these complications.

Although as adults we can synthesize L-carnitine, the diet seems to be an infant's only source of this amino acid. In the case of specific genetic disorders, such as organic aciduria, carnitine supplementation is necessary.

Since L-carnitine can both be found in foods and manufactured in our bodies under normal conditions, there is no RDI for this nutrient.

*Food Sources:* L-carnitine is found only in animal foods. We can synthesize carnitine provided that we have enough L-lysine—which is predominantly found in animal foods—as well as the other nutrients required for its synthesis.

## SUPPLEMENTS

The *L* forms of this nutrient, such as L-carnitine and acetyl-L-carnitine, are the most biologically active forms, and are the only forms found in foods and synthesized by our bodies. When carnitine is chemically synthesized, both the *L* and *D* forms are produced. Although supplements generally contain the *L* forms, be sure to avoid ones containing the *D* form, since they may actually inhibit the action of L-carnitine in metabolic processes.

L-carnitine and acetyl-L-carnitine are available as supplements at this time. Other forms of carnitine are generally used for research purposes, but may eventually find their way into the supplement market.

## OPTIMUM DAILY INTAKE—ODI

There is no Optimum Daily Intake for carnitine. Studies have generally used 1 to 5 grams of carnitine orally. Higher levels have been used in studies that administered the supplement intravenously.

*Remember:* If you have a medical condition, please consult your physician before taking supplements.

## TOXICITY AND ADVERSE EFFECTS

There is no known toxicity of carnitine, even with very high doses. In studies in which 5 to 6 grams were taken orally, some gastrointestinal side effects, such as bloating and flatulence, were noted. These can be avoided by starting with smaller doses and gradually increasing the dose over time.

# Chapter 39

# MELATONIN

Although melatonin is popularly regarded as a nutritional supplement, it is really a hormone secreted by the pineal gland, a tiny aspirin-sized organ buried deep in the brain. Not to be confused with the skin pigment melanin, melatonin is a potent chemical found in every cell of every living organism.

## FUNCTIONS AND USES

The hormone melatonin is responsible for regulating biological rhythms both in humans and in animals. In many animals, it insures that breeding and coat-shedding occur at the optimum time of the year. In humans, the release of melatonin—which occurs when our eyes register darkness—is what makes us feel drowsy at night.

Much of the data that has been gathered on melatonin relates to its role as timekeeper and its resulting ability to induce sleep, reduce jet lag, and untangle confused body rhythms induced by shift work. Other exciting research suggests that melatonin has a far wider range of actions. These include anticancer, antiaging, and antioxidant effects, as well as effects on fertility, sex drive, and the immune system.

### Insomnia

Researchers have found that insomniacs of all ages generally have decreased levels of melatonin in their blood, as do all elderly people. Several studies have demonstrated that melatonin may correct sleep disturbances such as difficulty in falling asleep and/or staying asleep, particularly in the elderly. Since our bodies synthesize melatonin from the amino acid tryptophan and the brain chemical serotonin, melatonin supplementation may be particularly useful in people who previously found tryptophan supplements to be a successful sleep aid. (Tryptophan supplements are currently available only by prescription as 5-hydroxytryptophan.) Unlike sleeping pills, melatonin, when taken in appropriate doses, generally does not produce a drugged feeling in the morning. In addition, melatonin supplements may improve the sleep disruption caused by drugs such as beta-blockers and benzodiazepines, which are known to alter melatonin production in the body. Melatonin may also correct sleep disturbances in blind people, who have little or no perception of light.

## Jet Lag

Like the insomnia studies, studies using melatonin to prevent jet lag have yielded good results. Both in experiments and anecdotally, many people report that they recover more quickly, have more energy, feel more alert, and sleep better when they use this supplement. Researchers have been uncertain as to the best dosage and timing of the melatonin. However, the greatest results were achieved in a study in which airplane crew members took 5 milligrams of melatonin on the day of arrival of the flight, and continued dosage for five consecutive days thereafter.

## Aging

As we get older, the production of melatonin tapers off. Researchers feel it may be no coincidence that as melatonin becomes scarce, the incidence of degenerative diseases and immune disorders begins to rise. There is, in fact, some evidence that melatonin may act as an antiaging hormone. Perhaps this is due in part to its role as a powerful antioxidant and free-radical scavenger. Oxidative damage from free radicals is linked with many degenerative conditions, including cancer, heart disease, and cataracts. Melatonin neutralizes one of the most damaging free radicals, and does so five times more effectively than the antioxidant enzyme glutathione, and twice as effectively as vitamin E. Unlike most other antioxidants, melatonin is found in every part of the cell. Maintaining levels of melatonin may prove to be just as important in retarding the aging process, protecting against degenerative diseases, and increasing longevity, as is maintaining optimal levels of other antioxidants, such as vitamins C and E, and selenium.

In one experiment using mice, researchers surgically switched the pineal glands of young and aging mice. The young mice with the old glands aged and died rapidly, but the older mice lived 30 percent longer than expected. In another study, the supplementation of rats with melatonin improved the texture and luster of their fur; prevented cataracts; improved digestion; increased strength, energy, and muscle tone; and prolonged sexual interest and capacity until the end of their lengthened lives.

In other animal studies, removal of the pineal gland raised cholesterol levels to 30 percent higher than normal by the time the animals reached adulthood. Whether or not this means that melatonin supplements can reduce heart disease in humans awaits further study. However, a recent study showed that melatonin was significantly lower in patients with coronary heart disease than in healthy individuals. Furthermore, because melatonin is able to enter the brain, it may protect that organ too, so there are hopes that it will help prevent or alleviate Alzheimer's and Parkinson's disease.

## PMS and Other Hormone-Related Problems

Melatonin is itself a hormone, and it plays a complex role in harmonizing other hormones in the body, particularly those related to reproduction. In both humans and animals, melatonin appears to be involved in the regulation of steroid hormone synthesis by the ovaries. In addition, animal data indicates that melatonin stimulates the parathyroid gland, which regulates bone mineralization. Thus, melatonin levels in the blood may be a marker for susceptibility to postmenopausal osteoporosis. Menopause is associated with a substantial decline in melatonin secretion, and it is possible that some of the symptoms of menopause, such as deranged sleep cycles and fatigue, may respond to melatonin supplementation.

The melatonin-hormone connection has implications for younger people, too. Human studies have shown that women who suffer from premenstrual syndrome (PMS) have lower melatonin levels, especially during the week preceding menstruation. Excess melatonin, however, lowers fertility, which is why this hormone is being studied as a contraceptive in Europe.

## Cancer

In test-tube and animal experiments, melatonin has been found to prevent both the initiation and the promotion of cancer cells, to slow the growth of some tumors, and to strengthen the immune system. Several studies have shown that low blood levels of melatonin seem to be associated with cancer growth.

Melatonin appears to block estrogen from binding onto the estrogen receptors of cells, including those of breast cancer cells, which are stimulated by estrogen. In a study of women whose cancers continued to grow despite being given the anti-estrogen drug tamoxifen, 28.5 percent of those who received melatonin in addition to the tamoxifen achieved tumor regression. Most patients also felt less anxious and experienced less toxicity from the tamoxifen. Furthermore, melatonin reduced an insulin-like growth factor that promotes breast cancer. In test tubes, melatonin has blocked the growth of breast cancer cells by 75 percent, and has blocked that of prostate cancer cells by 50 percent.

In a study involving people with advanced liver cancer, which usually responds poorly to treatment, patients were given melatonin along with interleukin 2, a substance used in immunotherapy. The results were remarkable. Tumors shrank in 36 percent of the subjects, the treatment was well tolerated, and the treatment's toxicity was low. Patients with advanced gastric cancer given melatonin with interleukin 2 also benefited, with 21 percent achieving tumor regression and reduced toxicity.

Another study included twenty-one people whose advanced kidney cancer had progressed despite treatment. When researchers administered melatonin plus interferon, seven of the patients—33 percent—achieved remission. In nine, the disease stabilized, and only five progressed. Again, the toxicity of the interferon was mild, and the side effects usually associated with this treatment were rare.

There is no known effective treatment for metastasized nonsmall-cell lung cancer. Patients with this disease who did not respond to chemotherapy were given melatonin along with supportive care. When compared with patients who received supportive care only, the one-year survival rate was significantly higher for the melatonin group. These patients also were generally able to function better.

The results of these remarkable studies demonstrate that adding melatonin to conventional cancer treatment improves the outcome of the treatment while reducing its toxicity. The studies suggest that melatonin may extend the lives of cancer patients whose disease is progressing even with medical treatment.

## RDIs AND DEFICIENCIES

Some of the daily stresses of modern life can create imbalanced cycles of light and dark. Since our body's production of melatonin is stimulated by darkness and inhibited by light, these stresses can adversely affect melatonin production. Such stresses may include travel across time zones, an erratic sleep schedule (such as sleeping late on weekends), changes in work shifts, working in a windowless environment, and even turning on a bright light upon awakening in the middle of the night. Exposure to electromagnetic fields, which are emitted by power lines and appliances such as electric blankets, has also been reported to reduce melatonin levels. Finally, many common drugs, including beta-blockers, calcium channel-blockers, ibuprofen, tranquilizers, and even aspirin, caffeine, alcohol, and tobacco, are known to depress melatonin levels.

No RDI has been established for melatonin.

*Food sources:* Melatonin is found in small amounts in rice, barley, corn, and a few other foods.

## SUPPLEMENTS

Melatonin is available in health food stores and drug stores in the form of pills, capsules, and liquid, in dosages beginning at one milligram. To obtain lower potencies, either use the liquid or crush the pills into smaller pieces.

## OPTIMUM DAILY INTAKE—ODI

There is no ODI for melatonin. Since it is a hormone, I suggest using this supplement cautiously and judiciously, and taking the lowest possible dose needed to get the desired effect. Not everyone benefits from daily supplementation; apparently, the response varies from person to person, and depends on the dose. I have had patients over the age of fifty who felt terrific after starting a program of exercise, dietary changes, and supplements. When they tried melatonin on their own, some of them felt headachy and reported feeling less well than they had before beginning supplementation. These patients probably didn't really need a melatonin supplement, because their lifestyle had enhanced their melatonin production sufficiently. Or perhaps they just needed a smaller amount than the 6 to 7 milligrams they were taking.

Because there have been no long-term studies on melatonin supplementation, I do not recommend that healthy people use it on a long-term basis. When used in the doses recommended below it may be helpful, and it appears safe for occasional use for insomnia and jet lag. I recommend starting with .1 milligram (a tenth of a one-milligram capsule), and increasing the dose until you have corrected your sleep problem. If you are taking it for preventive purposes, I also recommend starting with the lowest dose and increasing it slowly up to 3 milligrams. Use your judgment and monitor how you feel. Even better, ask your physician to measure your melatonin level to see if it is low. Melatonin should always be taken in the evening.

| Condition | Suggested Dosage |
|---|---|
| Aging-related problems | 1–3 mg daily |
| Cancer | 10–50 mg daily (only under professional supervision) |
| Insomnia | 1–8 mg (best if taken 1–2 hours before bedtime) |
| Jet lag | 1–8 mg (best if started upon arrival at destination and continued for 5 days) |

## TOXICITY AND ADVERSE EFFECTS

In some studies, doses of up to 6,000 milligrams of melatonin have produced no adverse effects. However, as is the case with any hormone, an excess can affect the actions of other hormones. For example, some studies suggest that excess melatonin may diminish libido or hamper fertility; as mentioned earlier, it may prove to be a valuable contraceptive. Excess melatonin may increase the level of the hormone prolactin, which decreases sex drive in men and could theoretically accelerate the growth of prolactin-sensitive breast cancers. Some people have reported experiencing wakefulness, nightmares, morning grogginess and headaches, or mild depression when taking melatonin. Melatonin supplements should be avoided—or taken only under professional supervision—by children, pregnant or nursing women, people trying to conceive, people with hormonal imbalances, people taking steroids, people who have severe allergies or other autoimmune disorders, and people with immune system cancers such as lymphoma or leukemia. Some researchers recommend that people with a tendency toward depression or who are on antidepressants also avoid taking this supplement. Many physicians, myself included, suggest taking melatonin only under professional supervision.

# Chapter 40

# DHEA

Like melatonin, discussed in the previous chapter, DHEA (dehydroepiandrosterone) is popularly viewed as a nutritional supplement, but is actually a hormone. One of the many steroid hormones secreted by the adrenal gland, DHEA was discovered in 1934. However, it is a precursor hormone—a hormone that is converted into several other hormones by the body—and for some time was thought to be less important than these metabolized end products. We now know that that this hormone has many functions, including support of the immune system; repair and maintenance of tissues; reduction of allergic reactions; and, possibly, the prevention of certain forms of age-related diseases, as well as a slowing of the aging process itself.

## FUNCTIONS AND USES

To understand how DHEA works within the body, it is important to first know that after DHEA is secreted by the adrenal glands, it is metabolized into DHEAS (dehydroepiandrosterone sulfate) in the liver, and then further converted to male hormones known as androgens (testosterone, dihydrotestosterone, and androstenedione), and female hormones known as estrogens (estrone and estradiol). Although the mechanism by which this conversion takes place isn't exactly known, it appears to be influenced by age, gender, and age-related diseases.

There are conflicting reports as to how much DHEA is made by the body. It is estimated that we have, on average, a range of 1 to 2 milligrams of DHEA and 10 to 15 milligrams of DHEAS circulating in the blood.

### Aging

As we age, our levels of DHEA and the male and female hormones significantly decline, along with those of other hormones, including the growth hormone. It is estimated that by age sixty, DHEA levels are a third or less of those in young adults. At age eighty, people have between 80 and 90 percent less DHEA in their blood than they had at the age of twenty-five. Many researchers believe that these reduced hormone levels are closely associated with aging-related problems, such as shrinkage of muscle mass, diminished immune function, and memory loss. In fact, the majority of human studies on DHEA have focused on aging and the diseases associated with aging.

In one study, men and women of ages forty to seventy were given 50 milligrams of DHEA daily for a six-month period. Within two weeks of the start of DHEA therapy, DHEA and DHEAS levels were restored to those of young adults. This supplementation resulted in a remarkable increase in perceived physical and psychological well-being for 67 percent of the male subjects and 84 percent of the female subjects, without any reported side effects.

Other studies have shown that DHEA or DHEAS given in appropriate replacement doses increases muscle strength and lean body mass, activates immune function, and enhances the quality of life in aging men and women, with no significant adverse effects. In year-long trials with elderly men and women, subjects reported enhanced overall feelings of wellness, improved sleep, and diminished joint soreness. Moreover, in animal studies, DHEA has been shown to restore memory function by encouraging neurite growth in the brain.

### Immune Function

Often, the influenza vaccine does not benefit those it is targeted to help—the elderly. The reason is that many individuals over the age of sixty no longer have the immune response necessary to make the antibodies to the vaccine.

In one study of subjects, ages sixty-five and older, one group received oral DHEAS before receiving a flu vaccine. The immune response to the vaccine was greater in the group that received DHEAS than in the supplemented group, suggesting that DHEAS supplementation may be a useful adjunct to the flu vaccine. However, in a similar study, supplementation with DHEAS did not enhance the immune response to a tetanus injection. Therefore, the ability of DHEAS to bolster the immune response to vaccines appears to be specific, and must be tested for each vaccine.

In another study, researchers evaluated the effects of DHEA on immune function in postmenopausal women. Women who received the DHEA supplement demonstrated improved levels of the cells needed for immune response. This beneficial action may account for the clinical and experimental evidence of DHEA's anticancer effect.

Many AIDS patients are using high levels of DHEA, as in advanced stages of AIDS, patients have extremely low DHEA blood levels. Although anecdotal reports indicate that DHEA may strengthen the immune system, relieve fatigue, and build muscle, experimental studies do not exist at this time.

Another immune-related disorder that has responded to DHEA supplementation is a condition known as hereditary angioneurotic edema (HAE). HAE is characterized by an allergic reaction that results in swelling of subcutaneous (beneath the surface of the skin) or submucous (beneath the mucous membrane) tissues. These patients have a deficiency of the C1 esterase inhibitor protein, which is the part of the immune response that normally protects against such attacks and inflammation. Eight patients with severe attacks of HAE were given DHEAS for three to twenty-eight months. Supplementation resulted in a dramatic improvement of clinical symptoms and a moderate increase in C1 inhibitor protein concentrations.

## Cancer

Animals studies have demonstrated that DHEA has anticancer properties. For example, when mice were exposed to chemicals that would normally induce breast cancer as well as other types of cancer, those animals that received DHEA did not develop cancer. Other animal studies have demonstrated that DHEA supplementation inhibits skin and lung cancer, as well.

## Cardiovascular Disease

Both human and animal studies have indicated that DHEA plays a role in cardiovascular health. In one study, a group of men received 50 milligrams of DHEA or a placebo for twelve days. The results suggested a natural "blood thinning" effect that may help prevent heart disease. In a twelve-year follow-up study of 143 middle-aged men, those subjects with high DHEAS levels in their blood suffered half as many cases of heart disease as did those with low DHEAS levels. However, the women with higher DHEA levels had a slightly higher risk of heart disease.

## Diabetes

As we age, we generally experience a decline in insulin sensitivity that causes glucose to remain in the blood in high levels. Thus, aging is associated with an increased incidence of diabetes.

In one study, a group of postmenopausal women were given 50 milligrams of DHEA daily for three weeks. Their insulin tissue sensitivity increased and their serum triglycerides were lowered, indicating improved glucose handling. Some researchers theorize that since DHEA levels are very low in patients with insulin-dependent diabetes, replacement of DHEA may prevent or even treat the atherosclerosis (hardening of the arteries) that is often associated with this type of diabetes.

## Lupus

DHEA has been shown to be beneficial in women with systemic lupus erythematosus. In one study, female patients given 200 milligrams of DHEA for three to six months experienced overall clinical improvement, enabling them to reduce their medication. DHEA may hold promise as a safe, effective treatment for lupus patients.

## RDIs AND DEFICIENCIES

There are no established RDIs for DHEA, and no deficiency symptoms have been identified.

*Food Sources:* At this time, no food sources of DHEA have been identified.

## SUPPLEMENTS

Although some studies have used DHEA while others have used DHEAS, only DHEA is available as a dietary supplement. You will generally find it in the form of tablets and capsules in doses beginning at 5 milligrams. Sprays and liquids of lower doses are also available.

## OPTIMUM DAILY INTAKE—ODI

There is no ODI for DHEA. Since DHEA is a hormone that can influence the production of androgens and estrogens, both I and other practitioners feel it is imperative that DHEA be used only under professional advice. Before beginning supplementation, it is best to have your physician first run a blood test of the following: DHEA; DHEAS; estradiol, estrone, and estriol, the three types of estrogen; and serum and free testosterone. Men with prostate conditions should have a physician measure their levels of dihydrotestosterone and PSA (prostate specific antigen, a marker for prostate cancer). DHEA should be used with extreme caution in men with prostate conditions, since it may raise levels of the androgens, which are the culprits in prostate disease. The same is true of women with disorders related to excessive estrogen. Once supplementation begins, all hormone levels should be retested within three weeks to evaluate the effects of the DHEA supplement in order to adjust the dosage as necessary.

The purpose of using DHEA is to raise levels of the measured hormones so that they fall *within* normal ranges. You do not want to take so much DHEA that your hormone levels *exceed* the normal reference range. It is best to start with low doses of DHEA—5 milligrams for women, and 10 milligrams for men—and slowly increase the levels by 5 to 10 milligrams each week until the desired result is achieved. Use the lowest dosage of DHEA needed to achieve results. Maximum doses are usually 25 milligrams for women and 50 milligrams for men. In studies, much higher doses have been used for some medical conditions, such as lupus. However, I still recommend starting with a lower dose and increasing slowly over time. Keep in mind that most studies have examined the effects of DHEA in individuals over the age of sixty—individuals who have comparatively low levels of DHEA.

*Remember:* If you have a medical condition, please consult your physician before taking supplements.

## TOXICITY AND ADVERSE EFFECTS

Serious side effects of DHEA supplementation have not been reported in human studies. Since high levels of DHEA stimulate the production of androgens, some side effects associated with high androgen levels have been reported, including acne and excessively oily skin, hair growth in women, deepening of the voice, and mood changes. These side effects are reversible when DHEA is discontinued. Only one animal study demonstrated liver cancer in rats given DHEA in doses far above what would normally occur in the animal.

# Part Five

## APPENDIXES AND NOTES

# SUMMARY OF VITAMINS, MINERALS, AND OTHER NUTRIENTS

The basic Optimum Daily Intake (ODI) is designed to enhance general health and prevent disease. Some individuals may wish to use higher levels, depending upon risk factors such as pollution, stress, and personal and family history.

Please note that for some nutrients—boron, for example—RDIs and ODIs have not yet been determined. For these nutrients, I have indicated a recommended range—in the case of boron, 3 to 6 milligrams—followed by an asterisk (*) to indicate that this dosage is not an ODI.

## QUICK-REFERENCE TABLE

| Nutrient | Major Uses | Food Sources | RDI | ODI |
|---|---|---|---|---|
| **Fat-Soluble Vitamins** | | | | |
| Vitamin A and Beta-carotene | Antioxidant.<br>Prevents night blindness and other eye problems.<br>May be useful for acne and other skin disorders.<br>Enhances immunity.<br>Cancer prevention.<br>May heal gastrointestinal ulcers.<br>Protects against pollution.<br>Needed for epithelial tissue maintenance and repair. | Fish liver oils, animal livers, green and yellow fruits and vegetables. | 5,000 IU | 5,000–50,000 IU (in a mixture of A and beta-carotene) |
| Vitamin D | Required for calcium and phosphorus absorption and utilization.<br>Prevention and treatment of osteoporosis.<br>Enhances immunity. | Fish liver oils, fatty saltwater fish, vitamin D-fortified dairy products, eggs. | 400 IU | 400–800 IU |
| Vitamin E | Antioxidant.<br>Cancer prevention.<br>Cardiovascular disease prevention.<br>Improves circulation.<br>Tissue repair.<br>May prevent age spots.<br>Useful in treating fibrocystic breasts.<br>Useful in treating PMS. | Cold-pressed vegetable oils, whole grains, nuts, dark-green leafy vegetables, legumes. | 30 IU | 400–1,200 IU |
| Vitamin K | Needed for blood clotting.<br>May play a role in bone formation.<br>May prevent osteoporosis. | Green leafy vegetables. | 80 mcg | 80 mcg |
| **Water-Soluble Vitamins** | | | | |
| Biotin | Needed for metabolism of protein, fats, and carbohydrates.<br>Not enough data available, but deficiencies may be implicated in high serum cholesterol, seborrheic dermatitis, and certain nervous system disorders. | Meat, cooked egg yolk, yeast, poultry, milk, saltwater fish, soybeans, whole grains. | 300 mcg | 300 mcg |

| Nutrient | Major Uses | Food Sources | RDI | ODI |
|----------|------------|--------------|-----|-----|
| Choline and Inositol | Involved in metabolism of fat and cholesterol, and absorption and utilization of fat.<br>Choline makes an important brain neurotransmitter. | Egg yolk, whole grains, vegetables, organ meats, fruits, milk. | None | 25–500 mg |
| Folic acid | Works closely with $B_{12}$.<br>Involved in protein metabolism.<br>Needed for healthy cell division and replication.<br>Prevention and treatment of folic acid anemia.<br>Stress may increase need.<br>May be useful for depression and anxiety.<br>May be useful in treating cervical dysplasia.<br>Oral contraceptives may increase need. | Beef, lamb, pork, chicken liver, whole wheat, bran, green leafy vegetables, yeast. | 400 mcg | 400–1,200 mcg |
| PABA | Needed for protein metabolism.<br>Needed for folic acid metabolism.<br>Used topically as a sunscreen. | Liver, kidney, whole grains, molasses. | None | 25–500 mg |
| Pantothenic acid | Needed in fat, protein, and carbohydrate metabolism.<br>Needed for synthesis of hormones and cholesterol.<br>Needed for red blood cell production.<br>Needed for nerve transmission.<br>Vital for healthy function of the adrenal glands.<br>May be useful for joint inflammation.<br>May be useful for depression and anxiety. | Eggs, saltwater fish, pork, beef, milk, whole wheat, beans, fresh vegetables. | 10 mg | 25–500 mg |

| Nutrient | Major Uses | Food Sources | RDI | ODI |
|---|---|---|---|---|
| Vitamin B Complex $B_1$ (thiamin); $B_2$ (riboflavin); $B_3$ (niacin, niacinamide); $B_6$ (pyridoxine) | Maintains healthy nerves, skin, eyes, hair, liver, mouth, muscle tone in gastrointestinal tract.<br>B vitamins are coenzymes involved in energy production.<br>Emotional or physical stress increases need.<br>May be useful for depression or anxiety. | Unrefined whole grains, liver, green leafy vegetables, fish, poultry, eggs, meat, nuts, beans. | $B_1$: 1.5 mg<br>$B_2$: 1.7 mg<br>$B_3$: 20 mg<br>$B_6$: 2.0 mg | 25–300 mg |

$B_1$: High-carbohydrate diet increases need.

$B_2$: May be useful with $B_6$ for treatment of carpal tunnel syndrome. May prevent cataracts. Increased need with oral contraceptives. Increased need with strenuous exercise. Antioxidant.

$B_3$: Useful for circulatory problems. Lowers serum cholesterol and triglycerides.

$B_6$: May be useful in preventing oxalate stones. May be used as mild diuretic. May be useful for PMS. Increased need with oral contraceptives. May be useful in treating asthma.

| Nutrient | Major Uses | Food Sources | RDI | ODI |
|---|---|---|---|---|
| Vitamin $B_{12}$ (cobalamin) | Needed for fat and carbohydrate metabolism.<br>Prevention and treatment of $B_{12}$ anemia.<br>Maintains proper nervous system function.<br>May be useful for anxiety and depression. | Kidney, liver, egg, herring, mackerel, milk, cheese, tofu, seafood. | 6 mcg | 25–500 mcg |
| Vitamin C (ascorbic acid) | Growth and repair of tissues.<br>May reduce cholesterol.<br>Antioxidant.<br>Cancer prevention.<br>Enhances immunity.<br>Stress increases requirement.<br>May reduce high blood pressure.<br>May prevent atherosclerosis.<br>Protects against pollution. | Green vegetables, berries, citrus fruit. | 60 mg | 500–5,000 mg (higher during stress or illness) |

**Minerals**

| Nutrient | Major Uses | Food Sources | RDI | ODI |
|---|---|---|---|---|
| Boron | Prevents bone loss.<br>May enhance bone density. | Fruits, vegetables. | None | 3–6 mg* |

| Nutrient | Major Uses | Food Sources | RDI | ODI |
|----------|-----------|--------------|-----|-----|
| Calcium | Needed for healthy bones and teeth. Needed for nerve transmission. Used for muscle function. May lower blood pressure. Osteoporosis prevention. | Dairy foods, green leafy vegetables, salmon, sardines, seafood. | 1,000 mg | 1,000–1,500 mg |
| Chromium | Required for glucose metabolism. May prevent diabetes. May reduce cholesterol. | Brewer's yeast, beer, meat, cheese, whole grains. | 120 mcg | 200–600 mcg |
| Copper | Involved in blood formation. Needed for healthy nerves. Needed for taste sensitivity. Used in energy production. Needed for healthy bone development. | Widely distributed in foods. Also derived from copper cookware and plumbing. | 2 mg | Generally available through foods: 0.5–2 mg |
| Iodine | Needed for healthy thyroid gland. Prevents goiter. | Iodized salts, seafood, kelp, saltwater fish. | 150 mcg | 150–300 mcg (0–150 mcg for those who use iodized salt) |
| Iron | Vital for blood formation. Needed for energy production. Required for healthy immune system. | Meat, poultry, fish, liver, eggs, green leafy vegetables, whole grain or enriched breads and cereals. | 18 mg | 15–30 mg |
| Magnesium | Needed for healthy bones. Involved in nerve transmission. Needed for muscle function. Used in energy formation. Needed for healthy blood vessels. May lower blood pressure. | Widely distributed in foods, especially dairy foods, meat, fish, seafood. | 400 mg | 500–750 mg |

| Nutrient | Major Uses | Food Sources | RDI | ODI |
|---|---|---|---|---|
| Manga-nese | Needed for protein and fat metabolism. Used in energy formation. Required for normal bone growth and reproduction. Needed for healthy nerves. Needed for healthy blood sugar regulation. Needed for healthy immune system. | Nuts, seeds, whole grains, avocado, seaweed. | 2 mg | 15–30 mg |
| Phos-phorus | Necessary for healthy bones. Needed for production of energy. Used as a buffering agent. Needed for utilization of protein, fats, and carbohydrates. | Available in most foods; sodas can be very high. | 1,000 mg | Generally available through foods: 200–400 mg |
| Potassium | May lower blood pressure. Needed for energy storage. Needed for nerve transmission, muscle contraction, and hormone secretion. | Dairy foods, meat, poultry, fish, fruit, legumes, whole grains, vegetables. | None | 99–300 mg |
| Selenium | Cancer prevention. Heart disease prevention. | Depending on soil content, may be in grains and meat. | 70 mcg | 50–400 mcg (50–100 mcg for those who live in high-selenium areas) |
| Zinc | Needed for wound healing. Maintains taste and smell acuity. Needed for healthy immune system. Protects liver from chemical damage. | Oysters, fish, seafood, meats, poultry, whole grains, legumes. | 15 mg | 22.5–50 mg |
| **Other Nutrients** | | | | |
| Coen-zyme Q$_{10}$ (CoQ) | Cell energy and metabolism. Prevents cell damage. May be useful in cardiovascular diseases such as angina, congestive heart failure, arrhythmia, and high blood pressure. May protect heart muscle and promote faster recovery from heart attack and heart surgery. | None | None | 50–300 mg* |

| Nutrient | Major Uses | Food Sources | RDI | ODI |
|---|---|---|---|---|
| DHEA | Antiaging properties.<br>May strenthen immune system.<br>May inhibit cancer.<br>May help prevent cardiovascular disease.<br>May increase insulin tissue sensitivity.<br>May help treat lupus. | None | None | Use only when needed |
| EPA | Prevents heart disease.<br>May lower blood pressure.<br>May lower triglycerides.<br>May lower cholesterol.<br>Prevents excess blood clotting.<br>May relieve inflammatory and allergic reactions.<br>May inhibit cancer.<br>May enhance immune system. | Cold-water fish. | None | 250–3,000 mg* |
| Flavonoids | Antioxidant.<br>May lower cholesterol.<br>May prevent cardiovascular disease.<br>May inhibit cancer.<br>Needed to maintain healthy blood vessels.<br>Helps fight viral infections. | Fruits, vegetables, grains, nuts, seeds, soybeans, tea, coffee, wine. | None | 250–1,000 mg |
| Garlic | May lower blood pressure.<br>May enhance immune system.<br>May prevent heart disease.<br>May lower triglycerides.<br>May lower cholesterol.<br>Antibacterial, antiviral, antifungal.<br>Prevents excess blood clotting.<br>May prevent cancer.<br>Antioxidant. | Garlic. | None | 200–1,200 mg* |
| GLA | May prevent heart disease.<br>Relieves allergic reactions.<br>Relieves eczema.<br>Relieves arthritis.<br>Relieves PMS symptoms.<br>May assist in weight loss. | Evening primrose oil, borage oil, black currant oil. | None | 70–240 mg* |

| Nutrient | Major Uses | Food Sources | RDI | ODI |
|---|---|---|---|---|
| Glutathione and NAC | Antioxidant. Helps fight viral infections. May inhibit cancer. Helps maintain healthy immune system. Protects against environmental and drug toxicity. | Fruits, vegetables, meat. | None | Glutathione: 500–5,000 mg* NAC: 1,000–3,000 mg* |
| L-Carnitine | Needed for fat metabolism. May inhibit muscle fatigue diseases. May alleviate or prevent heart conditions. Helps body detoxify drugs. | Animal foods. | None | 1,000–5,000 mg* |
| Melatonin | Regulates biological rhythms. Relieves insomnia. Prevents jet lag. Antiaging properties. Relieves some hormone-related problems. May inhibit cancer. | Found in small amounts in rice, barley, corn. | None | For short-term use, only when needed. |

# DRUG-INDUCED VITAMIN AND MINERAL DEFICIENCIES

Many drugs—both prescription and over-the-counter—have the potential to affect nutritional status. A large number of drugs can alter food intake by decreasing appetite; by changing the sense of taste; or by causing dry mouth, nausea, or, in some cases, vomiting. In addition, drugs may interact adversely with the nutrients that you take (vitamins, minerals, and food supplements), reducing absorption, distribution, activation, or utilization, and possibly increasing nutrient excretion. For this reason, nutrient replacement can greatly benefit the patient who is taking these drugs.

The following table is a listing of the vitamin and mineral deficiencies that may result when you take some of the most commonly used drugs. Naturally, before increasing your nutrient intake, you should discuss the proper dosage with your health care provider.

## DRUG-NUTRIENT INTERACTION TABLE

| Drug Class or Drug | Possible Deficiency Vitamin(s) | Possible Deficiency Mineral(s) |
|---|---|---|
| **Acetaminophen** (e.g., Tylenol) | C | |
| **Alcohol** | $B_1$, $B_2$, Folic Acid | Zinc |
| **Antacids:** Aluminum Hydroxide Preparations (e.g., Maalox, Mylanta), Sodium Bicarbonate | A, $B_1$, Folic Acid | Calcium, Copper, Iron, Phosphorus |

| Drug Class or Drug | Possible Deficiency Vitamin(s) | Possible Deficiency Mineral(s) |
|---|---|---|
| **Antibacterial Agents:** Boric Acid, Isoniazid, Rifampin, Trimethoprim | $B_2$, $B_3$, $B_6$, Folic Acid, Niacin, D | |
| **Antibiotics:** Chlortetracycline, Gentamicin, Neomycin, Tetracycline | $B_2$, Biotin, Folic Acid, Niacin, C, D | Calcium, Iron, Magnesium, Potassium, Zinc |
| **Anticancer Drugs:** Adriamycin, Cisplatin, Methotrexate | $B_{12}$, Folic Acid, E | Iron, Magnesium |
| **Anticoagulants:** Warfarin | Avoid Vitamin K | |
| **Anticonvulsants:** Phenobarbital, Phenytoin (e.g., Dilantin), Primidone (e.g., Mysoline), Valproic Acid (e.g., Depakene) | $B_6$, $B_{12}$, Folic Acid, D, K | Calcium, Magnesium, Carnitine |
| **Antihypertensive Agents:** Hydralazine | $B_6$ | Manganese |
| **Anti-Inflammatory Agents:** Aspirin, Colchicine, Prednisone, Sulfasalazine | $B_6$, $B_{12}$, Folic Acid, C, D | Calcium, Iron, Phosphorus, Potassium, Zinc |
| **Antimalarials:** Chloroquine, Pyrimethamine (e.g., Fansidar) | Folic Acid | |
| **Antipsychotic Agents:** Haldol, Mellaril, Stelazine, Thorazine | $B_2$, $B_{12}$, D | |
| **Digoxin** | | Calcium, Magnesium |

| Drug Class or Drug | Possible Deficiency Vitamin(s) | Possible Deficiency Mineral(s) |
|---|---|---|
| **Diuretics** | $B_2$ | Magnesium, Potassium, Sodium, Zinc |
| **H-2 Receptor Antagonists:** Cimetidine, Ranitidine | $B_{12}$ | |
| **Hypocholesterolemic Agents:** Cholestyramine (e.g., Questran), Colestipol | A, $B_{12}$, Folic Acid, D, E, K | Calcium, Iron |
| **Indomethacin** | C | Iron |
| **Laxatives:** Mineral Oil, Phenolphthalein | A, Carotene, D, E, K | Calcium, Potassium |
| **Levodopa** | Restrict $B_6$ to less than 5 mg unless taking Sinemet. | |
| **Methyldopa** | $B_{12}$, Folic Acid | |
| **Oral Contraceptives:** | $B_1$, $B_2$, $B_3$, $B_6$, $B_{12}$, Folic Acid, C | Calcium, Magnesium, Zinc |
| **Penicillamine** | $B_6$ | Copper, Iron, Zinc |
| **Premarin** | $B_2$, $B_6$, $B_{12}$, Folic Acid | Magnesium, Zinc |
| **Tobacco Products** | B6, C | |

# WORKSHEET

## HOW TO USE THE WORKSHEET

Begin by determining your ODIs. You may use the basic ODIs given in the following worksheet, which are in the low to middle range. These can provide many people with optimum general physical and mental health and will prevent most illnesses. Note, though, that your own ODIs may differ. Most of the ODIs given in the individual chapters on vitamins and minerals is expressed as a dosage range. Based on the information in the individual nutrient chapters and in Part One, decide whether your own ODI should be in the lower, middle, or upper level of the range. The ODI listed on the worksheet may be all you need.

Some people need to take higher amounts of certain specific nutrients. There may be factors in your life, such as your personal or family health history, that place you at a higher risk for certain diseases and disorders. If so, you may want to use supplements to provide an additional margin of safety. The worksheet illustrates and summarizes the most frequently encountered of these concerns.

For example, if cancer runs in your family, you would take higher ODIs of vitamins A, B, C, D, and E, and of manganese and selenium. If you are concerned about heart disease, your ODIs for vitamin C, vitamin E, chromium, and selenium would be higher than the basic ODIs. If you have more than one concern, do not add one specific ODI to another; simply use the upper range. For example, if you are concerned about cardiovascular disease prevention and are under great emotional stress, your ODI for vitamin C would be 5,000 milligrams, *not* 10,000 milligrams.

If a particular concern of yours is not listed in the worksheet, refer to the individual vitamin and mineral chapters for the ODI range and enter it in one of the columns marked "Other." For example, some women might be concerned about PMS (premenstrual syndrome).

Enter your starting ODI in the worksheet, and date it. As time goes by, evaluate the way you feel and adjust your ODIs accordingly.

## SAMPLE WORKSHEET

| Nutrient | Basic ODI | Emotional Stress | Enhance Immunity | Cardiovascular Disease Prevention |
|---|---|---|---|---|
| Vitamin A | 10,000 IU | | 10,000–100,000 IU | |
| B complex | 50 mg | 25–300 mg | 50 mg | |
| Vitamin C | 1,000 mg | 1,000–5,000 mg | 1,000–5,000 mg | 500–3,000 mg |
| Vitamin D | 400 IU | | | |
| Vitamin E | 400 IU | | | 400–800 IU |
| Vitamin K | 80 mg | | | |
| Boron | 3 mg | | | |
| Calcium | 1,000 mg | | | |
| Chromium | 200 mcg | | | 400 mcg |
| Copper | 2 mg | | | |
| Iodine | 150 mcg | | | |
| Iron | 15 mg | | | |
| Magnesium | 500 mg | | | |
| Manganese | 15 mg | | | |
| Phosphorus | Obtained from food source | | | |
| Potassium | Obtained from food source (reduce salt) | | | |
| Selenium | 50 mcg | | | 100–300 mcg |
| Zinc | 22.5 mg | | 30–50 mg | |
| Coenzyme $Q_{10}$ | 50 mg | | | |
| EPA | 250 mg | | 250–3,000 mg | 1,000–3,000 mg |
| Flavonoids | 250 mg | | | |
| Garlic | 200 mg | | 200–1,200 mg | 200–1,200 mg |
| GLA | 70 mg | | 70–240 mg | 70–240 mg |
| Glutathione | 500 mg | | | |
| L-carnitine | 1,000 mg | | | |
| NAC | 1,000 mg | | | |

| Cancer Prevention | Skin Problems | Diabetes Prevention | Osteoporosis Prevention | Other | Your ODI and Date |
|---|---|---|---|---|---|
| 50,000–200,000 IU | 50,000–200,000 IU | | | | |
| 50–150 mg | | | | | |
| 5,000–10,000 mg | 3,000–5,000 mg | 1,000–3,000 mg | | | |
| 400 IU | | | 400–800 IU | | |
| 400–800 IU | | | | | |
| | | | | | |
| | | | 3–6 mg | | |
| | | 1,200–2,000 mg | 1,500–2,000 mg | | |
| | | 400–600 mcg | | | |
| | | | | | |
| | | | | | |
| | | | | | |
| | | | 500–1,000 mg | | |
| 15–30 mg | | 20–30 mg | 15–30 mg | | |
| | | | 200–400 mg | | |
| | | | | | |
| 200–400 mcg | 200 mcg | | | | |
| | | | | | |
| | | | | | |
| 250–3,000 mg | 1,000–3,000 mg | | | | |
| | | | | | |
| 200–1,200 mg | | | | | |
| 70–240 mg | 70–240 mg | | | | |
| | | | | | |
| | | | | | |
| | | | | | |

# DAILY SUPPLEMENT SCHEDULE

Use the handy chart on the following page to serve as a guide when you buy supplements, and to help you keep track of your supplement schedule. Make sure to read the labels on your supplements to avoid duplication and double-dosing. For example, if you use a multivitamin supplement with 50 milligrams of B complex, you don't need to take a separate B complex 50. You may, however, want to buy a separate supplement of an individual B vitamin to use for a specific purpose. The same holds true for minerals and other nutrients.

Remember that if you are taking large doses of supplements, they should be divided as evenly as possible throughout the day. Simply write down the number of tablets of each supplement that you take after meals in the appropriate column, and keep the guide displayed for easy reference. (You may want to make a copy of the guide rather than tear it out of the book.) Eventually, taking your supplements will become such a habit that you won't need to refer to the schedule. For example, I take my multivitamin-mineral supplement after breakfast and lunch, and take whatever extra individual supplements I need after dinner.

# DAILY SUPPLEMENT SCHEDULE

| Supplement | Potency | Morning | Afternoon | Evening |
|---|---|---|---|---|
| Multivitamins | | | | |
| Multiminerals | | | | |
| Vitamin A | | | | |
| Beta-carotene | | | | |
| B complex | | | | |
| Other B vitamins: | | | | |
| | | | | |
| | | | | |
| | | | | |
| Vitamin C | | | | |
| Bioflavonoids | | | | |
| Vitamin D | | | | |
| Vitamin E | | | | |
| Boron | | | | |
| Calcium | | | | |
| Chromium | | | | |
| Copper | | | | |
| Iodine | | | | |
| Iron | | | | |
| Magnesium | | | | |
| Manganese | | | | |
| Selenium | | | | |
| Zinc | | | | |
| Other: | | | | |
| | | | | |
| | | | | |
| | | | | |
| | | | | |
| | | | | |
| | | | | |

# REFERENCE ABSTRACTS FOR VITAMINS, MINERALS, AND OTHER NUTRIENTS

In some cases, the following abstracts provide more detailed information on the studies discussed in the chapters, and refer you to the source of the material, should you decide to read it in its entirety. In other cases, the abstracts refer to studies that are not mentioned in the chapter, but that either support the points made in the text or reveal additional benefits of the nutrient. For the sake of simplicity, in some instances we have chosen not to cite all of the studies mentioned within the chapter.

## CHAPTER 1: WHAT ARE VITAMINS AND MINERALS?

For a thorough compilation of evidence on the safety levels of a wide range of intakes of vitamins and minerals, see *Safety of Vitamins and Minerals: A Summary of the Findings of Key Nutrients* (Washington, DC: Council for Responsible Nutrition, 1991).

For a report on current evidence of the potential benefits from the regular use of vitamin and mineral supplements, see *Benefits of Nutritional Supplements* (Washington, DC: Council for Responsible Nutrition, 1993).

## CHAPTER 2: THE RDIs—THE MINIMUM WAGES OF NUTRITION

### Marginal Vitamin Deficiencies

This editorial examines the importance of vitamin intake and notes that frank vitamin deficiency is rare in the U.S., but that there is compelling evidence that large segments of the population are consuming suboptimal levels of several micronutrients. The authors cite national surveys that show that many Americans fall far below the recommended intakes of several vitamins, and then mention evidence suggesting that such low intakes have serious health consequences, such as neural tube defects, cancer, and heart disease. They conclude that vitamin supplementation at the RDA levels may be beneficial for large segments of the population, especially elderly individuals and women of childbearing age. *Journal of American Medical Association* 270 (December 8, 1993): 2,726–2,727.

At a 1994 American College of Cardiology meeting, two thirds of the audience of approximately 700 physicians acknowledged that they themselves took antioxidant supplements daily. *Family Practice News* (March 1, 1994): 10.

## The Caveman Diet

The diet of Paleolithic humans was higher than the modern diet in many nutrients, including calcium and vitamin C. *The New England Journal of Medicine* (January 31, 1985): 283–289.

## Use of Supplements

This article discusses the pros and cons of supplementation. It notes that 40 percent of the population is consuming supplements, and that several economists have estimated that increasing our intake of vitamins and minerals would reduce health care costs by 25 percent for cardiovascular disease, 16 to 30 percent for a variety of cancers, and 50 percent for cataracts. *Journal of the American College of Nutrition* 13 (1994): 113–115.

Dr. Verlangieri, of the University of Mississippi, believes that everyone should take supplements, and recommends antioxidant vitamins C and E, and vitamin A or beta-carotene in excess of the RDAs. *Modern Medicine* 60 (July 1992): 15–18.

## Antioxidants

Oxidant by-products of normal metabolism result in extensive damage to DNA, protein, and lipids. This damage is probably a major contributor to aging-related and degenerative diseases such as cancer, cardiovascular disease, immune system decline, brain dysfunction, and cataracts. Antioxidant defenses include vitamins C and E and the carotenoids. Low intakes of fruit and vegetables—rich sources of antioxidants—can double the risk of most types of cancer when compared with high intakes. Only 9 percent of the American population consumes the recommended 5 servings of fruits and vegetables each day. *Proceedings of the National Academy of Sciences* 90 (September 1993): 7,915–7,922.

This study evaluated 413 individual case-controlled pairs of individuals, and is the largest study done to date of dietary factors and lung cancer risk in nonsmokers. The results suggest that dietary beta-carotene, raw fruits and vegetables, and vitamin E supplements reduce the risk of lung cancer in nonsmokers. *Journal of the National Cancer Institute* 86 (January 5, 1994): 33–38.

The Alliance for Aging recommends supplements of C, E, and beta-carotene far in excess of the RDA to prevent many conditions associated with aging. This article also quotes Jeffrey Blumberg, M.D., of Tufts University, who believes that we know enough at this time to make recommendations about supplementation. *Medical Tribune* 1 (March 24, 1994).

In a double-blind placebo-controlled study on the effect of vitamin E supplementation on the immune response of healthy elderly individuals, the majority of subjects who received 800 international units of vitamin E showed significant enhancement of their immune system. *Nutrient Modulation of the Immune Response* (New York: Marcel Drecker, 1993), 223–238.

The risk of cataract was 45 percent lower among women who used vitamin C supplements for 10 or more years. *British Medical Journal* (August 8, 1992): 335–339.

In a study of 30,000 people living in a single province of China, the overall death rate from cancer was less in the groups that took vitamin supplements than it was in groups that took "dummy" pills. *Journal of the National Cancer Institute* (September 1993): 1,446–1,447.

## CHAPTER 3: THE OPTIMUM DAILY INTAKES (ODIs)

### Antioxidant Supplementation

What follows is a sampling of the many articles published on the potential benefit of antioxidant supplements. For a fuller discussion of free radical damage and the role of antioxidants, see Nancy Bruning, *The Natural Health Guide to Antioxidants* (New York: Bantam, 1994).

Healthy subjects were supplemented with 15 milligrams of beta-carotene (25,000 international units), 30 milligrams of vitamin C, and 15 milligrams of vitamin E. These amounts stimulated free radical scavenging activity. This study confirmed the well-known antioxidant effects of these vitamins, with maximum protection occurring after 30 days. This type of supplementation would be an easy and rapid way to increase the oxidative stress defenses in various diseases in which free radicals occur. *The Annals of Pharmacotherapy* 27 (November 1993): 1,349–1,350.

Gladys Block has written many articles that support the role of antioxidants in reducing cancer risk. In this review article, Dr. Block argues that based on all of the available scientific literature, antioxidants do in fact demonstrate a protective defense against cancer in studies looking at food consumption and supplementation. For example, of approximately 130 studies that examined supplemental vitamin C, beta-carotene, or vitamin E, *or their rich food sources*, 120 have found statistically significant reduced risks of cancer of the lung, larynx, esophagus, oral cavity, pancreas, stomach, cervix, rectum, colon, ovary, endometrium, breast, and bladder. The level of intake is determined in part by the level of oxidative stress. Individuals, or populations, vary in the level of such stressors, which include nitrosamines, smoking, alcohol, ozone, and other environmental pollutants; infections; vigorous exercise; chronic disease; and sunlight exposure. No single level of intake is "right" at all times. *Nutrition Reviews* 50 (July 1992): 207–213.

In Linxian, China, approximately 30,000 adults, ages 49 to 69, received a daily vitamin and mineral supplement at dose ranges one to two times the RDA. There was significantly lower mortality in those receiving supplementation with the antioxidants beta-carotene, vitamin E, and selenium. The reduction was mainly due to lower cancer rates, especially stomach cancer, with reduced risk beginning to arise one to two years after supplements were started. *Journal of the National Cancer Institute* 18 (September 15, 1993): 1,492–1,498.

## Antioxidants and Cardiovascular Disease

This article reviews the relationship of antioxidants and atherosclerosis. It discusses evidence to support the theory that oxidative stress and inflammation lead to this condition, and the various roles of antioxidant nutrients vitamins C and E, beta-carotene, and the glutathione system. *Heart Disease and Stroke* 3 (1994): 52–57.

These two Harvard School of Public Health studies showed a reduced risk of heart disease for both men and women who took beta-carotene and vitamin E supplements. *The New England Journal of Medicine* 20 (May 20, 1993): 1,444–1,487. (See also Chapters 6 and 8.)

## Other Antioxidant Studies

**Exercise:** Antioxidant supplementation has been shown to reduce oxidative stress and speed recovery from muscle soreness after exercise. In one study, subjects took supplements containing 592 milligrams of vitamin E, 1,000 milligrams of vitamin C, and 30 milligrams of beta-carotene. These supplements significantly reduced exercise-induced oxidative stress. *Journal of Applied Physiology* 74 (1993): 965–969.

**Infection and Cataracts:** Two Canadian studies showed lower rates of infectious disease and cataracts among elderly people who took antioxidant vitamins. *Medical Tribune* (March 24, 1994): 1.

**Life Span:** This study showed that men who consume 300 milligrams of vitamin C daily (through food and supplements) had a 40-percent lower death rate from heart disease and other causes than those whose intake was less than 50 milligrams. *Epidemiology* 3 (1992): 194–202.

**Overall Health:** In this study, people who ingested less than 100 milligrams of vitamin C per day experienced the greatest number of clinical signs and symptoms, while those who ingested 200 milligrams per day had the least symptoms. Moreover, 50-year-olds who consumed the highest levels of vitamin C were clinically similar to 40-year-olds. *Journal of Advancement in Medicine* 7 (Spring 1994): 31–34.

**Eye Disorders:** This article reviews the role of nutrition in eye disorders. In the Nurses' Health Study, for example, women in the highest fifth of total carotene intake (14,500 international units per day) had a lower risk of cataracts compared with those in the lowest fifth. Vitamin C supplementation for over 10 years reduced the risk of cataracts by 45 percent. Regarding the intake of antioxidants vitamin C, vitamin E, beta-carotene, and riboflavin, those who were in the highest fifth had a 40-percent lower risk of cataracts. The carotenoid family in general was associated with a highly significant reduced risk of macular degeneration. The recommended amounts of antioxidants to achieve this protection are in considerable excess of the RDIs. *Journal of Nutritional Biochemistry* 5 (February 1994): 66–76.

## Multinutrient Studies

Many studies have examined the effects of several nutrients at once. Many of these looked at antioxidant nutrients in particular. The following is a selection of the most significant of these multinutrient studies.

### Cancer

This article reviews the use of vitamin and mineral supplementation in cancer treatment. It discusses the benefits of folic acid, folinic acid, vitamin K, and multivitamin and -mineral supplements in enhancing the effects of chemotherapy and radiation, as well as the possible antitumor effects of the nutrients themselves. It also discusses a study that evaluated 65 patients with bladder cancer, in a randomized comparison of BCG therapy along with multivitamins in the RDA range versus the same RDA-multivitamin plus megavitamin therapy. The megavitamin therapy included 4,000 international units of vitamin A, 100 milligrams of B6, 2,000 milligrams of C, 400 international units of E, and 90 milligrams of zinc. BCG therapy did not significantly reduce tumor recurrence. Recurrence after 10 months was markedly reduced in patients receiving the megadose vitamins. The 5-year estimates of tumor recurrence were 91 percent in the RDA group, and 41 percent in the megadose group. Overall recurrence was 24 of 30 patients in the RDA group and 14 of 35 in the megavitamin group. *Adjuvant Nutrition in Cancer Treatment*, 1992 Symposium Proceedings. Patrick Quillin, Ph.D., R.D., R. Michael Williams, M.D., Ph.D., editors, Cancer Treatment Research Foundation, Arlington Heights, IL, 1992.

This article gives a general overview of the randomized controlled large-scale worldwide prevention and treatment trials with respect to cancer. Daily dose ranges in these trials for vitamin A are approximately 25,000 international units; beta-carotene, 30 to 180 milligrams; vitamin C, 1,000 milligrams; vitamin E, 400 milligrams; calcium, 1,200 milligrams; and omega-3 fatty acids, 10 grams. *Annals of Medicine* 26 (1994): 73–78.

### Premenstrual Syndrome

A double-blind, randomized study on 44 women with PMS was conducted assessing the efficacy of a nutritional supplement. Subjects received 6 tablets of the supplement, 12 tablets of the supplement, or a placebo. Significant treatment effects were noted in three subgroups of the 6-tablet group and in all four subgroups of the 12-tablet group. The results of this study suggest that this nutritional supplement may play a role in the management of PMS. *American Journal of Clinical Nutrition* 10 (1991): 494–499.

## Skin

This article reviews the role of nutrients and skin disorders. Vitamin A may help prevent the development of chemical and UV light-induced skin cancers in animals. Oral retinoids may provide some benefit in patients with some types of skin cancers. Vitamin A supplementation at 25,000 international units in seriously injured patients enhanced wound healing and resistance to infection. Selenium is useful in protecting against UV-induced tanning, sunburn, and skin and other cancers. Vitamin C may be beneficial in the prevention of UV skin damage. Melanoma cell growth inhibition has been seen with vitamin $B_6$, C, D, and E. For the severely ill patient, 1 to 2 grams of vitamin C daily are recommended to enhance recovery. Topical zinc may be used for acne; fish oil, evening primrose oil, and Chinese herbal teas may be useful in atopic dermatitis. Vitamins A and D may be useful in the treatment of psoriasis. *Journal of the American Academy of Dermatology* 29 (1993): 447–461.

## Life Span

Antioxidant defenses are sufficient to allow a life span of 70 to 100 years. The amounts required of antioxidants to achieve these protective effects are in considerable excess of the RDI. The author recommends daily supplements of 200 to 400 international units of vitamin E, 100 to 250 milligrams of vitamin C, and 25 milligrams of beta-carotene. *Journal of Nutritional Biochemistry* 5 (February 1994): 66–76.

## CHAPTER 4: HOW TO DESIGN YOUR OWN NUTRITIONAL SUPPLEMENT PROGRAM

A researcher with the National Institute on Aging discusses research studies on the relationship between free radicals and longevity. *Antioxidants: Chemical, Physiological, Nutritional and Toxicological Aspects* (Princeton, NJ: Princeton Scientific, 1993), 151–161.

A University of California at Los Angeles researcher studied nearly 12,000 people, ages 25 to 74, for 10 years. The men who took an average 300 milligrams of vitamin C per day in food and supplements experienced a 42-percent lower death rate from heart disease and other causes than did the men whose intake was less than 50 milligrams. The women in the study did not see similar benefits. *Epidemiology* 3 (1992): 194, 202.

## CHAPTER 5: YOUR TOTAL HEALTH PLAN

This excellent, comprehensive article reviews the effects of the protective factors found in plant foods such as fruits and vegetables. These include beta-carotenes, vitamin C, sulfur-containing compounds, protease inhibitors, and many others. *Nutrition Action Health Letter* 21 (April 1994): 7–13.

In evaluating over 200 studies for the relationship between fruit and vegetable consumption and cancer, it was found that there was a significant protective effect in 128 of the 156 dietary studies. Low fruit and vegetable intake resulted in twice the risk of most cancers compared with high intake. *Nutrition and Cancer* 18 (1992): 1–29.

## CHAPTER 6: VITAMIN A AND BETA-CAROTENE

### Overviews

Vitamin A is required for vision, reproduction, and maintenance of epithelial tissue. It is beneficial in the treatment of acne, psoriasis, and other skin disorders, and may be important in cancer prevention and in treating precancerous conditions. *The New England Journal of Medicine* 310 (April 19, 1984): 1,023–1,031.

The authors review evidence regarding the possible mechanisms for the three major recognized functions that are dependent on vitamin A: cell growth and differentiation, reproduction, and vision. *Proceedings of the Society for Experimental Biology and Medicine* 172 (1983): 139–152.

### Immunity and Infections

In this study, 24 nonsmoking healthy males, ages 19 to 39, received 30 milligrams of beta-carotene per day or a placebo while on a low-carotenoid diet. Subjects received 12 exposures to UV-A/B light over 16 days. Follow-up was continued for 28 days. Delayed hypersensitivity test responses were significantly suppressed in the placebo group. There was no significant suppression in the beta-carotene group. The authors conclude that beta-carotene protects against photosuppression of immune function. *American Journal of Clinical Nutrition* 56 (1992): 684–690.

In a review of single nutrients and immunity, animal studies show there is an enhanced immune response when excesses of vitamin A are given. Conversely, there is an increase in susceptibility to infection when there is a vitamin A deficiency. *American Journal of Clinical Nutrition* (Supplement) 35 (February 1982): 428–430.

Carotenoids, including beta-carotene, can enhance immune function and can act directly as antimutagens and anticarcinogens. *Journal of Nutrition* 119 (1989): 135–136.

In laboratory mice treated with cyclophosphamide and prednisolone—drugs that suppress the immune system—vitamin A supplementation restored immune response to normal levels or better. *Pharmacology* 30 (April 1985): 181–187.

### Cardiovascular Disease

The predominant antioxidants protecting the LDL molecule against oxidative stress (free radicals) are vitamin E, vitamin A, and beta-carotene. Vitamin C is the first line of defense and also regenerates vitamin E. Antioxidants appear to protect the LDL molecule from increased lipid peroxidation, and thereby slow the atherosclerotic process. *Archives of Internal Medicine* 155 (1995): 241–246.

As part of the ongoing Physicians' Health Study, a group of 333 men with a history of cardiovascular disease were studied. Those who took 50 milligrams (85,000 international units) of beta-carotene every other day had half as many heart attacks, strokes, and deaths related to heart disease as those who did not take supplements. *Circulation* 82 (1992): Suppl. III: 202.

This article reviewed literature with respect to beta-carotene and vitamin E supplementation in men who smoke or consume alcohol. In one study, the highest carotene intake resulted in a 29-percent reduction in the risk of developing coronary heart disease. Among smokers, men with the highest carotene intake had a 70-percent reduction in coronary risk. *Nutrition Report* 11 (1993): 73, 80.

## Ulcers

In a 4-week study of 40 patients with chronic gastric ulcers, the number of patients whose ulcers completely healed or shrank was highest in the group that received 150,000 international units of vitamin A daily. The authors suggest that since gastric ulcers may be thought of as a precancerous condition, vitamin A may have a role in the prevention of cancer from gastric ulcers. *The Lancet* (October 16, 1982): 876.

Rats fed either a standard diet or one supplemented with 25 times the RDA for vitamin A were then given a substance that induces duodenal ulcers. In the unsupplemented group, 74 percent developed ulcers, compared with 32 percent of the supplemented group. The authors suggest that vitamin A may be useful in the prevention and treatment of duodenal ulcers in humans. *Journal of Parenteral and Enteral Nutrition* 10 *(January–February 1986): 74–77.*

## Cancer Prevention

Many studies show a correlation between high consumption of beta-carotene and/or higher vitamin A (retinol) blood levels, and lowered incidence of these cancers: lung, endometrium, bronchus, bladder, breast, cervix, rectum, and the skin cancer melanoma. Such studies have been conducted all over the world including the United States, England, Finland, Japan, Norway, and Poland. What follows is a representative sampling.

Designer food programs are underway to include food protective phytochemicals in food products. Diet supplementation with nontoxic doses of vitamin A and carotene may help prevent breast cancer. Three different carotenoids that may prevent breast cancer include beta-carotene, apo-carotenal, and canthaxanthin. Carotenoids appear to be the most active in preventing the activation of chemical carcinogens, while retinoids alter the promotional stage of carcinogenesis. The role of phytoestrogens, flavonoids, fiber, and other compounds are also reviewed. *Primary Care and Cancer* 14 (February 1994): 10–11.

In a 5-year study, 8,278 Norwegian men showed a threefold decrease in lung cancer with an increase in vitamin A consumption. Beta-carotene was the major source of this vitamin. *International Journal of Cancer* 15 (1975): 561–565.

In a 10-year follow-up study of 265,118 Japanese men, the risk of lung cancer was 1.4 times greater in the men who did not eat beta-carotene-rich vegetables. *Nutrition and Cancer* 1 (1979): 67–81.

In a 19-year study, the incidence of lung cancer among 2,107 men was inversely related to the intake of dietary beta-carotene. *Nutrition Reviews* 40 (September 1982): 265–268.

In a controlled study, a low carotene intake increased the odds of developing cancer of the larynx by twofold. A high carotene intake was found to be protective in men who had stopped smoking, but not in smokers. *American Journal of Epidemiology* 128 (1988): 980–988.

A large case-control study revealed that a higher carotene intake was associated with a lower risk of squamous and small cell lung cancer. *Cancer* 62 (November 15, 1988): 2,267–2,273.

People with low intakes of beta-carotene have a 30- to 220-percent higher risk of lung cancer than people with a high intake of beta-carotene. Evidence also suggests a protective effect of beta-carotene against cancers of the stomach, cervix, and breast, as well as other cancers. This protective effect may be due to its antioxidant properties as well as its enhancement of the immune system. *Nutrition Research* 8 (1988): 685–701.

In a controlled study, 200,000 international units of vitamin A were given weekly to subjects who regularly chewed betel, the leaves of an Asiatic plant. (Oral cancer is responsible for high cancer mortality among betel and tobacco chewers.) Subjects who received vitamin A experienced a pronounced remission of precancerous lesions, and prevention of new lesions. *Cancer Letters* 40 (1988): 93–101.

In a controlled study, higher levels of carotene in the blood reduced the risk of cancer of the cervix by approximately 80 percent. *Journal of National Cancer Institute* 80 (June 15, 1988): 580–585.

A large controlled study found an association between prostate cancer and low levels of vitamin A. *Cancer* 62 (November 1, 1988): 2,021–2,026.

In a controlled study, researchers found that men with prostate cancer had a lower intake of beta-carotene than did the control subjects. *Cancer Research* 48 (March 1, 1988): 1,331–1,336.

In a retrospective study of 28 patients with cancer of epithelial tissues (endometrium, lung, bronchus, bladder, and breast) and 53 patients with myeloma, a nonepithelial cancer, blood serum levels of vitamin A were lower in cancer patients than in healthy subjects, and particularly low in those with epithelial cancers. *European Journal of Cancer and Clinical Oncology* 18 (1982): 339–342.

In a study of 78 women with untreated cervical cancer, blood serum values for beta-carotene, folate, and vitamin C were significantly lower than in the 240 healthy women used for control subjects. In addition, after cancer surgery, the women's levels of beta-carotene, vitamin A, and several other nutrients dropped dramatically. *American Journal of Obstetrics and Gynecology* 151 (March 1, 1985): 632–635.

In a study conducted in England, the incidence of breast cancer was higher in women whose prediagnosis blood levels of beta-carotene (but not retinol) were lower than the levels of the control subjects who did not develop cancer. *British Journal of Cancer* 49 (1984): 321–324.

This study was the largest study to date of dietary factors and lung cancer risk in nonsmokers. The results suggest that dietary beta-carotene, raw fruits and vegetables, and vitamin E supplements reduce the risk of lung cancer in nonsmokers. *Journal of the National Cancer Institute* 86 (January 5, 1994): 33–38.

## Supplementation as Cancer Treatment

Some studies on animals and humans suggest that vitamin A or beta-carotene can affect the course of an already established cancer or precancer. These include the following:

After inoculating experimental mice with cancer cells, tumor metastasis (spread) was slower to appear in the group fed supplemental vitamin A. The authors conclude that vitamin A could be used to prevent metastases by confining tumor cells to the encapsulated area. *Cancer Research* 45 (July 1985): 3,311–3,321.

In a study using hamster cells, genetic damage of the type associated with carcinogenesis was significantly reduced in the cells that were treated with vitamin A. *Journal of Clinical Investigation* 75 (June 1985): 1,835–1,841.

This article reviews the potential benefit of beta-carotene and vitamin A derivatives in the treatment and prevention of oral leukoplakia and cervical cancer. High-dose vitamin A derivatives have resulted in a 50- to 90-percent regression of oral lesions; however, therapy is limited due to toxicity. Similar studies conducted using beta-carotene resulted in a 71-percent response and no toxicity. Topical application of vitamin A derivatives to the cervix has resulted in a 50-percent regression of lesions. Beta-carotene appears to have similar benefit with no toxicity. *Drug Therapy* (July 1992): 55–60. See also *The Female Patient* 17 (February 1992): 120–125.

In this study, 20 patients diagnosed with colon cancer were given 30 milligrams a day of beta-carotene for 6 months after surgery. Cancer cell proliferation was inhibited by 44 percent after 4 weeks of supplementation, and by 57 percent after 9 weeks of supplementation. It remained low for 6 months after supplementation was discontinued. *Cancer Research* 53 (1993): 3,723–3,725.

In this controlled, randomized study of 307 surgically-treated lung cancer patients, one group of subjects was given 300,000 international units of vitamin A daily for 12 months.

After a year, 37 percent of the supplemented group and 48 percent of the control group developed new primary tumors. Second primary tumors developed in 19 supplemented patients, but 29 of the control patients. *Journal of Clinical Oncology* 11 (1993): 1,216–1,222.

This review article states that all 13 of the published studies show a cancer-protective effect from the intake of carotenoids. Of these, 5 studies used beta-carotene alone. A recent multi-center study achieved a 55-percent response rate with beta-carotene, which was comparable to that achieved with the more toxic vitamin A. The author states, "In those that had an early primary head and neck cancer that was considered cured, the prevention of a second cancer may be accomplished with nontoxic agents such as vitamin E and beta-carotene." *The Nutrition Report* (October 1994) 12(10): 73–80.

High-dose vitamin A therapy (300,000 international units daily for 12 months) was tested on 307 patients whose lung cancer was removed surgically. After a year, 37 percent of the patients who received the supplement experienced a recurrence or new primary tumor, compared with 48 percent of the control group—a statistically significant difference. *Journal of Clinical Oncology* (July 1993) 11(7): 1,204–1,207.

## Supplementation as Complementary Cancer Treatment

In this Finnish study, researchers gave cancer patients a wide variety of vitamin and mineral supplements, including 15,000 to 40,000 international units of vitamin A and 10,000 to 20,000 international units of beta-carotene, along with their chemotherapy and radiation treatments. The supplemented group lived longer and suffered fewer side effects than did those who were unsupplemented. *Anticancer Research* 12 (May–June 1992): 599–606.

Breast cancer patients with higher blood levels of vitamin A responded twice as well to chemotherapy as did women with lower levels. The authors cite Scottish researchers who report an association between improved chemotherapy response and higher vitamin A levels for patients with cancer of the breast, cancer of the bowel, and melanoma. *Medical Tribune* 23 (March 1983): 23.

Of breast cancer patients whose blood levels of vitamin A are equal to or higher than those of a group of disease-free women, 83 percent responded to chemotherapy, 17 percent remained stable, and none progressed. Of the patients whose vitamin A levels were below those of the control group, only 36 percent responded to chemotherapy, while 24 percent remained stable and 40 percent progressed. *Proceedings of the American Association of Cancer Researchers* (1981) (22):184 (meeting abstract).

## Skin

In this review article, the authors point out that vitamin A has been used to treat acne since the early 1940s. In one series, 100 patients were given 100,000 international units per day. Of these, 97 were "cured or almost cured." A 1981 report indicated that doses of 50,000 to 100,000 international units were ineffective, but that intake of 300,000 international units daily for 3 to 4 months was highly efficacious. The researchers postulated that the risk of toxicity at the higher dosage range was exaggerated. *Drugs* 27 (1984): 148–170.

This is an extensive review of the protective effects of oral and topical antioxidant therapy as a defense against UV light exposure. The antioxidants reviewed include vitamin E, coenzyme $Q_{10}$, glutathione, vitamin C, and carotenoids. The reviewers feel that prophylactic antioxidant administration should start early and be used throughout the year to provide optimum conditions for protection. I. Emerit Basel, ed, *Free Radicals and Aging* (Switzerland: Birkhauser Verlag, 1992), 328–340.

This article reviews the role of nutrients and skin disorders. Vitamin A may help prevent the development of chemical and UV light-induced skin cancers in animals. Oral retinoids may provide some benefit in patients with some types of skin cancers. Vitamin

A supplementation at 25,000 international units in seriously injured patients enhanced wound healing and resistance to infection. *Journal of the American Academy of Dermatology* 29 (1993): 447–461.

Repeated exposure to ultraviolet (UV) light significantly reduced the carotenoids in the blood of volunteers. Since carotenoids protect against UV damage and cancer, lower levels caused by chronic UV exposure could increase UV-related tissue damage and cancer. *American Journal of Clinical Nutrition* 47 (May 1988): 879–883.

A statistically significant inverse relationship was found between the risk of skin cancer and a high intake of fish, vegetables, cruciferous vegetables, beta-carotene, and vitamin C-containing foods. Those subjects who developed skin cancer had lower beta-carotene and vitamin A levels than did the control subjects. *Nutrition and Cancer* 18 (1992): 237–244.

## HIV Infection and AIDS

In this study, 21 HIV-infected patients, most of whom were taking AZT, were given either 180 milligrams per day of beta-carotene or a placebo for 4 weeks in a crossover trial. Patients on beta-carotene had average elevations in their CD4 cells of approximately 17 percent, as well as improved levels of CD4 helper cells, in many cases. Total white blood cell counts increased only on beta-carotene. The vitamin therapy had no side effects. *Medical Tribune* 4 (February 25, 1993): 1.

Dr. Gregg Coodley and colleagues conducted a double-blind, placebo-controlled, crossover clinical study by giving participants either 180 milligrams per day (300,000 international units) of beta-carotene or a placebo. Beta-carotene supplementation was associated with an increase of total white blood cell count, of CD4 count, and of CD4/CD8 ratio. *Journal of Acquired Immune Deficiency Syndrome* 6 (1993): 272–276.

## Eye Disorders

In this study, researchers interviewed 112 subjects regarding their dietary and supplement intake, and measured plasma levels of beta-carotene. Those with the lowest plasma levels had 5 times the risk of developing cataracts of those with high levels. *Supplement to the American Journal of Clinical Nutrition* 53 (1991): 352S.

Dietary intake of beta-carotene was inversely associated with acute macular degeneration in patients ages 55 to 80. High vitamin C intake was associated with a marginal but significant decrease in developing acute macular degeneration. The authors conclude that increased intakes of antioxidants, beta-carotene, and vitamin C might decrease the risk of macular degeneration. *Investigative Ophthalmology and Visual Science* 34 (December 1993): 1,134.

## Bioavailability

In this study, 38 women randomly received 12 milligrams of beta-carotene from food (raw carrots or carrot juice) or from purified beta-carotene capsules after receiving a low carotenoid diet prior to and during the study. After 12 weeks, both goups had significant increases in their blood levels of beta-carotene, with the beta-carotene-capsule group having the greatest response. *Nutrition Research* 16 (1996): 565–575.

## Toxicity

In 2-year studies of rats, mice, and dogs, beta-carotene was added to the diet in amounts up to 1.7 million international units per kilogram of body weight. The authors concluded that beta-carotene can be given for long periods of time virtually without risk of toxicity. *Toxicology* 36 (August 1985): 91–100.

Animal studies have shown that beta-carotene is not carcinogenic, mutagenic, embryotoxic, or teratogenic and does not cause hypervitaminosis A. Adverse effects have not been reported in people who have taken high amounts of beta-carotene for several years for medical reasons. *Nutrition and Cancer* 11 (1988): 207–217.

In adults, vitamin A toxicity is uncommon at doses less than 100,000 international units per day. In most cases, when vitamin A is stopped, symptoms are relieved within a short amount of time. In humans, 5 cases of birth defects have been reported in which the mother took high doses of vitamin A during pregnancy. However, no clear cause-and-effect relationship was demonstrated in any of these cases. *American Journal of Clinical Nutrition* 49 (1989): 358–371.

## CHAPTER 7: VITAMIN D

### Overview

The author reviews what is known about the human requirement for vitamin D, the variables that influence the formation of $D_3$ in the skin, the symptoms of overdose, the diseases and drugs that may interfere with vitamin D metabolism, and the function of vitamin D. *Journal of the American College of Nutrition* 2 (1983): 173–199.

### Osteoporosis

In this study of 19 elderly women with and without vertebral fractures, both groups had low levels of calcium and vitamin D. After 7 days of treatment with vitamin D, bloodstream levels increased in both groups, but calcium absorption increased only in women without fractures. The authors suggest that pharmacologic doses of vitamin D may be necessary to increase calcium absorption in elderly women with vertebral fractures. *Clinical Science* 66 (1984): 103–107.

Studies indicate that a combination of the two forms of D3 may best mineralize the bone in patients with osteoporosis. Relatively lower doses of active D are required compared with inactive D, which may be toxic. The authors point out that D3 supplements may be preferable to estrogen therapy, which some physicians use to restore active $D_3$ concentrations, but more studies are needed. *Journal of Bone and Joint Surgery* 64-B:5 (1982): 542–560.

In this study of 3,000 elderly females, half were given 1,200 milligrams of calcium plus 800 international units of vitamin D, and half were given a placebo. The supplemented group had a 30-percent lower incidence of nonvertebral fractures and a 41-percent lower incidence of hip fractures compared with that of the placebo group. *Nutrition Reviews* 51 (1993): 183–185.

### Cancer Prevention

The diets of nearly 2,000 men were examined. During the subsequent 19 years, those who had the lowest intakes of calcium and vitamin D had 2.7 times the risk of colorectal cancer of those with the highest intakes. Other epidemiological studies have shown that sunlight exposure and milk intake reduce the incidence of colon cancer. The authors conclude that both calcium and vitamin D may have anticancer activity. *The Lancet* I (February 9, 1985): 307–309.

### Blood Pressure

In this study of over 300 women, younger women who consumed at least 400 international units of vitamin D per day had lower systolic blood pressure. (They also had significantly higher calcium and potassium intakes.) In older women, systolic blood pressure was significantly lower in those who consumed at least the RDAs of *both* calcium and vitamin D. The authors point out that this is the first report of a significant relationship between vitamin D and blood pressure, and that 50 to 75 percent of the women in the study had estimated vitamin D intakes of less than the RDA. *American Journal of Clinical Nutrition* 42 (July 1985): 135–142.

## Immunity

In this small study of the blood cells of adults, vitamin D was found to affect immune system function, with implications for treatment in some immunological diseases. *Life Sciences* 37 (July 8, 1985): 95–101.

Active vitamin D3 plays a role in the immune-regulatory processes. *The New England Journal of Medicine* 311:1 (1984): 47–49.

## Other Uses

The authors found that small oral doses and topical treatment of vitamin D improved symptoms of psoriasis, and that the lower the levels of vitamin D in the body, the more severe the disease. *Archives of Dermatology* 125 (1989): 231–234.

Vitamin D is the skin-derived endocrine messenger of sunlight, which attunes the body to the changing environment. The intensity and duration of light affects biological rhythms, mood, and behavior, partly through the effect of vitamin D. Vitamin D also affects adrenal hormones, the reproductive system, the digestive system, and the immune system. *Psychopharmacology* 97 (1989): 285–294.

## Intake and Requirements

Most patients with Crohn's disease have deficient levels of vitamin D. These patients are prone to osteomalacia, and should receive vitamin D supplements. *Nutritional Review* 41:7 (1983): 213–216.

Vitamin D requirements increase with age. A total supply of 600 to 800 international units from all sources (food, sunlight exposure, and vitamin D supplements) is recommended. *American Journal of Clinical Nutrition* 36 (November 1982): 1,014–1,031.

In this study, elderly individuals had significantly lower levels of vitamin D than did younger control subjects. The authors suggest that the elderly consider using a combination of moderate vitamin D supplementation and increased sunlight exposure to prevent subclinical vitamin D deficiency. *American Journal of Clinical Nutrition* 36 (1982): 1,225–1,233.

In a dietary survey of 270 healthy, highly educated elderly people of higher-than-average income, it was found that 74 percent of the women were getting less than 75 percent of the RDA for vitamin D, and 61 percent were getting less than 50 percent. Figures for men were comparable. The authors believe that low intakes of vitamin D are of particular concern to women. *American Journal of Clinical Nutrition* 36 (August 1982): 319–331.

## CHAPTER 8: VITAMIN E

## Overview

A prominent researcher discusses the clinical relevance of vitamin E and concludes that vitamin E has equivocal benefits in intermittent claudication, cutaneous ulcers, burns, wound healing, tardive dyskinesia, epilepsy, hemolytic anemia, and adult respiratory distress syndrome. Studies on its effect on platelets and LDL cholesterol oxidation support the benefits of vitamin E and cardiovascular disease. Regarding cancer, larger trials with higher doses of vitamin E are needed to determine its effect on cancer. Studies on vitamin E and immunity, especially in the elderly, are promising. *The Lancet* 345 (January 21, 1995): 170–175.

This overview of the medical uses of vitamin E discusses many aspects, including the advisability of supplementing diets high in PUFA with vitamin E; vitamin E as an effective antioxidant and protector against many toxic chemicals; the difficulty of detecting the subtle changes that may occur with vitamin E deficiency; and vitamin E and circulatory disease. *The New England Journal of Medicine* 308:18 (1983): 1,063–1,071.

This article discusses the popularity of vitamin E due to its role in preventing aging, cancer, heart disease, infertility, and chronic disease. The author estimates savings of $8 billion if Americans took vitamin E supplements. *Hippocrates* (November/December 1994): 46–53.

A prominent researcher concludes that we need at least 100 international units of vitamin E per day to counteract free radical damage to lungs from air pollution in our cities. *Annals of the New York Academy of Science* (September 30, 1992): 141-155.

Vitamin E supplementation reduced oxidative damage to platelets in smokers and nonsmokers. *American Journal of Clinical Nutrition* 60 (1994): 383–387.

## Antioxidant Powers

Vitamin E protects vitamins A and C against oxidation. It also reduces the oxidation of polyunsaturated fats and maintains the integrity of cell membranes. Corinne H. Robinson, *Normal and Therapeutic Nutrition*, 15th ed. (New York: Macmillan, 1977): 151–161.

Vitamin E is an effective antioxidant. In animals, it has provided protection against various toxic substances, including mercury, lead, benzene, and various drugs. *The New England Journal of Medicine* 308 (1983): 1,063–1,071.

In this study, animals fed heated vegetable oil showed a 38- to 97-percent decrease of vitamin E levels in their blood and tissues. *Nutrition Reports International* 32 (November 1985): 1,179–1,186.

Daily intakes of 100 milligrams of vitamin E are required to control fat oxidation in the body. Yet the RDA for vitamin E has been cut in half, from 30 international units to 15 international units, because 30 international units could not be easily obtained from a normal diet. Increasing the consumption of PUFA oils to achieve higher intakes of vitamin E would actually double the requirement of this vitamin by increasing the peroxidative potential of the tissues. The author concludes that an undesirable chronic level of cellular peroxidation is measurable—and can be ameliorated by supplementation of vitamin E. *Journal of Clinical Nutrition* 47 (June 1988): 1,088–1,089 (letter).

In this study of 100 healthy elderly people, higher levels of peroxides were found in those with lower levels of vitamins C and E. In people supplemented daily with 400 milligrams of C and/or 400 milligrams of E, peroxide levels decreased. The authors conclude that long-term supplementation of vitamins C and E can protect against free radical damage, which is thought to play a role in the aging processes and degenerative diseases. *Annals of Nutrition and Metabolism* 28 (May–June 1984): 186–191.

In a study of elderly subjects, 60 percent of the patients with dementia had below-normal blood levels of vitamin E. It has been suggested that the cell damage leading to dementia may be due to free radicals. Although vitamin E deficiency is not a likely cause of dementia, it could lower the age of onset or increase the rate of progression. *The Lancet* (April 5, 1986): 805–806.

## Cancer Prevention and Treatment

This study, conducted by the U.S. National Cancer Institute and Finland's Public Health Institute, involved 29,000 males, one group of which took supplements, including vitamin E. It was found that 50 milligrams of vitamin E per day reduced prostate cancer by 34 percent and colorectal cancer by 16 percent. However, it did not reduce lung cancer in smokers, as was hoped. *The New England Journal of Medicine* 330 (April 14, 1994): 1,029–1,035.

In this study of animal cells, the authors conclude that vitamin E can minimize genetic damage associated with carcinogenesis. *Journal of Clinical Investigation* 75 (June 1985): 1,835–1,841.

Low vitamin E intake may enhance the effect of selenium deficiency, which is associated with increased risk of fatal cancer. *British Medical Journal* 290 (February 9, 1985): 417–420.

In this animal study, rats were exposed to cigarette smoke. Of the group that was fed a diet deficient in vitamin E and selenium, 31 percent died. Of the group that was supplemented, only 8 percent died. The authors cite a previous study that showed that patients with lung cancer have lower vitamin E levels than healthy people. *Environmental Research* 34 (June 1984): 8–17.

In this study of over 5,000 women, the risk of breast cancer was found to be 5.2 times higher for women with the lowest vitamin E levels than for those with the highest levels. *British Journal of Cancer* 49 (1984): 321–324.

In a controlled study, women with low blood levels of vitamin E had a higher risk of cancer, especially epithelial cancers. *International Journal of Epidemiology* 17 (1988): 281–286.

Researchers found that the D-alpha tocopherol succinate form of vitamin E inhibits the proliferation of estrogen receptor-positive and estrogen receptor-negative human breast cancer cell lines in a dose-dependent manner *in vitro*. *Nutrition and Cancer* 19 (1993): 225–229.

The authors of this review article suggest that total fat is the most consistent dietary factor positively associated with breast cancer. PUFAs may be particularly implicated, while selenium and vitamin E are protective. *Clinical Nutrition* 4 (July–August 1985): 119–130.

The authors review the evidence relating vitamin E to breast cancer. Studies have shown that vitamin E reduces the incidence of cancer due to carcinogens. It also enhances the therapeutic effect of radiation treatment of cancer. One epidemiological study found that the group of women with the lowest blood serum vitamin E levels had five times the risk of cancer. *Journal of the American College of Nutrition* 4 (September–October 1985): 559–564.

Vitamin E was found to reduce the free-radical damage in experimental animals given anticancer chemotherapy. The authors conclude that this provides strong evidence for the protective use of vitamin E in cancer-free animals. They further suggest that its use during anticancer therapy is theoretically advisable because it may reduce the toxicity of some drugs, without reducing the drugs' effectiveness. The authors cite several other studies that report the benefits of large doses of vitamin E and other antioxidant vitamins to cancer patients. *Anticancer Research* 3 (1983): 59–62.

The antioxidants alpha-tocopherol and coenzyme Q inhibited lipid peroxidation due to the chemotherapy drug Adriamycin, but did not interfere with suppression of DNA synthesis in cancer cells. *Journal of Nutrition, Science, and Vitaminology* 31 (March–April 1985): 129–137.

In this study of over 400 males, vitamin E levels in the blood were lower in the group that developed lung and colorectal cancers than in the group that did not. *Journal of the National Cancer Institute* 73 (December 1984): 1,463–1,468.

## Cardiovascular Disease

This entire book is devoted to vitamin E. It discusses, among other studies, those which have suggested that vitamin E might prevent deposition and accumulation of cholesterol in the arterial wall. Several other studies have suggested that vitamin E plays an important role in both lipid synthesis and degradation in the arterial wall. Results from these studies may explain the accumulation of lipids in atherosclerotic lesions. Further experiments are still in progress. *Vitamin E: Biochemical, Hematological, and Clinical Aspects.* New York: Annals of the New York Academy of Sciences, vol. 393 (1982).

Rats that were fed a mixture of heated vegetable oils had enhanced platelet aggregation, when compared with rats fed unheated oils. The vitamin E in these oils, which were rich in polyunsaturated fats, was depleted 91 percent by the heat treatment. The consumption of diets rich in PUFA is generally recommended for the prevention of cardiovascular diseases. However, the use of these fats for cooking may ironically result in enhanced platelet aggregability. Provision of extra vitamin E may minimize this effect. *Lipids* 20 (July 1985): 439–448.

A significant decrease in the adhesiveness of platelets was noted after 2 weeks of supplementation with 400 international units of vitamin E. *Research* 49 (1988): 393–404.

Two landmark studies suggested that vitamin E supplementation reduces the rate of heart disease in women and men by 40 percent. Data from these two studies—the Nurses' Health Study and the Physicians' Health Study—were published in *The New England Journal of Medicine* 328 (May 20, 1993), 1,444–1,456 and 1,487–1,489.

Another landmark study, from the Center of Human Nutrition of the University of Texas Southwestern Medical Center, found that only groups of subjects who received at least 400 international units per day of vitamin E experienced a decrease of the susceptibility of LDL cholesterol to oxidation from free radicals. *Arteriosclerosis, Thrombosis and Vascular Biology.* 15 (1995): 190–198.

This article reviewed literature with respect to beta-carotene and vitamin E supplementation in men who smoke or consume alcohol. In one study of 40,000 men, those taking at least 100 international units of vitamin E per day for two or more years had a 40-percent reduction in the risk of coronary heart disease compared with men not taking supplements. *Nutrition Report* 11 (1993): 73, 80.

These letters to the editors argue that it is not premature to recommend vitamin E supplementation for the prevention of coronary artery disease, and that the reasons for withholding vitamin E therapy are not convincing. A substantial amount of physicians in the United States are taking vitamin E supplements themselves. The authors question, "If vitamin E is good enough for physicians, why is it not good enough for their patients?" *The New England Journal of Medicine* (November 4, 1993): 1,424.

In this study by prominent researcher Dr. Jialal, subjects were given 800 international units of vitamin E, 1,000 milligrams of C, and 30 milligrams of beta-carotene per day, and experienced a 40-percent decrease in the oxidation rate of blood lipids. A group that received 800 international units of vitamin E alone experienced similar results, leading the researchers to conclude that combining the three antioxidants was no better than using vitamin E alone. However, it should be noted that the amounts of the other two antioxidants may have been too low to exert any noticeable effect. *Circulation* 88 (December 1993): 2,780–2,786. See also *Journal of the American College of Nutrition* 12 (1993): 631–637.

## Wound Healing

The authors note that daily doses of 800 to 2,000 international units of vitamin E are recommended by some physicians to prevent postoperative problems in women who have undergone breast augmentation. *Plastic and Reconstructive Surgery* 69 (June 1982): 1,029–1,030.

## The Immune System

Rats were fed a purified diet containing 0, 7.5, 15, 50, 200, or 1,000 milligrams of DL-alpha tocopherol acetate per kilogram of feed. The higher the dosage of vitamin E, the better the immune response, suggesting that the vitamin E requirement for optimal immune responsiveness is higher than that for other commonly used indicators of vitamin E adequacy. *Journal of Nutrition* 116 (April 1986): 675–681.

The evidence seems clear that excesses of vitamin E have an often beneficial effect on resistance to disease in a variety of experimental animals. *American Journal of Clinical Nutrition* (Supplement) 35: 431–433.

In this study, 5 discoid lupus erythematosus patients given 800 to 2,000 international units of vitamin E daily made an excellent recovery, with no side effects. This disease is normally treated with thalidomide and immunosuppressants, which have considerable side effects. The author concludes that treatment of autoimmune diseases such as DLE with vitamin E would seem preferable to the use of potentially hazardous drugs. *British Journal of Dermatology* III (July 1984): 125–126 (letter).

Patients receiving 900 to 1,600 international units of vitamin E per day showed complete or almost complete clearing of lupus symptoms. Lower dosages of 300 international units had no benefit. *Cutis* 21 (1978): 321–325.

In this study, 7 rheumatoid arthritis patients who no longer responded to conventional therapy alone were also given 400 international units of vitamin E and 350 micrograms of selenium. In 4 of these patients, joint pain disappeared; in the remaining 3, pain lessened and joint mobility markedly increased. *Biological Trace Element Research* 7 (May–June 1985): 195–198.

## Neurological Disorders

Based on evidence from patients with disorders of fat metabolism leading to severe vitamin E deficiency, it is suggested that vitamin E is important for normal neurological function in humans. *The Lancet* (January 29, 1983): 225–228.

Children with vitamin E deficiency, often due to fat malabsorption, had neurological disorders that responded to vitamin E therapy. *Canadian Journal of Neurological Science* 11 (November 1984): 561–564.

Supplementation with large doses of vitamin E over a long period of time can stabilize neurological dysfunction and degeneration in older patients, and may prevent the development of neurological symptoms in young patients. Evidence suggests that vitamin E and other antioxidants may help retard the degeneration of the nerves that occurs in Parkinson's disease. *Free Radical Biology and Medicine* 6 (1989): 189–207.

## Women's Health

### Fibrocystic Breast Disease

In a study of 26 with breast disease and 8 controls, 85 percent (22 women) of those who received daily supplementation of 600 international units of vitamin E for 8 weeks responded to the treatment. In 10 women, there was a total disappearance of cystic lesions and breast tenderness, and in 12 women, lesions decreased in number and size. The authors suggest that vitamin E supplementation may be an inexpensive and safe way of treating this disorder. *Nutrition Research* 2 (1982): 243–247.

### Premenstrual Syndrome

Vitamin E has been reported to improve many symptoms of PMS. *Journal of the American College of Nutrition* 3 (1984): 351–356.

### Intrauterine Device Bleeding

The authors administered 100 milligrams of vitamin E every other day to 51 women who suffered excessive menstrual bleeding after insertion of an IUD. In almost every subject, blood loss was reduced to normal. *International Journal of Fertility* 28 (1983): 55–56.

## Oral Contraceptives

In this study, 200 milligrams of vitamin E were given to women taking oral contraceptives. The supplement reduced the tendency of blood platelets to aggregate excessively. *Contraception* 36 (September 1987): 347–358.

## Smoking

This study found that although the levels of vitamin E in the blood of smokers and nonsmokers were similar, smokers had significantly lower levels in the cells of their lungs. Smoking seems to produce oxidant lung injury, which may play a role in the development of emphysema. Since vitamin E is an antioxidant, the authors suggest a possible role for vitamin E in the lungs' defense against cigarette smoke. *Journal of Clinical Investigation* 77 (March 1986): 789–796.

# Other Uses

## Diabetes

In a study of 30 elderly patients with angina, daily supplementation with 900 international units of vitamin E for 4 months lowered fasting plasma insulin concentrations and triglycerides. The researchers conclude that high doses of vitamin E might be useful therapy for elderly insulin-resistant patients with coronary heart disease. *American Journal of Clinical Nutrition* 61 (1995): 848–852. A previous study with similar results was published by the same author in *American Journal of Clinical Nutrition* 57 (May 1993): 650–656.

## Cataracts

In comparing vitamin E effects on cataract prevention, there was a 56-percent decrease in cataract risk in subjects who took vitamin E supplements compared with those who didn't take supplements. *American Journal of Clinical Nutrition* (1991 Supplement) 53: 346S–351S.

## Hemodialysis-Related Anemia

Anemia is a major problem in kidney patients being treated with dialysis. In this controlled study, daily vitamin E supplementation of 600 milligrams brought about significant increases in the red blood cell count and other blood factors associated with reduction of anemia. *Nephron* 40 (August 1985): 440–445.

## Kidney Disease

In this study, 16 children with hemolytic uremic syndrome were treated with vitamin E. Of these, 94 percent recovered completely, compared with 36 to 50 percent of patients previously treated with other therapies. *Archives of Disorders in Children* 59 (May 1984): 401–404.

## Exercise and Muscle Damage

In this double-blind study, subjects who took 800 international units of vitamin E exercised at 75 percent of their maximum heart rate for 45 minutes. When they were compared with those who took a placebo, the supplemented subjects experienced less oxidative stress to their tissues after the exercise. The authors conclude that vitamin E may provide protection against oxidative injury after exercise. *The Nutrition Report* 264 (1993): R992–R998.

In this study, researchers from the USDA supplemented 21 men with either 800 international units of vitamin E or a placebo daily for 7 weeks. Vitamin E reduced exercise-induced oxidative damage in both young and old subjects. The researchers discovered that vitamin E blunted the immune signals that trigger inflammation. *Food Chemical News* 34 (September 28, 1992): 52.

## Toxicity and Absorbability

In a review of the literature, the authors found that vitamin E is not mutagenic, carcinogenic, or teratogenic. Very few side effects have been reported in humans even at doses of 3,200 milligrams per day. Side effects have been uncommon in other large trials. The adverse reaction reports have been mostly individual case reports or uncontrolled studies. *American Journal of Clinical Nutrition* 48 (September 1988): 612–619.

Natural vitamin E has been found to be more bioavailable than synthetic forms. *American Journal of Clinical Nutrition* 60 (1994): 397–402.

# CHAPTER 9: VITAMIN K

## Osteoporosis

Blood levels of vitamin K in patients with osteoporosis were approximately one third the levels of those in an apparently healthy control group. The authors concluded that low levels of the vitamin may be a factor in the development of osteoporosis. *Journal of Clinical Endocrinology and Metabolism* 60 (June 1985): 1,268–1,269.

## Behavior

Vitamin K-deficient animals became less active and suffered from general malaise. These results suggest that vitamin K deficiency may contribute to physical and psychiatric symptoms. *Physiology and Behavior* 34 (May 1985): 727–734.

## Cancer

Anticoagulant drugs have been demonstrated to reduce metastasis and improve survival in cancer patients. Since vitamin K is involved in coagulation, one would think it is contraindicated in cancer patients. However, vitamin K has unique antineoplastic properties alone, and also augments patient survival when used in conjunction with radiation therapy. Paradoxically, vitamin K also increases the antimetastatic capacity of anticoagulant therapy. *Adjuvant Nutrition in Cancer Treatment*, 1992 Symposium Proceedings, eds. Patrick Quillin, Ph.D., R.D., R. Michael Williams, M.D., Ph.D. (Arlington Heights, IL: Cancer Treatment Foundation, 1992).

# CHAPTER 10: VITAMIN B COMPLEX

## The Elderly

$B_{12}$ deficiencies in the elderly can result in neuropsychiatric disorders such as depression, personality changes, mood swings, cognitive impairment, memory loss, gait abnormalities, orthostatic hypotension, and optic and peripheral neuropathies. Folic acid deficiency may result in reduced DNA formation, failure of cell proliferation, demyelinization, and degeneration of the central nervous system. Hyperhomocysteinemia is more prevalent in the elderly due to subclinical deficiencies of $B_6$, $B_{12}$, and folic acid, and is a risk factor for heart attack. Hyperhomocysteinemia is treatable with these vitamins. Considering the high cost of treatment in a long-term care facility, the authors suggest it is both efficient and cost effective to assess the levels of these vitamins periodically. *Clinical Laboratory Sciences* 6 (September/October 1993): 272–274.

In a randomized, placebo-controlled, double-blind study, 14 geriatric patients suffering from depression were given antidepressant treatment with 10 milligrams each of $B_1$, $B_2$, and $B_6$. Within 4 weeks, supplemented patients demonstrated improved B-vitamin status and improved scores on ratings of depression and cognitive function, compared with the placebo group. The levels of B vitamins used in this study were 5 to 8 times the RDA. *Journal of the American College of Nutrition* 11 (1992): 159–163.

## HIV Infection

In a study of 296 HIV-infected men, those who took a multivitamin supplement were one-third less likely to develop full-blown AIDS, compared with those who did not take supplements. Those who had higher-than-average intakes of vitamins A, $B_1$, $B_2$, or niacin had higher CD4 counts. *Medical Tribune* (March 24, 1994): 18.

## CHAPTER 11: VITAMIN $B_1$ (Thiamin)

### Surgery

Elderly patients experienced a significant lowering of thiamin levels in the blood after surgery. The authors suggested that thiamin deficiency may be one factor in postoperative mental confusion and overall deterioration in this population, and that more attention should be paid to assessing their thiamin status. *Age and Aging* 11 (1982): 101–107.

### Thiamin Intake and Absorption

Although the classic signs of beriberi were absent, 28 percent of study subjects had low thiamin levels. This subclinical condition may not be a vitamin deficiency disease per se, but rather may be due to a high calorie intake that overtaxes the oxidative metabolism. High calorie diets with disproportionately low intakes of vitamins and minerals may be the source of widespread marginal malnutrition that is not being sufficiently recognized by physicians. *Journal of the American College of Nutrition* 7 (1988): 61–67.

Severe disease increasingly interferes with the dietary intake of thiamin, and alcoholism interferes with the absorption of thiamin in a major fashion. *American Journal of Clinical Nutrition* 36 (November 1982): 1,067–1,082.

### Immunity

In this study, thiamin-deficient experimental animals showed less response to immunization vaccinations. *Proceedings of the Society of Experimental Biology and Medicine* 77 (1951): 526–530.

### Psychiatric Disease

In a study of psychiatric patients, schizophrenics, and alcoholics, as a group, these subjects were significantly overrepresented in low-thiamin patients. *British Journal of Psychiatry* 141 (1982): 271.

A survey of 172 unselected psychiatric patients showed 30 percent to be biochemically deficient in thiamin, although only 1 of these had clinical symptoms of deficiency. An inadequate intake of vitamins, particularly B₁, can result in mental illness. *Clinical Neuro-pharmacology* 8 (July–September 1985): 286–293.

## Cancer

The authors speculate that thiamin supplementation (in this study, 100 milligrams per day) could help prevent cell damage, fibrinogenesis, and collagen breakdown in cancer patients. *Journal of Nutrition, Growth and Cancer* 1 (July–December 1984): 207–210.

## Toxicity

Toxicity of thiamin was seen only in cases in which doses were thousands of times larger than normal. There have been no toxic effects of thiamin administered by mouth reported in humans. Robert S. Goodhart and Maurice E. Shils, *Modern Nutrition in Health and Disease*, 6th ed. (Philadelphia: Lea and Febiger, 1980).

## CHAPTER 12: VITAMIN B₂ (Riboflavin)

### Sickle Cell Anemia

This study of sickle cell anemia patients suggested that nearly half were deficient in vitamin B₂. *American Journal of Clinical Nutrition* 38 (December 1983): 884–887.

### Anemia

Riboflavin administered with iron enhanced recovery from microcytic anemia in men and children. *Human Nutrition. Clinical Nutrition* 37C (1983): 413–425.

### The Immune System

Riboflavin deficiency in animals results in a diminished ability to produce antibodies in response to test antigens. *American Journal of Clinical Nutrition* (Supplement) 35 (February 1982): 421.

### Esophageal Cancer

In this animal study, nearly half the subjects fed a riboflavin-free diet developed precancerous or cancerous tumors of the esophagus. The authors concluded that riboflavin helps to maintain the lining of the mouth and esophagus, and that its deficiency may increase the susceptibility of these tissues to carcinogens. *Journal of the National Cancer Institute* 72 (April 1984): 941–948.

### Cataracts

A study of laboratory rats showed that a diet deficient in vitamin B₂ causes cataracts within 2 to 3 months. Other changes in the eye also occurred. *American Journal of Ophthalmology* 14 (1931): 1,005–1,009.

Riboflavin deficiency has been linked to cataract formation in some studies. Low riboflavin intake or impaired riboflavin utilization could lead to an increase in cataract formation. *American Journal of Clinical Nutrition* 34 (May 1981): 861–863.

In an experiment with rats, the results indicated that vitamin B₁₂ is fairly active in maintaining transparency of the lens of the eye. *International Journal for Vitamin and Nutrition Research* 53 (1983): 243–250.

## Nervous Symptoms

In a study of psychiatric patients, 53 percent were deficient in at least one of these vitamins: thiamin, riboflavin, and vitamin $B_6$. The authors concluded that a deficiency in one or several of these nutrients has a primary role in the cause of emotional disorder. *British Journal of Psychiatry* 141 (1982): 271–272.

## Carpal Tunnel Syndrome

A man with carpal tunnel syndrome was given 50 milligrams of riboflavin and 500 milligrams of pyridoxine ($B_6$) daily for a total of eight months. All of his CTS symptoms disappeared. *Proceedings of the National Academy of Science* 81 (November 1984): 7,076–7,078.

## Exercise

Riboflavin plays a role in energy production. The daily allowance for riboflavin is proportional to energy needs. Regular exercise has been shown to increase the daily needs of riboflavin. Mild deficiencies have been shown in athletes undergoing strenuous daily exercise. *Nutrition Research* 4 (1984): 201–208.

Weight-reducing women require more than the RDA of riboflavin during both periods of nonexercise and periods of exercise. *American Journal of Clinical Nutrition* 41 (February 1985): 270–277.

## Oral Contraceptives

In this study, riboflavin deficiency was found to be more prevalent in women taking oral contraceptives than in women who were not. *American Journal of Clinical Nutrition* 35 (March 1982): 495–501.

## Detecting and Alleviating Deficiencies

In an Indian study, 4 milligrams of riboflavin (the RDA) failed to correct deficiencies in half the subjects. *Nutrition Research* 2 (1982): 147–153.

The authors studied 42 adolescent boys with no clinical symptoms of riboflavin deficiency. Biochemical testing showed that 38 percent were deficient in this nutrient. *American Journal of Clinical Nutrition* 39 (May 1984): 787–791.

## CHAPTER 13: VITAMIN B₃ (Niacin and Niacinamide)

### Cardiovascular Disease

Both cholesterol and triglycerides may be lowered by 50 percent or more by niacin therapy. The authors believe that niacin is the agent of choice in many patients with hyperlipidemia. *Drug Therapy* (August 1984): 62–70.

Niacin was given in a time-release or unmodified form to patients with elevated triglyceride and/or LDL cholesterol levels. The unmodified form was a more effective therapy and resulted in fewer side effects than did the time-release niacin. Triglycerides were decreased by 42 percent (versus 1 percent), and LDL cholesterol was increased by 22 percent (versus 9 percent). *Metabolism* 34 (July 1985): 642–650.

When niacin (3 grams per day) and clofibrate were compared, niacin was found to be from 28 to 48 percent more effective in lowering cholesterol and triglycerides in the blood. Niacin also created a more desirable HDL/LDL ratio. *Atherosclerosis* 51 (1984): 251–259.

A previously untreated diabetic was treated with insulin and diet. His triglyceride level dropped from 258 to 158. This was sharply reduced further when niacin therapy was added. Other studies have shown that triglyceride levels can be lowered by more than 60 percent by nicotinic acid. *Postgraduate Medicine Journal* 57 (August 1981): 511–515.

When subjects were given 100 milligrams per deciliter of niacin and 200 milligrams per deciliter of chromium for 4 weeks, it significantly lowered their serum cholesterol. Supplementation for 4 months resulted in a further decrease in serum cholesterol. *Journal of Family Practice* 27 (December 1988): 603–606.

## Epilepsy

The authors discuss their study and previous studies, which show that nicotinamide—as well as vitamins E and B$_6$ and calcium pantothenate—may be useful in the treatment of epilepsy when used with anticonvulsants. They suggest that such combined treatment not only would give an anticonvulsant effect, but could also improve the nutrition and structural metabolism of the brain, a matter of great importance. *Byolleten Eksperimental noi Biologii i Meditsiny* 94 (9): 61–64.

## Cancer

In this animal study, only 14 percent of the subjects that were given niacinamide along with a potent carcinogen developed pancreatic cancer, as compared with 43 percent of those that were given the carcinogen alone. The authors concluded from this and previous research that niacinamide inhibits cancer at several sites, and that since niacin has low toxicity, it may be useful in cancer prevention. *Journal of the National Cancer Institute* 73 (September 1984): 767–770.

In mice with laboratory-induced breast cancer, the effectiveness of radiation therapy with or without the administration of niacin was assessed. The average size of the tumor in mice given niacinamide with radiation was decreased by 86 percent 2 weeks after treatment, and remained 79 percent lower after 4 weeks. The authors suggest that niacin sensitizes tissues to the effects of radiation and may have a role in the treatment of malignant tumors. *Cancer Research* 45 (August 1985): 3,609–3,614.

## Supplements

In this study, 120 patients with severe intermittent claudication received either 2,000 milligrams of IHN or a placebo. After 3 months, the IHN group had significantly larger changes in claudication times and in number of free-walking paces compared with the placebo group. In the whole patient population, IHN gave improvements in subjective and functional assessments of intermittent claudication that were statistically significantly greater than the placebo. The improvement was particularly marked in smokers. *British Journal of Clinical Practice* 42 (1988): 377–383.

In this study, 15 patients with Raynaud's disease were given 1 gram of IHN 4 times each day for 9 months. At the end of the trial, the Reactive Thermal Gradient was found to be significantly improved when compared with baseline values. Subjective ratings of cold, numbness, and pain significantly improved. General tolerance to IHN at this dosage was good; no side effects or adverse reactions were found. *Journal of International Medical Research* 9 (1981): 393–400.

## Toxicity

This article reviews four cases of niacin-induced hepatotoxicity. All patients were using sustained-release niacin preparations in a dose of at least 2.6 grams per day. *Southern Medical Journal* 30 (January 1994): 30–32.

## CHAPTER 14: VITAMIN B6 (Pyridoxine)

### Overview

A deficiency in vitamin B6 results in skin and nervous system disorders, kidney disorders, depression of immune responses, anemia, and carpal tunnel syndrome. Studies have shown deficiencies of and/or an increased need for B6 in oral contraceptive users and alcoholics; during certain situations such as exposure to radiation; and from certain drugs, cardiac failure, pregnancy, and lactation. American Journal of Medical Technology 49:1 (1983): 17–21.

### Emotional Illness

Of the psychiatric patients admitted to the hospital in this study, 53 percent were deficient in at least one of the following: B6, thiamin, or riboflavin. B6 is associated with depression and other emotional disorders, and the authors suggest that along with riboflavin, B6 deficiency has a primary role in the cause of emotional disorder. British Journal of Psychiatry 141 (1982): 271–272.

The authors conclude that the current data suggests that as much as 20 percent of a medically cleared population of outpatient depressives may suffer from a B6 deficit. They point out that nutrition, diet, and vitamin levels have received very little attention in the psychiatric literature, and implicate reducing diets as playing a possible role in depression. *Biological Psychiatry* 9:4 (1984): 613–616.

In this study of 11 psychiatric patients, 57 to 100 percent of the depressed patients and 25 to 50 percent of the obsessive-compulsive patients had inadequate levels of B6. The authors ask, "Does depressive illness cause vitamin B6 inadequacy, or vice-versa?" *Nutrition Reports International* 27 (April 1983): 867–873.

The authors describe how 500 milligrams of B6 were effective in treating an acutely schizophrenic patient who did not respond to other psychotropic medications. They recommend that B6 be considered as an alternative treatment for this disorder. *Biological Psychiatry* 18:11 (1983): 1,321–1,328.

### Carpal Tunnel Syndrome

A patient with carpal tunnel syndrome (CTS) who was given 500 milligrams of B6 and 50 milligrams of riboflavin supplements experienced complete disappearance of his symptoms. *Proceedings of the National Academy of Sciences* 81 (November 1984): 7,076–7,078.

In this small study, 4 out of 6 CTS patients claimed some partial relief after B6 supplementation. The authors note that a number of recent studies report that patients with CTS respond to pyridoxine treatment, but that a large double-blind controlled study is necessary to fully test the efficacy of this treatment. *Annals of Neurology* 15 (January 1984): 104–107.

### Childhood Epilepsy and Autism

Pyridoxine-dependent seizures (PDS) in infants, which should be suspected in every infant with convulsions before 18 months of age, were controlled by administration of B6. Failure to treat PDS with B6 promptly results in severe mental retardation or death. *Annals of Neurology* 17 (February 1985): 117–120.

Many forms of infant and childhood epilepsy respond to B6 treatment. All infants with refractory epileptic seizure must be given an adequate trial of B6. *Archives of Disease in Childhood* 58 (1983): 1,034–1,036 (letter).

The effects of vitamin B6 and magnesium supplementation on 60 autistic children were examined in a double-blind trial. The combination resulted in a significant improvement in many aspects of autistic behavior. *Biological Psychiatry* 20 (May 1985): 467–478.

## Premenstrual Syndrome

The researchers report overwhelming evidence in both their study and others that 100 milligrams per day of B6 appears to have a 60 to 80 percent success rate in the treatment of PMS. B6 has been effective in cases in which progesterone has failed. Owing to the low toxicity of B6, it is the authors' opinion that it should be tried as the first line of treatment in PMS. *The Practitioner* 228 (April 1984): 425–427.

## Pregnancy and Breastfeeding

During the last month of their pregnancy, the women in this study were shown to have consumed an average of only 50 percent of the RDA for B6. For breastfeeding women, intake rose after delivery, but only to 60 percent of the RDA. *Journal of the American Dietetic Association* 84 (November 1984): 1,339–1,344.

In a study of 24 mothers and their infants, only those who received supplements of 10 to 20 milligrams of B6 daily produced milk that met the American Academy of Pediatrics recommended concentration of B6. *American Journal of Clinical Nutrition* 41 (January 1985): 21–31.

In this double-blind trial, 52 pregnant women were given pyridoxine supplements. Those who received 7.5 to 20 milligrams per day delivered babies whose Apgar scores were significantly higher than those of infants of mothers who received only 2.6 milligrams. *Journal of Nutrition* 114 (May 1984): 977–988.

## Cardiovascular Disease

Based on the results of this controlled study of men with heart disease, the authors conclude that vitamin B6 deficiency may influence vascular connective tissue and thrombogenesis (clotting). *Atherosclerosis* 55 (June 1985): 357–361.

Experiments giving animals diets deficient in vitamin B6 have resulted in an enhanced risk of cardiovascular disease in the subjects. Other experiments suggest the same may be true for humans. The authors also point out that exposure to environmental pollution causes vitamin B6 deficiency. *Medical Hypotheses* 15 (December 1984): 361–367.

Patients with acute heart attacks had lower levels of PLP, an active metabolite of B6, than did controls. The authors suggest that low levels of B6 may increase the risk of heart attack. *American Journal of Cardiology* 63 (1989): 513–516.

## Asthma

In this study, 15 adult asthmatics had significantly lower pyridoxine levels than did 16 healthy controls. Those subjects who took 50 milligrams of B6 daily reported a dramatic decrease in the frequency and severity of wheezing or asthmatic attacks while taking the supplement. *American Journal of Clinical Nutrition* 41 (1985): 684–688.

## Sickle Cell Anemia

In this study, 16 patients with sickle cell anemia had pyridoxine levels significantly lower than those of 16 healthy controls. B6 has been shown to have anti-sickling properties, and these studies suggest that pyridoxine supplementation may have therapeutic benefits. *American Journal of Clinical Nutrition* 40 (August 1984): 235–239.

## Diabetes

According to the author of this letter, one quarter of adult diabetic patients have below-normal levels of pyridoxine. Diabetics may not metabolize $B_6$ normally and may need more than the RDA. Further research seems to be indicated. *American Journal of Clinical Nutrition* 39 (May 1984): 841–842.

## Chinese Restaurant Syndrome

This study shows that the symptoms of Chinese Restaurant Syndrome caused by monosodium glutamate sensitivity fail to recur after treatment with 50 to 200 milligrams of pyridoxine. *Hoppe-Seyler's Zeitschrift fur Physiologishe Chemie* 365:3 (1984): 405–414.

## Kidney Disease

In a study of humans with kidney disease, the average level of $B_6$ in the blood was significantly lower than that in the controls. The authors conclude that the development of immune dysfunction and cardiovascular disease in patients with kidney disease may be related to $B_6$ deficiency. *International Journal of Vitamin Research* 54 (October–December 1984): 313–319.

In this study, the administration of 25 to 200 milligrams of $B_6$ daily led to decreased oxalate secretion in patients with a form of hereditary kidney disorder. (Excess oxalate may lead to calcium deposits in the kidney, which may in turn lead to kidney failure and death.) *The New England Journal of Medicine* 312 (April 11, 1985): 953–957.

In a group of 22 patients with oxalate kidney stones, a dose of 250 to 500 milligrams of $B_6$ was found to be an effective treatment. *Canadian Medical Association Journal* 131 (July 1984): 14.

Based on his experience with a patient to whom he gave 500 milligrams of pyridoxine a day for 17 months, the author of this letter suggests that pyridoxine therapy can reverse the course of renal failure in certain infants. *The New England Journal of Medicine* 311 (September 20, 1984): 798–799.

## Melanoma

In animal experiments, topical injections of $B_6$ retarded the growth of malignant melanoma. In one study, the tumors of the treated mice weighed 62 percent less than those in untreated controls. In another, tumor growth was inhibited by 39 percent. *Nutrition and Cancer* 7 (January–June 1985): 43–52.

## The Immune System

In this overview, the authors point out that pyridoxine deficiencies cause more profound effects on immune system function than do deficiencies of any other B vitamin. Both human and animal studies have shown $B_6$ to be involved in a wide variety of organs and processes of the immune system. *American Journal of Clinical Nutrition* (Supplement) 35 (February 1982): 418–421.

In laboratory animals, vitamin $B_6$ deficiency impaired the immune response and increased the animals' susceptibility to a cancer-causing virus. *Journal of Nutrition* 114 (May 1984): 938–945.

In a study of humans who were undergoing hemodialysis, B6 levels were low and the immune system was impaired in over half the subjects. After the subjects were given B6 supplements, their immune systems were improved. *Nephron* 38 (September 1984): 9–16.

## Bioavailability

The authors studied the bioavailability of B6 from several foods and found that the amount of B6 in foods does not necessarily represent the amount of the vitamin available to humans. In fact, the bioavailability of B6 from natural sources is limited. *Journal of Nutrition* 113 (1983): 2,412–2,420.

## Toxicity

The authors report 7 cases of neurotoxicity resulting from massive intakes (2 to 6 grams per day) of B6. Symptoms of toxicity include unsteady gait, numb feet, and numbness and clumsiness of the hands. In most of the cases, B6 was the only nutritional supplement used by the patient. All patients improved substantially following withdrawal of B6. *The New England Journal of Medicine* (August 25, 1983): 445–448.

In this study, a group of 22 patients received doses of 250 to 500 milligrams of pyridoxine with no ill effects, and the authors concluded that these amounts are safe for long periods (up to 6 years). *Canadian Medical Association Journal* 131 (July 1984): 14.

There are many reports stressing the absence of toxic side effects of vitamin B6 at doses up to 500 milligrams. In the strictly scientific sense, no causal relationship between pyridoxine and neuropathy has been demonstrated. It would appear that long-term administration of up to 200 milligrams daily may still be considered safe. *International Journal for Vitamin and Nutrition Research* 58 (1988): 105–118.

## CHAPTER 15: VITAMIN B12 (Cobalamin)

### Subclinical Anemia

Even slightly decreased B12 levels are often important even though the classic hematological hallmarks may be absent. Of patients with pernicious anemia, only 64 percent had very low B12 levels, suggesting the need to pay close attention to all low B12 levels. *Archives of Internal Medicine* 148 (August 1988): 1,712–1,714.

### The Nervous System

The authors of this review recommend that the patient who fails to respond to treatment of any psychiatric symptom complex should be evaluated for B12 deficiency. *Biological Psychiatry* 16 (1981): 197–205.

Patients who do not have severe anemia may develop neurologic abnormalities before the underlying vitamin B12 deficiency is recognized. *Annals of Family Practice* 25 (January 1982): 111–115.

In one study, over 73 percent of elderly patients with organic psychiatric disorders had low blood levels of B12. Similar statistics have been noted in other studies. B12 deficiency has been shown to be significantly more frequent in patients with Alzheimer-type dementia than in others. The authors point out that the clarification of this observation may provide an important clue in our understanding of this disease, since prolonged low B12 levels may produce permanent neurological changes. *Age and Aging* 13 (1984): 101–105.

Vitamin B12 and folate levels were analyzed in patients with major depression and psychotic depression. The authors confirm previous findings that low B12 is associated with mental disturbance. Low $B_{12}$ levels may predispose the development of psychotic symptoms during a depressive episode. *British Journal of Psychiatry* 153 (August 1988): 266–267.

## Cancer Prevention

In this animal study, mice were implanted with tumor cells. Only 2 of the 50 that received $B_{12}$ and ascorbic acid developed tumors, while all 50 of the untreated mice developed tumors. Vitamin $B_{12}$ and vitamin C given separately in the same doses did not have the same effect. *IRCS Medical Science* 12 (September 1984): 813.

Smokers—especially smokers with precancerous changes in the bronchial tissues—were found to have low circulating levels of $B_{12}$ and folate. Supplementation decreased the number of patients with atypical cells, suggesting that this may be an effective form of early intervention. *Journal of the American Medical Association* 259 (March 11, 1988): 1,525–1,530.

## Nitrous Oxide

Prolonged excess exposure to nitrous oxide may result in $B_{12}$ anemia. *Journal of Clinical Pathology* 33 (1980): 909–916.

## Fatigue

In a double-blind study, 28 patients complaining of fatigue were given injections of $B_{12}$ or a placebo for 4 weeks. The group that received the placebo for the first 2 weeks and then $B_{12}$ for the next two weeks showed a favorable response with respect to general well-being and happiness only when given the $B_{12}$. The group that received the $B_{12}$ for the first 2 weeks and the placebo for the next 2 weeks did not notice any difference between the active and placebo treatments. This suggests that the effects of $B_{12}$ may persist for a period of at least 4 weeks. *Journal of Nutrition* 30 (1973): 277–279.

## CHAPTER 16: FOLIC ACID

### Cervical Dysplasia and Cancer

Oral contraceptives may cause localized rather than systemic folate deficiency, which could alter the susceptibility of cervical cells to cancer-causing substances. In this controlled study of oral contraceptive users with mild to moderate cervical dysplasia, those women supplemented with 10 milligrams of folic acid daily showed significant improvement over those who were unsupplemented. The authors concluded that localized changes in folate metabolism may be misdiagnosed as cervical dysplasia, or that these changes are an integral part of the condition and that dysplasia may be arrested or reversed with folic acid supplementation. *American Journal of Clinical Nutrition* 35 (1982): 73–82.

The author cites studies that suggest that folic acid supplementation may help reduce the risk of cervical cancer in women taking combination oral contraceptives. One study involved 89 women with mild to moderate cervical neoplasia who had been taking combination oral contraceptives for 6 months or longer. This double-blind random study concluded that folate (10 milligrams per day for 3 months) had a substantial beneficial effect on cervical epithelium. There was no change among the women in the placebo group. *Journal of the American Medical Association* 244:7 (1980): 633–634.

Oral contraceptives impair folate metabolism. In this study, the mean blood level of folate in women using the pill decreased, and it required up to 3 months for them to return to normal after the pill was stopped. *CMA Journal* 126 (February 1, 1982): 244–247.

## Pregnancy and Birth Defects

Mothers of children born with harelip received 10 milligrams of folic acid plus a multivitamin daily prior to or during the first trimester of their subsequent pregnancies. Only 1 of the supplemented mothers gave birth to another child with harelip; 15 of the unsupplemented group had children with this birth defect. The authors state that the results are highly suggestive that moderate supplementation may reduce the rate of recurrence of some birth defects. *The Lancet* (July 24, 1982): 217.

Pregnant guinea pigs were fed either an RDA-sufficient diet alone or one with folic acid and vitamin C supplements. In the unsupplemented group, 68.8 percent of the fetuses did not survive to midpregnancy, compared with 17.5 percent of the supplemented group. The authors conclude that during early pregnancy, intakes of these 2 nutrients well above the RDA may be needed for optimal reproductive performance in humans. *British Journal of Nutrition* 55 (January–February 1986): 23–35.

In a randomized controlled trial, 2,104 women who received multivitamin supplementation with trace minerals were compared with 2,052 women who received trace element supplements only. The multivitamin supplement contained 12 nutrients, including .8 milligram of folic acid, 4 minerals, and 3 trace elements. The trace element supplement contained copper, manganese, zinc, and low-dose vitamin C. The group that received the multivitamin plus trace element supplements had a significant decrease in the incidence of infants born with neural tube defects. *The New England Journal of Medicine* 327 (December 24, 1992): 1,832–1,835.

This is an editorial responding to the study cited above. The author notes that vitamin supplements containing both a multivitamin and trace elements supplement were used, so that one cannot be sure that the preventive effect was due to folic acid alone or an association with other nutrients. *The New England Journal of Medicine* 327 (December 24, 1992): 1,875–1,877.

This Irish study of more than 56,000 pregnant women demonstrated that the maternal levels of folic acid and $B_{12}$ associated with neural tube defects were not those usually associated with deficiency. The authors note that since food fortification has been made to include both $B_{12}$ and folic acid, the prevalence of neural tube defects has fallen from 4.7 to 1.3 per 1,000 individuals. *Quarterly Journal of Medicine* 87 (1993): 703–708.

## Depression

In this study, folic acid blood levels were significantly lower in depressed patients, leading the authors to conclude that a folic acid deficiency depression may exist. *Psychosomatics* 21 (November 1980): 926–929.

In this review article, the authors point out that depression is a common manifestation of severe folate deficiency. Depressed patients with folate deficiency had more severe illness and responded less well to conventional antidepressant therapy than those without this deficiency. In addition, those in whom the deficiency was treated made better recoveries than those with untreated folate deficiency. *The Lancet* II (July 28, 1984): 196–198.

## Mental Retardation

Large doses of folic acid (2 milligrams three times a day) have been reported to improve the behavior of adults with a chromosomal abnormality linked with mental retardation. Female carriers of the syndrome, who are apt to be mildly retarded, might also benefit from folate supplementation. *American Journal of Medicine* 77 (October 1984): 602–611.

## The Immune System

This overview cites studies indicating that deficiencies of folic acid lead to a reduction in the resistance to disease in humans and animals. Both antibody and white cell production are affected. *American Journal of Clinical Nutrition* (Supplement) 35 (February 1982): 421.

## Impaired Absorption and Metabolism of Folic Acid

Anticonvulsants and sulfasalazine (prescribed for inflammatory bowel disease) may interfere with folate absorption. Gastric surgery and intestinal conditions can also interfere. There is some evidence that the physiological process of aging influences the intestinal absorption of folate. *American Journal of Clinical Nutrition* 36 (November 1982): 1,060–1,066.

In this study, blood levels of folate in a healthy woman fell by 29 percent when she received therapeutic doses of aspirin. (However, the authors point out that it is not known whether tissue stores were affected.) *Journal of Laboratory and Clinical Medicine* 103 (June 1984): 944–948.

In animal studies it has been shown that folic acid is lost from the liver when nitrous oxide is administered as an anesthetic gas. *American Journal of Clinical Nutrition* 34 (1981): 2,412–2,417.

## Adverse Effects

Oral supplementation of folic acid lowers the plasma zinc levels and increases zinc excretion. Therefore, women with cervical dysplasia undergoing folic acid treatment may be particularly prone to zinc deficiency. This may be a hazard—especially in users of oral contraceptives, because this medication may also lower zinc levels. *Journal of the National Cancer Institute* 74 (January 1985): 263 (letter).

## CHAPTER 17: PANTOTHENIC ACID

## Emotional and Physical Stress

### Exercise

In this overview, the authors discuss why pantothenic acid has long been considered an antistress vitamin. They cite several studies of pantothenic supplementation, including: laboratory rats who showed a significant improvement in exercise tolerance and resistance to radiation-induced injury; humans who better withstood cold water stress; and the delay in the onset of fatigue. Human subjects consuming 10 grams of pantothenic acid per day significantly increased tolerance to cold water stress. Another study, testing a B-complex vitamin on exercise fatigue, concluded that 30 milligrams of pantothenic acid daily may act to delay the onset of fatigue. Only one study in the literature reported negative results with 20 milligrams per day. In the study conducted by the reviewers, 1 gram of pantothenic acid daily did enhance exercise endurance. *Journal of Sports Medicine* 24 (1984): 26–29.

### Wound Healing and Physical Injury

Experimental animals who were given pantothenic acid supplements before and after surgery healed better than did those who were unsupplemented. The authors conclude that such supplementation appears to have a beneficial effect on wound healing. *American Journal of Clinical Nutrition* 41 (March 1985): 578–589.

A drug combination containing a form of pantothenic acid was applied to animals before and after exposure to UV radiation. As a result, they experienced less skin inflammation and more rapid healing of skin inflammation. *Arzneimittelforshung* 32 (1982): 1,096–1,100.

A drug combination containing a form of pantothenic acid was applied to students with sports injuries. They experienced decreased swelling and increased joint mobility. *Arzneimittelforshung* 33 (1983): 792–795.

## The Nervous System

The authors point out that homopantothenic acid (HOPA), a naturally occurring substance, is now in widespread clinical use as a potent agent to improve epilepsy, postencephalitic sequelae, mental retardation, and mental and physical disorders in children. *Tohoku Journal of Experimental Medicine* 140 (1983): 45–51.

## The Immune System

In human and animal studies, pantothenic acid deficiencies depress antibody responsiveness to antigens. *American Journal of Clinical Nutrition* (Supplement) 35 (February 1982): 421.

In this overview, the authors point out that lower blood levels of pantothenic acid are associated with arthritis. They cite studies showing that pantothenic acid supplements have helped alleviate symptoms of this disease, and urge that further trials are indicated. *The Practitioner* 224 (February 1980): 208–211.

In this study, 30 out of 37 patients with chronic discoid lupus improved with massive doses of pantothenic acid (6 to 10 grams), followed by lower maintenance levels of 2 to 4 grams per day. *Journal of Investigative Dermatology* 15 (1950): 291.

## Cardiovascular Disease

In this study, 24 patients with Types IIA, IIB, or IV hyperlipidemia received pantethine in doses of 300 milligrams, 3 times daily. After 1 year, there was a significant decrease in serum cholesterol and triglyceride levels. *Clinical Therapies* 8 (1986): 537.

Pantethine was as effective as fenofibrate in lowering total and LDL cholesterol without the side effects of fenofibrate in hypercholesterolemic patients. These results suggest it is the therapy of choice for hypercholesterolemia. *Current Therapeutic Research* 38 (1985): 386–395.

Supplementation of pantethine resulted in normal serum values in 83 percent of hypercholesterolemic patients and 35.7 percent of hypertriglyceridemic patients. *Current Therapeutic Research* 34 (1983): 383–390.

Supplementation with pantethine in doses of 300 milligrams, 4 times daily, in hyperlipidemic patients demonstrated inhibition of platelet aggregation and thromboxane production. *Current Therapeutic Research* 35 (1984): 700.

## CHAPTER 18: BIOTIN

### The Nervous System

In this study, 8 patients experienced marked improvement in their hemodialysis-related neurologic disorders with daily supplementation of 10 milligrams of biotin. The authors conclude that biotin supplementation is effective in preventing and treating the neurological disorders that can result from chronic hemodialysis. They recommend that biotin therapy be started in patients with advanced renal failure before severe symptoms appear. *Nephron* 36 (1984): 183–186.

## Dermatitis

Treatment of the mothers of breast-fed infants with seborrheic dermatitis by injection of pharmacologic doses of biotin has been reported to have beneficial effects. *Nutrition in Health and Disease,* 6th ed. (Philadelphia: Lea and Febiger, 1980), 274–279.

## CHAPTER 19: CHOLINE, INOSITOL, AND PABA

### Cardiovascular Disease

#### Atherosclerosis

In this study, 9 men and 9 women with high triglycerides and cholesterol were given lecithin. Triglycerides, cholesterol, and platelet aggregation were all significantly decreased, and HDL cholesterol was increased. The authors conclude that lecithin may be a useful adjunct in the treatment of atherosclerosis. *Biochemical and Medical Metabolism and Biology* (January–February 1986): 31–39.

#### Cholesterol Levels

This study reports on over 153 patients with hyperlipidemia treated with inositol hexaniacinate at dosages from 600 to 1,800 milligrams per deciliter without reports of side effects or adverse reactions. The researchers concluded that inositol hexaniacinate is superior to nicotinic acid as an oral therapeutic agent. *International Record of Medicine* 174 (1961): 9–15. See also *Nutrition Reports International* 28 (1983): 899–911 and *British Journal of Clinical Practice* 42 (1988): 719–722.

In 10 Alzheimer's patients, extremely high doses of lecithin (35 grams daily) significantly lowered total cholesterol and LDL cholesterol and raised HDL cholesterol after 2 to 3 months in a double-blind crossover study. *American Journal of Psychiatry* 139 (1982): 1,633–1,634.

### Neurotransmitters

The rates at which neurons synthesize neurotransmitters such as serotonin, acetylcholine, and the catecholamines—norepinephrine and dopamine—depend on the availability of the precursors: tryptophan, choline, and tyrosine, respectively. The concentrations of precursors in the circulation and in neurons change rapidly after food consumption, depending upon what is eaten. Nutrient intake normally influences the synthesis of these neurotransmitters. These neurotransmitters participate in the control of a number of bodily functions and behaviors, such as hunger, food choice, sleep, alertness, sensitivity to environmental stimuli, and disease states. Dietary manipulations—or the consumption of individual nutrients—can thus be used as adjunctive tools in the treatment of some diseases of these neurons. *Journal of Neural Transmitters* 15 (1979): S69–S79.

### Learning Disabilities

This article reviews 2 case reports of young children with multiple neurodevelopmental delays. Both were followed from age 4 to age 8. At age 4, one child was given 2,400 milligrams of choline as a thick oil form of lecithin with noted results. Treatment was not continued. At age 5, treatment was resumed, first with 500 milligrams of choline, and then with an increased dose of 3,000 milligrams twice a day. Significant improvement was seen. He was also given fish oil for treatment of Raynaud's disease. The other child was also treated with choline. At age 4, the dose was 500 milligrams. This was increased to 1,000 milligrams over time. There was significant improvement. *Journal of the American College of Nutrition* 12 (1993): 239–245.

## CHAPTER 20: VITAMIN C (ASCORBIC ACID)

### Antioxidant Powers

In a study of 100 elderly people, in those who were supplemented with 400 milligrams of vitamin C and/or 200 milligrams of vitamin E, serum lipid peroxides declined to as little as 74 percent of initial levels after one year. The authors conclude that long-term supplementation of moderate amounts of these nutrients presumably protects against free radical damage, which may play a role in aging and the development of degenerative diseases. *Annals of Nutrition and Metabolism* 28 (May–June 1984): 186–191.

### The Immune System

Vitamin C has been shown to reduce symptoms experienced by asthmatics challenged with histamine or methacholine. Vitamin C significantly reduced airway reactivity to methacholine aerosol. *American Review of Respiratory Disease* 127 (February 1983): 143–147.

In a study of 44 pairs of twins living apart, there was an apparent protective effect of vitamin C. Among these pairs, the vitamin C group, as compared with the placebo group, developed 19 percent fewer colds, the total duration was 38 percent less, total severity was 22 percent less, and intensity was 20 percent less. *Acta Geneticae Medicae et Gemollologiae* 30 (1981): 249–255.

Vitamin C levels in serum and body tissues lower with age. Vitamin C enhanced the immune responsiveness in subjects who received doses of 500 milligrams. The authors conclude that vitamin C should be considered as a possibly successful nontoxic and inexpensive substance that may have some application in improving immune competence of the aging. *Gerontology* 29 (1983): 305–310.

This article reviews the 21 placebo-controlled trials that have been conducted since 1971 to evaluate vitamin C's effect on the common cold. Doses ranged from 1 to 4 grams per day, and in each of the studies, vitamin C reduced the duration of the cold and the severity of its symptoms by an average of 23 percent. The author concludes that it is reasonable to use vitamin C during a cold. *Scandinavian Journal of Infectious Diseases* 26 (1994): 1–6.

In this trial of 3 matched groups of 46 subjects, 1 group of marathon runners took 600 milligrams of vitamin C daily 21 days before a marathon, a sedentary control group also took vitamin C, and another group of runners took a placebo. The results suggest that vitamin C supplementation may enhance resistance to post-race upper respiratory infection, and that it may reduce the severity of infection in sedentary people. *American Journal of Clinical Nutrition* 57 (1993): 170–174.

### Life Span

This study showed that men who consumed 300 milligrams of vitamin C daily, through food and supplements, had a 40-percent lower death rate from heart disease and other causes than did those whose intake was less than 50 milligrams. *Epidemiology* 3 (1992): 194–202.

### Tissue Repair and Wound Healing

In this review article, the authors conclude that clinical studies provide evidence that wound healing in subjects judged not deficient in vitamin C can be significantly accelerated with supplements in daily dosages of 500 to 3,000 milligrams. The subjects of the studies reviewed included those recovering from surgery and other injuries, pressure sores, and leg ulcers. *Oral Surgery (March 1982): 231–236.*

## Cancer

In this famous study by Cameron and Pauling, 100 advanced cancer patients who received large supplemental doses of ascorbic acid lived from 4.2 to 20 times longer than the controls. The authors conclude that ascorbic acid is of definite value in the treatment of patients with advanced cancer. *Proceedings of the National Academy of Sciences* 73:10 (October 1976): 3,685–3,689.

In this follow-up study by Hoffer and Pauling, high-dose vitamin C (12 grams per day) was given with other nutrients to 101 cancer patients, and the results were compared with 31 cancer patients who did not receive supplements. Among the 80 percent of "good responders" in the supplemented group, the mean survival time was 122 months for patients with cancer of the breast, uterus, ovaries, and cervix, and 72 months for those with other types of cancer. By way of contrast, the mean survival time was only 5.7 months for patients who did not receive supplements. *Journal of Orthomolecular Medicine* 5 (1990) 3: 143–154.

Vitamin C has been effective in blocking the formation of nitrosamines and similar compounds. The author of this review article evaluates studies that give evidence of vitamin C's role in preventing bladder cancer, stomach cancer, colon cancer, cervical and uterine cancer, and esophageal and lung cancer. There are specific cases such as recurrent bladder cancer or achlorhydria (low stomach acid) in which vitamin C may prove useful at high doses. *Seminars in Oncology* 10 (September 1983): 294–298.

In a study of 78 women with cervical cancer, blood levels for vitamin C, beta-carotene, and folate were significantly lower than those levels in the 240 healthy women used for controls. *American Journal of Obstetrics and Gynecology* 151 (March 1, 1985): 632–635.

In a controlled study, high levels of vitamin C reduced the risk of cervical cancer by 60 percent. *Journal of the National Cancer Institute* 80 (June 15, 1988): 580–585.

In this animal study, a mixture of vitamin C and $B_{12}$ was given to mice implanted with tumor cells. All 50 of the unsupplemented mice developed tumors; but only 2 of the 50 supplemented mice had tumors, and these tumors were smaller than those in the controls. *IRCS Medical Science* 12 (September 1984): 813.

A statistically significant inverse relationship was found between the risk of skin cancer and a high intake of fish, vegetables, cruciferous vegetables, beta-carotene, and vitamin C-containing foods. *Nutrition and Cancer* 18 (1992): 237–244.

In an animal model, it was found that infusion of ascorbic acid before radiation therapy significantly protected healthy tissue against fatal radiation syndrome and the destruction of skin layers. The researchers discovered that much more radiation was required to produce the ill effects of radiation in the ascorbic acid-treated animals. The ascorbic acid did not protect the tumor or interfere with the radiation therapy in an adverse way. Extrapolating this to a human model, one might suggest that high-dose vitamin C therapy prior to radiation treatment might allow for the dose to be increased with an expected increase in tumor response, without increasing complications. *American Journal of Clinical Nutrition* 54 (1991): S1281–S1283.

Researchers developed a topical vitamin C solution that protects the skin against UV light exposure. It can deliver 20 times the amount of vitamin C normally found in skin, and it cannot be washed off. It is protective for as long as 3 days, and it is effective against UV-A and UV-B oxidative damage. The researchers note that if vitamin C levels are enhanced in the skin, premature aging, wrinkles, and even skin cancer may be prevented. *Journal of the National Cancer Institute* 83 (1991): 847–850.

## Cardiovascular Disease

In this review article, the author discusses studies of the beneficial effects of vitamin C on veins and arteries. In one study, the deep vein thrombosis rate was lowered by 50 percent in surgical patients given 1,000 milligrams of vitamin C daily. In another clinical trial, atherosclerotic patients given vitamin C could walk farther without feeling pain or breathlessness. Vitamin C may help to prevent cholesterol deposits by preventing and repairing damaged arterial walls and moving cholesterol away from the arterial wall to the liver. The author suggests that atherosclerosis is a long-term deficiency of vitamin C. *American Heart Journal* 88:3 (1974): 387–388.

High intakes of vitamin C or fruits and of green vegetables that are high in vitamin C have been related to lowered mortality from stroke and heart disease. The author suggests that ascorbic acid has a preventive effect on hypertension. *International Journal for Vitamin and Nutrition Research* 54 (1984): 343–347.

Two studies show that when people with high cholesterol were given 300 to 1,000 milligrams of vitamin C daily, their cholesterol levels dropped. *The Lancet* (October 20, 1984): 907.

Correlations between serum HDL cholesterol and vitamin C intake were positive and significant in women. In men, high levels of HDLs seem to be associated with very high vitamin C intakes. If an adequate supply of vitamin C is necessary for the maintenance of optimal HDL levels, then perhaps the requirements of men are substantially higher than those of women. *American Journal of Clinical Nutrition* 40 (December 1984): 1,334–1,338.

In a study of adult males, higher serum vitamin C and selenium levels were associated with lower blood pressure. This supports the hypothesis that antioxidants play a role in the development of hypertension. *American Journal of Clinical Nutrition* 48 (November 1988): 1,226–1,232.

Lipoprotein(a) is an independent risk factor for coronary heart disease. In 1989, Drs. Rath and Pauling discovered that lipoprotein(a) is a surrogate for vitamin C, and that optimal vitamin C intake prevents the deposition of lipoprotein(a) in the vascular wall. Linus Pauling Institute for Science and Medicine Newsletter (March 1992): 2.

In this study, 101 patients with chronic strokes were found to have significantly higher levels of lipoprotein(a). Serum lipoprotein(a) levels were significantly increased in young adults with stroke compared with patients over 45 years of age. The authors conclude that lipoprotein(a) is a genetic, independent, and critical risk factor for stroke, especially in young adults. *Stroke* 25 (1994): 74–78.

## HIV Infection and AIDS

This study reviews the synergistic effects of NAC and vitamin C on HIV suppression. NAC caused approximately a 2-fold inhibition of HIV reverse transcriptase activity and had a synergistic effect when tested simultaneously with ascorbic acid. The continuous presence of ascorbic acid was necessary for HIV suppression. These results support the potent antiviral effects of ascorbic acid and suggest its synergistic effect with compounds such as NAC. *American Journal of Clinical Nutrition* 54 (1991): S1231–S1235.

An evaluation of the micronutrient intake of 108 HIV-positive patients found that the highest levels of total intake of vitamin C, $B_1$, and niacin were associated with a significant decreased progression rate to AIDS. *American Journal of Epidemiology* 138 (1993): 937–951.

Taking vitamin C to bowel tolerance (40 to 100 grams daily) is reported to put AIDS into extended clinical remission. The author recommends that all at risk for AIDS take vitamin C to bowel tolerance. *Mental Hypothesis* 14 (August 1984): 423–433.

## Smoking

Smoking cigarettes raises the requirement for vitamin C. *American Journal of Clinical Nutrition* 34 (1981): 1,347–1,355.

This study revealed that smokers have lower bloodstream levels of vitamin C than do nonsmokers. Two to four times as many smokers as nonsmokers had vitamin C deficiencies in the near-scurvy range. Smokers have a special need for vitamin C, and a normal dietary intake may not adequately keep their vitamin C level within a normal range. *Federation Proceedings* 43 (1984): 861.

In this study, increases in blood pressure immediately following cigarette smoking were lowered by 400 milligrams of vitamin C. *Nutrition Research* 3 (1983): 653–661.

## Oral Contraceptives

Women taking long-term oral contraceptives eliminate vitamin C from their bodies at a higher rate. They may need increased daily doses of vitamin C. In addition, vitamin C has been shown to enhance the levels of certain hormones in the blood (estradiol), and it is possible that the dosage of estrogen in oral contraceptives may be reduced with vitamin C supplementation. *Annals of Nutrition and Metabolism* 28 (May–June 1984): 186–191.

## Eye Disorders

High dietary intake of vitamin C in patients ages 55 to 80 was associated with a marginal but significant decrease in the development of acute macular degeneration. The authors conclude that increased intakes of antioxidants, beta-carotene, and vitamin C might decrease the risk of macular degeneration. *Investigative Ophthalmology and Visual Science* 34 (December 1993): 1,134.

When rats were fed a high-sugar diet designed to cause cataracts, only 6 percent of the group supplemented with vitamin C developed cataracts, versus 69 percent of the unsupplemented control group. When the sugar was removed from the diets, all of those rats started on vitamin-C supplementation lost their cataracts, versus 67 percent of those who were unsupplemented. Even though rats synthesize their own vitamin C, supplementation delayed the progression of these cataracts and hastened their regression. *Nutrition Report International* 33 (April 1986): 665–668.

## Other Uses

### Birth Defects

Neural tube defects (spina bifida and anencephalous) are associated with low levels of vitamin C and folic acid. *Canadian Medical Association Journal* 129 (November 15, 1983): 1,088–1,091.

### Pregnancy Complications

In a study of 87 pregnant women, 74 percent of those with abruptio placentae had significantly lower blood levels of vitamin C than did those without this complication. The authors concluded that a deficiency of vitamin C could result in symptoms observed in this complication of pregnancy. *Human Nutrition and Clinical Nutrition* 39C (May–June 1985): 233–238.

## Male Infertility

Infertile men with lowered sperm counts were given 1,000 milligrams of vitamin C daily. Throughout the several weeks of the study, there was a continuous rise in the percentage of normal sperm, sperm viability, and sperm motility. *Journal of the American Medical Association* 249 (May 27, 1983): 2,747–2,748.

## Depression and Mania

In 2 studies, patients improved when treated with a low-vanadium diet or with high doses of ascorbic acid. *Nutritional Review* 40:10 (October 1982): 293–295.

## Schizophrenia

This article reviews several clinical studies in which ascorbic acid supplementation improved symptoms in schizophrenic patients. One gram per day of ascorbic acid supplementation significantly improved depressive, manic, and paranoid symptoms; 8 grams per day improved 10 out of 13 patients on stable neuroleptic regimens; 2 grams of ascorbic acid plus haloperidol was more beneficial than haloperidol alone; 2 to 6 grams per day improved patients on medications while 1 patient achieved full remission within one week. *The Nutrition Report* 8 (September 1990): 65, 72.

## The Elderly

Vitamin C therapy of 1,000 milligrams per day given to institutionalized elderly led to an improvement of their nutritional status and a reduction in petechial hemorrhages (pin-sized red dots under the skin). *American Journal of Clinical Nutrition* 34 (1981): 871–876.

## Hospital Patients

The vitamin C levels of 199 elderly hospital patients were measured upon admission. Those with low vitamin C levels had a mortality rate of 45 percent during the study, but only 27 percent of those with higher vitamin C levels died, although the severity of illness was the same in both groups. In addition, half were given 200 milligrams of vitamin C daily; half were given a placebo. Those with low initial levels of vitamin C who received the supplement tended to improve more than did those given the placebo. The authors conclude that supplementation of patients who have low vitamin C levels may improve their prognosis. *International Journal for Vitamin and Nutrition Research* 54 (January–March 1984): 65–74.

## Drug Hepatotoxicity

In laboratory mice given large doses of acetaminophen or cocaine, ascorbic acid decreased damage to the liver by about 80 percent. The authors conclude that vitamin C may be a safe and effective agent for preventing the liver toxicity of some drugs. *Drug and Nutrient Interaction* 3 (January–March 1984): 33–41.

## Lung Protection

In this study of 2,526 adults, those with a higher intake of vitamin C had better lung function. The authors conclude that vitamin C protects the lungs. This effect was not limited to smokers, but was more evident in asthmatic and bronchitis patients. *American Journal of Clinical Nutrition* 59 (1994): 110–114.

## Optimum Vitamin C Intake

The author arrived at an estimated body pool of vitamin C of 5,000 milligrams for a 70-kilogram person. An intake of 200 milligrams daily would maintain this level. This refers to people who are free from stress. Individuals who have high levels of physical activity or who experience strain from pregnancy, mental stress, diabetes, injury, infection, cancer, atherosclerosis, pollution, or medications may require much higher dosages. *Nutrition and Health* 1 (1981): 66–77.

Human beings are genetically programmed to consume the diet that was available to our ancient hunter-gatherer ancestors, who evolved 40,000 years ago. The authors estimate that these people consumed a diet containing almost 400 milligrams of vitamin C each day. *The New England Journal of Medicine* 312 (January 31, 1985): 283–289.

In a study of adolescent boys, the group that was given 70 milligrams of vitamin C daily improved their aerobic work capacity by 10 percent. The authors conclude that the optimal intake of vitamin C is 80 to 100 milligrams a day. *International Journal for Vitamin and Nutrition Research* 54 (January–March 1984): 55–60.

Rats maintain a vitamin C body pool that is 5 times greater than the pool calculated for humans. *Journal of Biological Chemistry* 230 (1958): 923.

The author reviews data concerning the synthesis of vitamin C in animals and the ingestion of vitamin C in nonvitamin C-producing animals, both under normal conditions and under stress. He concludes that this data suggests that the optimum daily intake of vitamin C for humans is between 250 and 4,000 milligrams. *Proceedings of the National Academy of Sciences* 71:11 (1974): 4,442–4,446.

The author notes that most animals produce their own vitamin C at the rate of up to 275 milligrams per kilogram daily, and that this is much higher than the RDA for humans, which is .9 milligrams per kilogram. In animals that must obtain vitamin C from the diet, about 10 times this amount, necessary to prevent scurvy, was needed to maintain health, and up to 40 milligrams per kilogram was needed to survive the stresses of long-term captivity. Research suggests that the amount of vitamin C necessary to prevent scurvy is less than that required for maximal enzyme activity. *The New England Journal of Medicine* 314 (April 3, 1986): 892–902.

An in-hospital depletion-repletion study was conducted on 7 healthy volunteers for a period of 4 to 6 months. Participants consumed a diet containing under 5 milligrams of vitamin C daily. The authors looked at bioavailability, plasma saturation, and neutrophil, monocyte, and lymphocyte saturation of varying amounts of vitamin C. Based on the data from this study, the researchers conclude that the RDA of 60 milligrams should be increased to 200 milligrams. *Proceedings of the National Academy of Science* 93 (1996): 3,704–3,709.

## Toxicity and Adverse Effects

Based on 2 studies in which adults were supplemented with 3,000 to 10,000 milligrams of vitamin C daily, the authors conclude that the probability of oxalate stone formation due to ingestion of vitamin C is very small. *International Journal for Vitamin and Nutrition Research* 54 (April–September 1984): 245–249.

In a 2-year toxicity study, experimental mice and rats were given very high doses of ascorbic acid—up to 2,800 and 13,800 milligrams per kilogram of body weight, respectively. No evidence of toxicity was found. *Journal of Toxicology and Environmental Health* 14 (October 1984): 605–609.

Previous studies have suggested that high doses of vitamin C destroy $B_{12}$ in the body.

More recent studies, using superior techniques, have shown no significant evidence of destruction of B12 body stores with up to 2,000 milligrams of vitamin C. *Scottish Medical Journal* 27 (1982): 240–243.

The authors reviewed human and animal studies and found that the few case reports of possible rebound scurvy are anecdotal and not well-founded. They conclude that there is no basis for the belief that high-dose vitamin C consumption leads to rebound scurvy in humans. *Nutrition Research* 8 (1988): 1,327–1,332.

Vitamin C supplementation of 250 or 300 milligrams per day did not adversely affect zinc or copper levels. *Nutrition Report International* 37 (June 1988): 1,307–1,317.

When comparing kits used by physicians to determine oxalate levels in the urine, the authors of this study found that ascorbic acid interferes with those kits using oxidase, but less so with those using decarboxylase. *Clinical Biochemistry* 26(2) (April 1993): 93–96.

# CHAPTER 21: CALCIUM

## Overview

This article discusses those who may be at risk for inadequate calcium intake from poor diet, problems with absorption and utilization such as age, physical activity, estrogen deficiency, phosphorus-calcium balance, and diets high in protein, fat, and fiber. It is suggested that calcium balance can be maintained either by estrogen replacement therapy *or* by increased calcium intake. *American Journal of Clinical Nutrition* 36 (November 1982): 986–1013.

## Blood Pressure

This review article discusses various epidemiological and clinical studies correlating high calcium intakes with low blood pressure in men and in pregnant and nonpregnant women. For example, in one clinical trial, 1,000 milligrams of calcium given daily to hypertensives produced a 48-percent reduction in systolic blood pressure. *Nutrition Reviews* 42:6 (1984): 205–213.

In a controlled, double-blind, randomized study, 48 hypertensives were given 1,000 milligrams of calcium per day for 8 weeks. Of these, 21 (44 percent) achieved a therapeutically meaningful reduction in their blood pressure. Of the responders, 14 had previously required therapy with antihypertensive drugs to achieve similar results. Oral calcium therapy was remarkably well tolerated. *Annals of Intestinal Medicine* 103:6 (1985): 825–831.

During a 4-year controlled study of 81 women, half of them were given 1,500 milligrams of calcium per day. Of the hypertensive women, those who took the supplement experienced a significant reduction in systolic blood pressure. In the unsupplemented women, systolic blood pressure continued to rise, even though they were given hypertensive medication. *American Journal of Clinical Nutrition* 42 (July 1985): 12–17.

In this study, the diets of over 10,000 adults were examined. Of the 17 nutrients examined, low calcium was most consistently associated with high blood pressure. Intakes of potassium, sodium, and vitamins A and C were also lower in people with higher blood pressure, while cholesterol intake was not consistently different. The authors concluded that diets that restrict the intake of calories, sodium, or cholesterol may also reduce the intake of calcium and other nutrients that may be protective against hypertension. *Science* 224 (June 29, 1984): 1,392–1,398.

In this study, 12 normal men consumed a high-salt diet (6.6 grams per day) for 2 weeks. They experienced an increase in excretion of calcium and phosphorus. Those who consumed a low-calcium diet also excreted more phosphorus. Men with the higher calcium intake had lower blood pressure. The authors suggest that sodium intake may influence blood pressure through its effects on calcium and potassium excretion, and that these effects may be more pronounced in people with low calcium intake. *American Journal of Clinical Nutrition* 41 (January 1985): 52–60.

In a review of the effect of calcium on blood pressure, the authors discuss recent findings that low sodium intake is related to high blood pressure, and that the antihypertensive effect of calcium may depend on adequate salt intake. Severe sodium restriction may actually *exacerbate* high blood pressure, as well as reduce calcium intake by limiting consumption of dairy products. They suggest that calcium may be safe and effective as a treatment for both essential and pregnancy-related hypertension, and as a preventive measure. *Nutrition Reviews* 42 (June 1984): 205–213.

Oral calcium supplementation can lower blood pressure in hypertensive individuals. It appears that salt-sensitive hypertensives may benefit the most. *Journal of Nutrition* 117 (1987): 1,806–1,808.

## Cancer

This article reviews several studies of the relationship between vitamin D, calcium, and colon cancer. The incidence of colon cancer in Scandinavian countries was correlated with the intake of milk. In Southern California, where there is high exposure to sunlight and milk is fortified with vitamin D, an association was found between high milk consumption and a lowered risk of colon cancer. Yogurt has been shown to explicitly convey colonic bacterial flora that inhibits the effects of known colonic carcinogens. *Nutrition Reviews* 43:6 (1985): 170–172.

Researchers examined the cells lining the colons of 10 patients with family histories of colon cancer, and found that they had a proliferation pattern characteristic of high-risk individuals. After supplementation with calcium, the cells were less proliferative and were almost the same as those in people at low risk for colon cancer. *The New England Journal of Medicine* 313 (1985): 1,381–1,384.

A group of nearly 2,000 men was followed for 19 years. Those who developed colorectal cancer were found to have consumed significantly less calcium and vitamin D than those who did not. Men with the lowest intake had 2.7 times the risk of those with the highest intake. The authors concluded that both vitamin D and calcium may have anticancer activity. *The Lancet* I (February 9, 1985): 307–309.

A study that evaluated 2,591 Dutch adults, ages 40 to 65, found that women with the lowest calcium intake had an increased risk of gastrointestinal cancer. Both men and women with a lower-than-average intake of calcium had a higher risk of colorectal mortality. *International Journal of Cancer* 54 (1993): 20–25.

## Osteoporosis

Calcium supplements of 1,000 milligrams per day were given to 14 postmenopausal women. The results of this study led the authors to conclude that calcium therapy, which has no serious side effects, decreases bone resorption in cases of postmenopausal osteoporosis. Previous studies have shown that 1,000 to 2,500 milligrams of calcium per day reduce the incidence of vertebral fracture by 50 percent, and that 1,000 milligrams of calcium daily protect healthy menopausal women against osteoporosis. *American Journal of Clinical Nutrition* 39 (June 1984): 857–859.

In a study of 26 healthy women ages 47 to 66, bone density increased with calcium supplementation *with or without* estrogen therapy. *New York State Journal of Medicine* 75 (1975): 326–336.

The author of this article suggests that the only rational approach to osteoporosis is prevention. Current data indicates that osteoporotic patients consume less calcium, require more dietary calcium to achieve calcium balance, lose more bone mass per day, and have lower vitamin D hormone levels than do controls. According to one study, postmenopausal women with osteoporosis require 1,500 milligrams per day of calcium to attain calcium balance, compared with 1,000 milligrams in premenopausal controls. *Nutrition Reviews* 41:3 (1983): 83–85.

Calcium intake was found to be lower in both men and women with subsequent hip fracture than in those without hip fracture. A daily intake of over 765 milligrams of calcium was associated with a 60-percent reduction in the risk of hip fracture. *The Lancet* II (November 5, 1988): 1,046–1,049.

Severe skeletal bone loss in mature men and women may exist before it is manifested by clinical symptoms or biochemical changes. *Nutrition Reports International* 38 (July 1988): 211–219.

The authors conclude that within 10 years of menopause, in normal postmenopausal women whose calcium intake is below 1,000 milligrams, increasing intake to 1,400 milligrams reduces the rate of bone loss. *Journal of Clinical Nutrition* 117 (1987): 1,929–1,935.

In a study of menopausal women, the calcium intake contributing to maximal bone values was 500 to 800 milligrams per day, and only the highest level of physical activity was associated with increased bone mass. *American Journal of Clinical Nutrition* 49 (1989): 534–541.

In women 25 to 35 years of age, those with intakes of calcium higher than the RDA had greater bone mineral density than women taking less than the RDA. There was an additive relationship between the effects of exercise and calcium. The authors suggest that the optimal intake of calcium for premenopausal women is 800 to 1,000 milligrams per day. *Journal of Bone and Mineral Research* 3 (1988): 145–149.

This article reviews the role of calcium supplementation in the treatment of bone loss in postmenopausal women. It points out that calcium supplementation results in a significant slowing of bone loss, with no side effects, at a cost similar to that of some forms of hormone replacement therapy. *Pharmacoeconomics* 5 (1994): 1–4.

This article reviews the importance of copper, manganese, and zinc supplementation, in addition to calcium, for increasing mineral density in postmenopausal women. In a 2-year double-blind placebo-controlled trial including 200 postmenopausal women, the group taking calcium had no significant bone loss, but the group taking 1,000 milligrams of calcium, 15 milligrams of zinc, 2.5 milligrams of copper, and 5 milligrams of manganese experienced an *increase* in bone density. *Journal of the American College of Nutrition* 12 (1993): 384–389.

In this study of 3,000 elderly females, half were given 1,200 milligrams of calcium plus 800 international units of vitamin D, and half were given a placebo. The supplemented group had a 30-percent lower incidence of nonvertebral fractures and a 41-percent lower incidence of hip fractures compared with the placebo group. *Nutrition Reviews* 51 (1993): 183–185.

A study of 118 women who had recently gone through menopause showed that calcium supplementation alone was less effective than estrogen, progesterone, and calcium given together. However, calcium alone still resulted in a significant slowing of bone loss, and the authors believe that calcium supplementation should be encouraged to help prevent bone loss during the early part of menopause. *Annals of Internal Medicine* 120 (January 15, 1994): 97–103.

This double-blind, placebo-controlled trial included 137 women age 65 or older. Some subjects were supplemented with 1,000 milligrams a day of calcium citrate malate, or with the same amount of calcium plus 2.5 milligrams of copper, 5 milligrams of manganese, and 1.25 milligrams of zinc. In the placebo group, spinal bone density decreased after 2 years. The women who took the calcium with trace minerals experienced an increase in spinal bone density. *Geriatrics* 46 (July 1991): 67.

## Calcium Intake and Absorption

In an article that considers the nature and current implications of Paleolithic nutrition, the authors determine that our early ancestors consumed approximately 1,600 milligrams of calcium per day. *The New England Journal of Medicine* 312:5 (1985): 283–289.

In this article, the author reviews factors that influence calcium intake and absorption, and may therefore contribute to the development of osteoporosis. These include age; high phosphorus intake; and the use of drugs such as glucocorticoids (steroids), diuretics, tetracycline, and aluminum-containing antacids. Depending on age, two thirds to three fourths of U.S. females ingest less than the RDA; fully one fourth ingest less than 300 milligrams. The author notes that a large percentage of patients with osteoporosis had a calcium imbalance with a calcium intake of 800 milligrams per day, and concluded that the RDA of 800 milligrams cannot be sufficient for the entire population. *American Journal of Clinical Nutrition* 36 (October 1982): 776–787.

In a study of 98 postmenopausal women, the authors found that malabsorption of calcium was an important risk factor for osteoporosis, probably owing to the mobilization of bone to maintain blood calcium levels. *Journal of Clinical Endocrinological Metabolism* 60 (April 1985): 651–657.

Absorption of calcium is normally only 20 to 40 percent of intake. A vegetarian diet contains acids that may bind 360 milligrams of calcium per day. However, over 80 percent of these acids are fermented in the intestine so that much of the calcium may be released and become available for absorption. *American Journal of Clinical Nutrition* 35 (April 1982): 783–808.

Calcium absorption may be impaired in postmenopausal women owing to inadequate stomach acid. In this population, calcium citrate is better absorbed (45 percent) than calcium carbonate (5 percent) on an empty stomach. If taken with food, calcium carbonate absorption is essentially the same as it is in normal people (over 20 percent). *The New England Journal of Medicine* 313 (July 11, 1985): 70–73.

Calcium malabsorption was discovered and correlated with rheumatoid arthritis activity in 20 women with this disease. Osteoporosis may result. *Annals of Rheumatoid Disease* 44 (September 1985): 585–588.

In this study, a group of women who were given 700 to 800 milligrams of calcium plus 375 international units of vitamin D experienced an increase in bone density. The other group of women took a balanced supplement consisting of calcium, vitamin D, and the RDA of 15 other vitamins and minerals. The latter group experienced a 2 to 3 times greater increase in bone density than the former group. *Nutrition Reports International* 31 (March 1985): 741–755.

The authors of this study found that an average of 15 percent of calcium citrate was absorbed compared with 8 percent of calcium phosphate. *American Journal of Clinical Nutrition* 47 (May 1988): 884–888.

### Antacids as a Source of Calcium

Adverse effects of aluminum-containing antacids include high levels of calcium secreted in the urine, bone resorption, impairment of fluoride absorption, and phosphorus depletion—all of which may contribute to bone disease. *Gastroenterology* 76 (1979): 603–606.

### Toxicity and Adverse Effects

In a study of 200 ulcer patients and 200 normal controls, the authors suggest that the slightly higher risk of kidney stone formation in ulcer patients (7 versus 1 percent) was due to milk-alkali syndrome. This occurs when patients drink 2 to 5 quarts of milk per day, in addition to taking antacids. *American Journal of Gastroenterology* 68 (1977): 367–371.

## CHAPTER 22: PHOSPHORUS

### Overviews

This chapter discusses the uses of phosphorus in the body, including its role in the bone and its many soft-tissue functions. According to the Food and Nutrition Board, the average daily intake of phosphorus is 1,500 to 1,600 milligrams. Committee on Dietary Allowances, *Recommended Daily Allowances,* 9th ed. (Washington, D.C.: National Academy of Sciences, 1980), 133–134.

The author describes the uses of phosphorus in the body, and points out that although it is recommended that the intake of calcium and phosphorus be equal, in most diets the phosphorus intake exceeds the calcium intake. Corinne H. Robinson, *Normal and Therapeutic Nutrition,* 15th ed. (New York: Macmillan, 1977), 108–109.

### Phosphorus/Calcium Balance

In this study, 34 men and women were tested for calcium and phosphorus intakes. It was found that the intakes for both minerals were higher for men than for women—1,075 milligrams and 1,533 milligrams versus 695 milligrams and 1,095 milligrams. However, both groups were in negative balance. The authors discuss the contribution that high phosphorus intake makes to the eventual decrease in bone mass. They suggest that diets high in protein, soft drinks, and phosphorus additives are responsible for the undesirable calcium-to-phosphorus ratio. *American Journal of Clinical Nutrition* 40 (December 1984):1368–1379.

In a survey of a large number of women, the frequency of skeletal fractures was increased by a factor of 2.3 in athletic women who consumed carbonated beverages. This relationship seems to apply to phosphate contained in carbonated soft drinks rather than dietary phosphorus. *Journal of Nutrition* 118 (1988): 657–660.

## CHAPTER 23: MAGNESIUM

### Osteoporosis

This study revealed that almost 75 percent of the women who took 250 to 750 milligrams of magnesium daily for 2 years had bone density increases of 1 to 8 percent. *Medical Tribune* (July 22, 1993): 1.

### Fibromyalgia and Chronic Fatigue

Leading health researchers are recommending magnesium malate (magnesium plus malic acid) supplements for the treatment of chronic fatigue. In particular, fibromyalgia pain may be reduced within 48 hours while fatigue may take 2 weeks. The therapeutic dose of 6 tablets generally contains 300 milligrams of magnesium and 1,200 milligrams of malic acid. *Health Watch* 3 (Spring 1993): 1,3.

In this study, 15 patients with fibromyalgia were treated with an oral dosage of 6 to 12 tablets of magnesium malate supplying 1,200 to 2,400 milligrams of malate and 300 to 600 milligrams of magnesium, respectively. Subjective improvement in symptoms occurred within 48 hours of supplementation. Subjective worsening of muscle pain occurred within 48 hours of placebo ingestion. *Journal of Nutritional Medicine* 3 (1992): 49–59.

### Psychiatric Disorders

Of 41 unmedicated psychiatric patients, 11 women who attempted suicide had significantly lower cerebrospinal fluid levels of magnesium than nonsuicidal patients and controls. The authors hypothesize that magnesium may be required to maintain normal serotonergic (neurotransmitter) activity in the central nervous system. *Biological Psychiatry* 20 (February 1985): 163–171.

In this study, 165 boys who had been admitted to a psychiatric hospital were compared with normal boys. Patients with low magnesium blood levels had significantly more symptoms of depression, schizophrenia, and sleep disturbances. The authors concluded that low blood magnesium is associated with depressive and schizophrenic symptoms in children. *Biological Psychiatry* 19 (June 1984): 871–876.

The effects of vitamin $B_6$ and magnesium supplementation on 60 autistic children were tested in a double-blind trial. Neither supplement, when used alone, had any significant effect. A combination of the 2, however, resulted in significant improvement. *Biological Psychiatry* 20 (May 1985): 467–478.

When hair samples from 28 autistic children were taken, mean calcium and magnesium levels were found to be well below normal and significantly less than in controls. Although vitamin $B_6$ has also been found to be low in autistic children, $B_6$ supplementation when given without magnesium worsened the symptoms of some of the children in this study. *Orthomolecular Psychiatry* 13 (April–June 1984): 117–122.

## Cardiovascular Disease

### Blood Pressure

Magnesium may modify blood pressure by interacting with other electrolytes known to affect blood vessel and smooth muscle tone, such as sodium, potassium, and calcium. *American Journal of Clinical Nutrition* 42 (1985): 1,331–1,338.

In this study, hypertensives had significantly less magnesium in their blood cells than did normal people. The authors point out that previous studies have shown magnesium supplementation to be an effective hypotensive agent in some types of blood pressure. *Proceedings of the National Academy of Science* 81 (October 1984): 6,511–6,515.

### Angina

Previous studies have shown that magnesium is significantly lower in patients with angina. This study treated 15 patients who had 5- to 15-minute angina attacks with intravenous magnesium. During 41 occasions, the attacks ended within .5 to 2 minutes after treatment. Four patients who had daily attacks were treated daily for 5 days and had no further attacks. The authors contend that magnesium deficiency may be an important factor in the production of coronary vasospasm, which, in turn, can cause angina. *Magnesium* 3 (January–February 1984): 46–49.

### Retinopathy

In this study, 8 young men with untreated hypertension and abnormal blood vessels of the retina were found to have low levels of magnesium. When supplemented with 450 milligrams of magnesium for 3 months, the blood vessels returned to normal. *Magnesium* 3 (May–June 1984): 159–163.

A group of 71 insulin-treated diabetics all had low levels of magnesium. Those with the lowest levels had the severest degree of retinal disease. The author concluded that inadequate magnesium appears to be an additional risk factor in the development and progress of this complication. *Diabetes* 27 (1978): 1,075–1,077.

## Pregnancy Complications

In a study of 534 women with threatening premature labor, the group of patients who received magnesium supplementation experienced a reduction in the proportion of prematurity and intrauterine growth retardation. The researchers concluded that a certain percentage of these conditions are due to magnesium deficiency and can be averted with supplementation. *Magnesium* 4 (January–February 1985): 20–28.

## Diarrhea

After receiving radiation therapy, 20 cervical cancer patients developed diarrhea so severe that they required hospitalization. In the 10 patients who were treated with magnesium, diarrhea disappeared within 3 days. In the group that was treated conventionally, it took 2 to 6 weeks for symptoms to clear. Radiation caused decreases in blood levels of magnesium, and the authors suggest that pretreatment with magnesium might prevent this side effect. In addition, magnesium has been found to reduce diarrhea due to malnutrition, Crohn's disease, and other conditions. *Magnesium* 4 (January–February 1985): 16–19.

## Drug Interactions

In this study, 12 bone marrow transplant patients who were treated with the drug cyclosporine experienced neurological symptoms. All patients had low magnesium levels at the onset of symptoms. These symptoms resolved or did not recur after magnesium levels were restored. The authors suggest that the neurotoxicity of this drug is due to magnesium depletion, and that supplementation would reduce the risk of these side effects. *The Lancet* II (November 17, 1984): 1,116–1,120.

## Deficiencies

Magnesium deficiency results in thrombosis, and oral contraceptive use has been found to lower blood levels of magnesium. This offers a possible clue to the higher incidence of clotting disorders among women on oral contraceptives. *Medical World News* (September 13, 1974): 32.

A group of "Type A" behavior men and a group of "Type B" behavior men were given a stressful task. The results of the experiment led the authors to postulate that stress causes the release of magnesium from the cells, which is then excreted in the urine. Eventual magnesium depletion can increase the risk of hypertension, coronary vasospasm (angina), and damage to the heart. *Journal of the American College of Nutrition* 4 (April–June 1985): 165–172.

The levels of magnesium in the red blood cells of women with premenstrual tension (PMT) were significantly lower than those of the controls. This may be due to decreased intake/absorption or increased excretion. Since PMT patients often complain of nervous tension, the magnesium may also be depleted because of stress. The author suggests that magnesium therapy may be beneficial to PMT patients with low red cell magnesium. *American Journal of Clinical Nutrition* 34 (November 1981): 2,364–2,366.

Magnesium in the blood serum and urine was measured in 25 patients who were hospitalized with Crohn's disease. Evidence of magnesium deficiency was found in 84 percent of the patients. *Journal of the American College of Nutrition* 4 (September–October 1985): 553–558.

## CHAPTER 24: ZINC

### Overviews

The authors discuss the possible symptoms of a marginal zinc deficiency in adults and children, including impaired wound healing, impaired growth, and loss of taste acuity. *Pediatric Clinics of North America* 30:3 (June 1983): 583–596.

This article reviews the possible causes of low zinc levels, including malabsorption syndromes and chronically debilitating diseases. The signs of chronic zinc deficiency include growth retardation, male hypogonadism, skin changes, poor appetite, mental lethargy, and delayed wound healing. Zinc has a wide variety of functions, including protection of the liver from carbon tetrachloride, a possible direct effect on free radicals, and the alleviation of the toxic effects of cadmium and lead. *Nutrition Reviews* 41:7 (July 1983): 206.

### Growth, Pregnancy, and Development

Pregnant women with the lowest levels of zinc in their blood had more complications than did women with the highest levels of zinc. *American Journal of Clinical Nutrition* 40 (September 1984): 496–507.

This study found that pregnant women take in marginal amounts of zinc (8.6 milligrams per day) and copper (0.95 milligrams), resulting in poor body retention. Supplements containing 10 to 12 milligrams of zinc and 2 milligrams of copper combined with normal dietary intakes are sufficient to achieve positive balances during pregnancy. The authors point out that prenatal zinc and copper deficiencies in animals have been shown to cause birth defects. *American Journal of Clinical Nutrition* 42 (June 1985): 1,184–1,192.

Data shows that women with zinc malabsorption and/or low blood levels of zinc have an increased risk of having a malformed child. The authors point out that few prenatal supplements contain zinc. *American Journal of Clinical Nutrition* 38 (December 1983): 943–953.

The offspring of zinc-deficient monkeys were fed a diet deficient in zinc after they were weaned. They developed bone abnormalities similar to those found in rickets. *American Journal of Clinical Nutrition* 40 (December 1984): 1,203–1,212.

Recent U.S. studies indicate that zinc deficiency in infants and preschool children is not uncommon. Earliest signs of deficiency include slowing of physical growth, poor appetite, and diminished taste acuity. The authors suggest that calcium carbonate in hard tap water may interfere with zinc absorption or utilization. *American Journal of Clinical Nutrition* 37 (January 1983): 37–42.

Zinc levels in the sweat of dyslexic children were only 66 percent as high as those in controls. Since dyslexia tends to be a family trait, further studies on zinc levels and the effects of supplementation before conception, during pregnancy, and in childhood are urgently needed. *British Medical Journal* 296 (February 27, 1988): 607–609.

### Taste, Vision, and Smell

There is strong evidence to support the connection between zinc depletion and the development of night blindness and loss of taste acuity. It is likely that impaired color discrimination and smell acuity may also develop. Other investigators have suggested that such impairments may be better indicators of zinc depletion than are the traditional blood tests, which are notoriously unreliable. *Annals of Internal Medicine* 99 (1983): 227–239.

The highest concentration of zinc in the human body is in the eye. It is well established that zinc is an essential component of many parts of the eye, including the retina, choroid, cornea, and lens. Zinc deficiency causes functional impairment in various parts of the eye, and there is a growing body of evidence that this deficiency is related to many conditions, such as night blindness, cataract formation, and optic neuritis. *Survey of Ophthalmology* 27:2 (September–October 1982): 114–122.

The authors found that zinc and copper levels were lower in patients with cataracts when compared with controls. Since zinc and copper are required for superoxide dismutase (SOD) to protect the lens from oxidation damage, diets chronically deficient in these nutrients may impair this important mechanism. *Nutrition Reports International* 37 (January 1988): 157–163.

The authors treated 12 chronic hemodialysis patients with zinc. Sensitivity to 4 taste qualities was significantly heightened, and the authors suggest that zinc replacement may be an effective therapy for loss of taste acuity in dialysis patients. *Kidney International* 24: Supplement 16 (December 1983): S315–S318.

## Physical and Mental Stress

The author notes that in many patients, an upper respiratory infection with fever has been associated with a zinc deficiency. In addition, patients with severe burns have low zinc levels and severe loss of appetite, which improve with zinc supplementation. Corinne H. Robinson, *Normal and Therapeutic Nutrition*, 15th ed. (New York: Macmillan, 1977), 117–118.

The data from this study supports other reports that injury results in zinc depletion. The average zinc levels in injured subjects in this study were significantly lower than those in controls for at least 4 days after hospital admission. *Nutrition Research* 5 (1985): 253–261.

Diabetics were found to have lower zinc levels than did controls. This may be related to several common complications of diabetes, including impaired immune function, low testosterone levels, slow healing of ulcers, and neurosensory changes. *Nutrition Research* 8 (1988): 889–897.

In an 8-week study, 18 patients with arterial or venous leg ulcers were treated with compresses of zinc oxide. In addition, 19 controls were treated with unmedicated compresses. Of the treated group, 83 percent improved, versus 42 percent of the untreated group. Four weeks after the end of the treatment, 61 percent of the zinc oxide-treated ulcers were healed, compared with 2 percent of the untreated group. The authors note that previous studies have shown that zinc given orally for 1 to 2 months improves the healing of similar ulcers in patients with low zinc levels. *British Journal of Dermatology* 111 (October 1984): 461–468.

The authors review the effectiveness of topical zinc applications in treating types 1 and 2 herpes virus lesions. Solutions of zinc have been shown to relieve pain, tingling, burning, and itching; to shorten healing time by 40 to 60 percent; and to reduce recurrence rates from 100 percent in controls to 0 to 14 percent in treated patients. For facial and upper body skin infections and genital infections, solutions can be applied as warm rinses, wet dressings, douches, or wet vaginal sponges. For oral lesions and colds due to nasal herpes, lozenges can be used. *Medical Hypotheses* 17 (June 1985): 157–165.

In a study of 20 "Type A" personalities and 19 "Type B" personalities, the "Type A" personalities had higher levels of zinc in their red blood cells and lower levels in their urine. After a 20-minute stressful task, urinary zinc was increased in both groups, but more so in the "Type A." "Type A" personalities appear to deplete zinc most rapidly in stressful situations. *Journal of the American College of Nutrition* 4 (April–June 1985): 165–172.

In a study of 9 healthy male runners, it was found that strenuous running led to significant losses of chromium and zinc. *Biological Trace Element Research* 6 (1984): 327–336.

## The Immune System

In this study, 83 normal human subjects were given 660 milligrams of zinc sulfate daily for one month. When compared with 20 untreated controls, the zinc-supplemented group experienced significantly increased lymphocyte responses. This beneficial effect does not result from a correction of latent zinc deficiency. The authors note that the supplementation of an excess of zinc had no effect on serum copper. They suggest that since the treatment is so well documented, nontoxic, and inexpensive, their findings encourage additional studies in various conditions associated with immune deficiencies. *American Journal of Clinical Nutrition* 34 (1981): 88–93.

Zinc deficiencies in animals have been shown to impair a variety of immune functions and defense mechanisms, including function of the thymus, spleen, and lymph nodes; depressed killer cells; and antibody responsiveness. These were corrected by zinc supplementation. *American Journal of Clinical Nutrition* (Supplement) 35:2 (1982): 449–451.

The author notes that zinc deficiencies have been reported in many malignant conditions, and that this is frequently associated with a high copper-to-zinc ratio. A significant survival advantage was demonstrated for patients with squamous cell lung cancer who had high zinc concentrations in their blood. *Progress in Clinical and Biological Research* 129 (1983): 1–33.

The authors studied 88 healthy people, ages 1 month to 85 years, and 72 people with Down's syndrome, ages 10 days to 25 years. They found that biologically active thymic hormone (involved in immunity) decreased with age in normal subjects, and was low in most Down's syndrome subjects, regardless of age. When zinc was added to samples of their blood plasma, thymic hormone activity increased to levels found in healthy young people. *The Lancet* I (May 5, 1984): 983–986.

In a study involving kidney disease patients, the authors found that supplementation with zinc improved their lymphocyte function. *Nephron* 40 (May 1985): 13–21.

The author proposes that zinc deficiency may be a factor in the development of AIDS (Acquired Immune Deficiency Syndrome). Zinc deficiency has been associated with acquired immune deficiency states of other types. Since semen contains a remarkable quantity of zinc, sexually overactive men will have a large loss of zinc. *Journal of the American Medical Association* 252 (September 21, 1984): 1,401–1,410.

People with AIDS had much lower zinc levels than did control subjects, and nearly undetectable thymulin. When zinc was added to blood samples, thymulin increased to the same levels as those found in controls. Some of the immune deficiency observed in AIDS may be the result of poor zinc status, and supplementation may correct some of the immune derangement. *Journal of the American Medical Association* 259 (February 12, 1988): 839–840.

## Anorexia Nervosa

The authors studied 8 women with anorexia nervosa and 8 healthy women. Zinc levels after meals were significantly lower in anorexic women than in the controls. The authors hypothesize that food restriction may lead to reduced zinc levels, which, in turn, may result in impaired small intestinal metabolism and zinc absorption. *The Lancet* I (May 4, 1985): 1,041–1,042 (letter).

In this case history, a 13-year-old girl with anorexia nervosa was found to have an impaired sense of taste, which is a common early symptom of zinc deficiency. She was given a total of 30 milligrams of zinc per day for 2 weeks, and then 150 milligrams daily for 4 months. She regained her appetite and sense of taste and overcame her depression. Ten months after zinc supplements were stopped, she showed signs of recurrence. When supplements were resumed, she returned to normal. *The Lancet* II (August 11, 1984): 350.

In this randomized double-blind placebo-controlled trial, 35 female anorexia nervosa patients received either 100 milligrams of zinc gluconate or a placebo. The rate of increase in body mass in the supplemented patients was twice that in the unsupplemented group. The authors conclude that zinc supplementation may improve the rate of weight gain in anorexia nervosa patients. *International Journal of Eating Disorders* 15 (1994): 251–255.

## The Prostate Gland

Zinc inhibits the specific binding of androgens to the prostatic cytosol and nuclear androgen receptors. *Acta Endocrinologia* 105 (1984): 281–288.

Zinc supplementation reduced the size of the prostate and BPH (benign prostatic hypertrophy) symptomatology in the majority of patients. *Federation Proceedings* 35 (1976): 361.

In one study, 19 patients took 150 milligrams of zinc sulfate (supplying 34 milligrams of elemental zinc) for 2 months, followed by 11 to 23 milligrams of elemental zinc. All patients reported symptomatic improvement, and 14 out of 19 patients experienced shrinkage of the prostate. *Zinc and the Prostate,* presentation at the annual meeting of the American Medical Association, Chicago, 1974.

## Lead and Cadmium Accumulation

In a study comparing hair mineral concentrations of normal and hypertensive women, researchers found that hypertensives had 5 times as much cadmium, 2.5 times as much lead, and almost 3 times as much zinc as did the controls. They suggest that enhanced dietary zinc might prevent the hypertensive effect of cadmium. *Bulletin of Environmental Contamination and Toxicology* 32 (May 1984): 525–532.

## Behavioral Changes

Experimental monkeys were marginally deprived of zinc from conception and compared with controls. In the deprived monkeys, the amount and variety of problem behaviors were significantly less than in the controls (10 to 71 percent). These and other results suggest that syndromes of lethargy, apathy, and slowed activity are characteristic behavioral effects of marginal zinc deprivation in primates. *American Journal of Clinical Nutrition* 42 (1985): 1,229–1,239.

## Osteoporosis

This article reviewed the importance of copper, manganese, and zinc supplementation, in addition to calcium, for increasing mineral density in postmenopausal women. In a 2-year double-blind placebo-controlled trial involving 200 postmenopausal women, the group taking 1,000 milligrams of calcium (as calcium citrate-malate) had a bone mineral density (BMD) of -.50 percent, compared with the placebo group, which had a BMD of -2.23 percent. This demonstrated that the calcium supplement clearly slowed bone loss. However, the group that received 1,000 milligrams of calcium along with 2.5 milligrams of copper, 5 milligrams of manganese, and 15 milligrams of zinc had a BMD of +1.28 percent, indicating an *increase* in BMD. *Journal of the American College of Nutrition* 12 (1993): 384–389.

## Absorption

Normal subjects were given zinc after an overnight fast. The absorption ranged from 40 to 86 percent. Patients with a wide variety of diseases exhibit decreased zinc absorption. *American Journal of Clinical Nutrition* 34 (1981): 2,648–2,652.

In this study, 3 groups of healthy young men were given radiolabeled zinc after eating either 20 grams of coarse bran or Rice Krispies, or nothing. Seven days later, it was found that the group that received no food with the zinc retained the most zinc. Those who ate bran absorbed the least. *Human Nutrition. Clinical Nutrition* 38C (November–December 1984): 433–441.

Laboratory rabbits were given 3 different forms of zinc. Zinc sulfate and zinc pantothenate appeared to be absorbed and utilized similarly. Zinc orotate was absorbed more slowly than these 2. There were no significant differences in the zinc concentrations in the blood. *European Journal of Drug Metabolism and Pharmacokinetics* 7:3 (1982): 233–239.

## Deficiencies

The authors surveyed 58 people of over 62 years of age and found that average zinc intake was only 7 milligrams—less than half the RDA. Lower taste acuity was also found in these patients, which is a symptom of zinc deficiency. These findings indicate that this population is at risk for zinc deficiency. *Journal of the American Dietetic Association* 82 (February 1983): 148–153.

The author studied 40 geriatric patients, 20 of whom had senile purpura. The mean plasma level of the patients with purpura was below the lowest zinc level in patients without this condition. The author concludes that senile purpura may be due to a zinc deficiency, possibly combined with deficiencies in other trace minerals. *Journal of Clinical Pathology* 38 (1985): 1,189–1,191.

The authors note that recent "advances" in food production and an increase in the consumption of highly refined foods have led to a reduction of zinc and other important nutrients in the modern diet. They further note that nutritional deficiency states for some of these trace elements have been reported in certain population groups. *British Journal of Nutrition* 48 (1982): 241–248.

Certain diuretics used to control hypertension cause increased zinc excretion, which may lead to zinc deficiency. Side effects of these drugs, such as impotence, may be linked to zinc depletion rather than to the drugs themselves. Diuretic therapy before or after myocardial infarction may contribute to a zinc deficiency, which might slow the healing of the heart. *South African Medical Journal* 64 (December 1983): 936–941.

Zinc levels were low and prolactin levels were high in 32 men with end-stage kidney disease who had been undergoing hemodialysis. Zinc has been shown to inhibit prolactin synthesis *in vitro*. Zinc deficiency may be the cause of high prolactin levels in these patients. *The Lancet* II (October 5, 1985): 750–751.

Zinc deficiency has been found in people with malabsorption syndromes such as Crohn's disease, celiac disease, short bowel syndrome, and jejunoileal bypass. Diarrhea is a symptom of zinc deficiency and can also cause zinc losses. Subtle signs of zinc deficiency such as loss of appetite, impaired night vision, and depressed immune and mental functions may appear in these patients. *Journal of the American College of Nutrition* 4 (January–March 1985): 49–64.

Zinc blood levels were found to be significantly lower in 54 patients with Crohn's disease than in 19 healthy control subjects. The more severe the disease, the lower the levels. The authors conclude that high disease activity leads to deficiencies of zinc, and that supplementation may be beneficial. *Hepatogastroenterology* 32 (January–February 1985): 34–38.

In this study, healthy men given 400 micrograms of folic acid daily excreted more zinc and had lower blood levels of zinc than did controls. The authors express concern that women treated with folic acid to reverse cervical dysplasia (see Chapter 16) could develop zinc deficiency. This may be a hazard, especially for users of oral contraceptives, which decrease folic acid and zinc. The authors recommend that people receiving folic acid supplements be monitored for zinc status. *Journal of the National Cancer Institute* 74 (January 1985): 263 (letter).

When blood samples from 450 pregnant women were tested, it was found that women with the lowest levels of zinc had significantly higher pregnancy complications, including infection and miscarriage, than did those with the highest zinc levels. *American Journal of Clinical Nutrition* 40 (September 1984): 496–507.

## Skin Disorders

In this study, 3 patients with folliculitis had significant improvement with combination therapy of oral fusidic acid plus zinc sulfate. It is noted that zinc is also used in acrodermatitis enteropathica, acne vulgaris, alopecia areata, and leg ulcers. *ACTA Dermato-Venereologica* 72 (1992): 143–145.

## Toxicity and Adverse Effects

A 57-year-old man who had been taking 450 milligrams of zinc a day for 2 years developed severe anemia, which appears to have been caused by impaired copper metabolism. *Annals of Internal Medicine* 103 (September 1985): 385–386.

In this study, 9 healthy young men were fed a high-protein diet that was supplemented with copper sulfate and various amounts of zinc. Based on the results of this study, the authors conclude that short-term daily intake of 18.5 milligrams of zinc results in increased copper excretion. *American Journal of Clinical Nutrition* 41 (February 1985): 285–292.

In a study of 25 men, the group that received 50 milligrams of zinc per day for 6 weeks did not have their blood levels of copper affected. Copper and zinc superoxide dismutase levels did decrease, which may suggest that zinc supplements decreased copper status. *American Journal of Clinical Nutrition* 40 (October 1984): 743–746.

The authors studied 11 men who were given 150 milligrams of zinc twice a day. None of the subjects showed evidence of untoward side effects. However, there was impairment of some immune functions, which returned to normal when supplements were stopped. There was also a significant decrease of HDLs and a slight increase in LDL levels. *Journal of the American Medical Association* 252 (September 21, 1984): 1,443–1,446.

The authors gave 23 healthy men 50 milligrams of zinc per day for 6 weeks along with a diet marginal in copper. During this time, diastolic blood pressure decreased, and there was a tendency for cholesterol to decrease and HDL cholesterol to increase. *Nutrition Reports International* 32 (August 1985): 373–382.

In a study involving 270 healthy elderly people taking a zinc supplement, it appeared that the zinc abolished the beneficial effects of exercise on increasing serum HDL cholesterol. *Metabolism* 34 (June 1985): 519–523.

Over 200 milligrams per day of zinc were given to 2 patients with Wilson's disease accompanied by severe neurological symptoms. After 2 years of the zinc treatment, liver copper content was reduced by 40 percent in one patient and 57 percent in the other. Their neurological symptoms almost completely disappeared. The authors note that there were no side effects in these patients nor in others taking zinc for up to 25 years. *British Medical Journal* 289 (August 4, 1984): 273–276.

## CHAPTER 25: IRON

### Fatigue and Behavioral Changes

A double-blind study on iron therapy was conducted in chronically fatigued nonanemic women. The researchers found that there is a possibility that some chronically fatigued women may be suffering from iron deficiency even though their hemoglobin value is within the accepted normal range. These patients' individual norm for hemoglobin must be above average. *Annals of Internal Medicine* 52 (1960): 378–381.

Iron-deficient women experience cold sooner, but so do women with low to normal hemoglobin levels. Iron supplementation improves cold tolerance. This suggests that nonanemic women can be symptomatically iron-deficient, and that noniron-deficient women may be experiencing other symptoms as well as cold intolerance, such as effects on attention span and learning, and minor sleep disturbances. *Journal of the American Medical Association* 260 (August 5, 1988): 607.

The authors suggest that iron-deficient nonanemic runners suffer from diminished endurance exercise performance, which can be prevented by oral iron therapy. *American Journal of Diseases of Children* 142 (February 1988): 165–169.

Adolescent runners with low iron levels run the risk of developing iron deficiency and anemia during the running season, and should be treated with iron supplementation. *Journal of Pediatrics* 114 (April 1989): 657–663.

In a group of 69 normal university students, iron status was significantly related to cognitive performance. *American Journal of Clinical Nutrition* 39 (1984): 105–113.

In a study of 78 iron-deficient children and 41 nonanemic children, it was found that the iron-deficient children responded to supplementation with significantly higher school achievement scores. *American Journal of Clinical Nutrition* 42 (1985): 1,221–1,228.

The mental development scores for anemic infants were lower than those for a group of infants with no iron deficiency, and lower than those for a group with iron deficiency but no anemia. After iron supplementation, the anemic infants improved significantly in relation to mental development, cooperativeness, and attention span. Six of the iron-deficient, nonanemic infants also showed significant improvement. The authors suggest that the effect of iron deficiency on behavior may be present during mild iron deficiency and in some cases before overt anemia. *Journal of Pediatrics* 102 (April 1983): 519–522.

## The Immune System

Iron deficiency is one of the likeliest forms of single micronutrient deficiency to occur. Iron is one of the most important micronutrients in terms of its influence on immune system functions and on other aspects of host defense, including increased susceptibility to infection, reduced white blood cell counts, and impaired antibody production. *American Journal of Clinical Nutrition* (Supplement) 35:2 (February 1982): 442–449.

## Angular Cheilosis

Of 156 cases of angular cheilosis observed in a dental practice, 19.2 percent were due to iron deficiency, and only 5.8 percent to vitamin B deficiencies. In 17 of the 30 iron-deficient patients, the condition was accompanied by smooth tongue and difficulty swallowing, which represents a premalignant condition called Plummer-Vinson syndrome. *Journal of Oral Medicine* 39 (October–December 1984): 199–206.

## Triglycerides

In a study involving laboratory rats, the group that was iron-deficient showed liver triglyceride levels 8 times as high as those of the iron-sufficient controls. *Journal of Nutrition* 115 (January 1985): 138–145.

## Salt Craving

A hypertensive 33-year-old woman had a salt craving that caused her to consume a half pound of salt per week. After treatment with large amounts of iron, her craving decreased dramatically. The authors note that pica, the compulsive consumption of particular substances, occurs in about 50 percent of iron-deficient patients, half of whom eat ice. Salt craving is recognized as a symptom of several conditions, but has not been previously reported in connection with iron deficiency. *American Journal of Kidney Diseases* 5 (January 1985): 67–68.

## Low Intakes

The authors studied the diets of 74 female college students. Based on 4-day dietary records, they found that only 6 of the 74 met the RDA for iron. *Nutritional Reports International* 31 (February 1985): 281–285.

Iron deficiency is the most common single nutrient deficiency in the world. The authors note that even in the absence of anemia, iron deficiency may have detrimental effects on behavior and learning. *The New England Journal of Medicine* 313 (November 7, 1985): 1,239–1,240.

The actual foods eaten by lacto-ovo vegetarian women were analyzed, and it was found that their average iron intake was 11 to 14 milligrams per day. These women had normal hemoglobin values, and were not considered to be anemic. However, they also did not appear to have enough iron stores to cope with heavy menstrual losses or pregnancy without possible jeopardy to their iron nutritional status. *Nutrition Report International* 27 (January 1983): 199–206.

## Sports Anemia

Blood tests were performed on 43 male athletes who ran 50 to 200 kilometers (30 to 125 miles) per week, and on 119 men with ordinary levels of physical activity. Some of the tests indicated that the runners showed signs of anemia, but other tests showed that inadequate iron was not the cause. The authors postulate that the runners' false anemia was due to mechanical injury of red blood cells, not to decreased iron. *Acta Medica Scandinavica* 216:2 (1984): 157–164.

## Toxicity and Adverse Effects

The authors studied the effect of iron supplementation on zinc status in 291 healthy infants. They found no evidence that the iron supplements compromised zinc absorption. *American Journal of Clinical Nutrition* 42 (October 1985): 683–687.

The author provides specific arguments against the suggestion that high stores of iron in the body are a risk factor for cancer, and comments that numerous studies have failed to support the hypothesis. *The New England Journal of Medicine* 320 (April 13, 1989): 1,012–1,014.

The author comments on the low correlation between high iron in the body and increased risk of cancer. *The New England Journal of Medicine* 319 (October 20, 1988): 1,047–1,052.

This is a commentary on the role of iron in heart disease. A 3-year Finnish study of 1,391 men, ages 42 to 60, showed an increased risk in heart attack with serum ferritin levels of at least 200 micrograms per deciliter. Two follow-up studies found no link between serum ferritin and heart attack. No link between dietary iron intake and heart disease has been found. *Medical Tribune* (April 8, 1993): 7.

This study assessed the relation of serum iron, dietary iron, and the use of iron supplements to the risk of heart attack in thousands of patients. Although an association between serum iron levels and heart attack was found, there was no association found with dietary iron or iron supplements. The association of higher serum iron with heart attack was not explained by iron intake. *Epidemiology* 5 (1994): 243–246.

## CHAPTER 26: COPPER

### Bone Density

This article reviewed the importance of copper, manganese, and zinc supplementation, in addition to calcium, for increasing mineral density in postmenopausal women. In a 2-year double-blind placebo-controlled trial involving 200 postmenopausal women, the group taking 1,000 milligrams of calcium (as calcium citrate-malate) had a bone mineral density (BMD) of -.50 percent, compared with the placebo group, which had a BMD of -2.23 percent. This demonstrated that the calcium supplement clearly slowed bone loss. However, the group that received 1,000 milligrams of calcium along with 2.5 milligrams of copper, 5 milligrams of manganese, and 15 milligrams of zinc had a BMD of +1.28 percent, indicating an *increase* in BMD. *Journal of the American College of Nutrition* 12 (1993): 384–389.

### Immunity

Experimentally induced deficits or excesses of copper have each been reported to increase the severity of infection in laboratory animals. *American Journal of Clinical Nutrition* (Supplement) 35:2 (February 1982): 455.

### Copper Compounds

Copper complexes have been shown to be effective anti-inflammatory, anti-ulcer, anti-convulsant, anticancer, and antidiabetic agents. *Biological Trace Element Research* 5 (1983): 257–273.

Copper complexes of antiarthritic drugs are more potent as anti-inflammatory agents, are less toxic than parent compounds, and have potent anti-ulcer activity. *Inflammation* 1:3 (1976): 317–331.

Copper complexes of anti-arthritic drugs are more potent than the parent drugs, and are used to treat a wide range of degenerative diseases, such as rheumatoid arthritis, ankylosing spondylitis, and lupus erythematosus. *Inflammation* 2:3 (1977): 217–238.

Urinary copper was measured in 5 patients with chorea and in 22 controls. In 4 of the chorea patients, copper was markedly depressed. When copper supplements were given to a chorea patient, her symptoms began to lessen within 3 weeks, and she improved steadily over the next 3 months. When a placebo was substituted, her shoulder and arm jerking returned within 4 days. The authors suggest that copper deficiency could be an underlying abnormality in some patients with chorea. *Biological Psychiatry* 19 (December 1984): 1,677–1,684.

### Cholesterol

Copper and other trace minerals have been shown to lower cholesterol in experimental animals and humans. A copper deficiency is associated with increased cholesterol levels, and the mean copper intake in United States diets is approximately half the RDA. Copper deficiency is suspected to occur in the United States population and abroad. *Federation Proceedings* 41 (September 1982): 2,807–2,812.

A healthy 29-year-old man was given a copper-depleting diet for 105 days. The total cholesterol in his blood plasma increased from 202 to 234 milligrams. In addition, 6 abnormal heartbeats were recorded near the end of depletion. When his copper was replenished over a period of 39 days, his cholesterol levels returned to normal. The authors conclude that diets inadequate in copper lead to high cholesterol and abnormal ECG patterns, and may be important in the development of ischemic heart disease. *Metabolism* 33 (December 1984): 1,112–1,118.

## Pregnancy and Oral Contraceptive Use

This study found that pregnant women take in marginal amounts of zinc (8.6 milligrams per day) and copper (0.95 milligrams), resulting in poor body retention. Supplements containing 10 to 12 milligrams of zinc and 2 milligrams of copper combined with normal dietary intakes are sufficient to achieve positive balance during pregnancy. The authors point out that prenatal zinc and copper deficiencies in animals have been shown to cause birth defects. *American Journal of Clinical Nutrition* 42 (June 1985): 1,184–1,192.

In 259 pregnant women being screened for fetal abnormalities, the average blood copper level was lower in pregnancies that ended in spontaneous abortion and in which fetal abnormalities were discovered. The authors suggest that decreased copper levels in the mother may be associated with the development of spontaneous abortion and neural tube defects. *Clinical Chemistry* 30 (October 1984): 1,676–1,677.

Blood copper levels were significantly elevated during oral contraceptive treatment in experimental monkeys. *American Journal of Clinical Nutrition* 35 (1982): 1,408–1,416.

## Absorption and Depletion

Copper absorption was measured in patients with celiac disease (inability to digest the gluten in cereal grains) and in healthy controls. The controls absorbed 67 percent more copper than the celiac patients. The authors conclude that patients with intestinal disease have a reduced uptake of copper, zinc, and perhaps other minerals, and may have signs of deficiency. *Science of the Total Environment* 42 (March 15, 1985): 29–36.

A 36-year-old woman complained of difficulty walking and had other signs of copper deficiency, including anemia. After 3 weeks of copper therapy, her symptoms improved. She had been taking an antacid that contained aluminum, magnesium, sodium, and other oxides for 6 years. The authors conclude that use of antacids should be considered a risk factor for copper deficiency. *Nutrition Reviews* 42 (September 1984): 319–321.

## Copper Toxicity From Tap Water

This article reports on a family in Vermont who acquired copper intoxication from drinking water from their faucet, indicating that tap water must be taken into consideration when determining copper intakes. *Pediatrics* 74:6 (1984): 1,103–1,106.

## CHAPTER 27: MANGANESE

### Overview

The author reviews the functions of manganese in the body, including normal bone growth and development, enzyme activation, normal lipid metabolism, reproduction, and nerve function. Corinne H. Robinson, *Normal and Therapeutic Nutrition*, 15th ed. (New York: Macmillan, 1977), 119–120.

## Osteoporosis

This article reviewed the importance of copper, manganese, and zinc supplementation, in addition to calcium, for increasing mineral density in postmenopausal women. In a 2-year double-blind placebo-controlled trial involving 200 postmenopausal women, the group taking 1,000 milligrams of calcium (as calcium citrate-malate) had a bone mineral density (BMD) of -.50 percent, compared with the placebo group, which had a BMD of -2.23 percent. This demonstrated that the calcium supplement clearly slowed bone loss. However, the group that received 1,000 milligrams of calcium along with 2.5 milligrams of copper, 5 milligrams of manganese, and 15 milligrams of zinc had a BMD of +1.28 percent, indicating an *increase* in BMD. *Journal of the American College of Nutrition* 12 (1993): 384–389.

## Birth Defects

A total of 61 infants and their mothers were tested for manganese levels. Infants with congenital malformations (including central nervous system defects, cleft lip and palate, and hermaphroditism) and their mothers both had much lower levels of manganese than did normal infants and their mothers. The authors conclude that low levels of manganese could be a factor in the development of birth defects. *American Journal of Clinical Nutrition* 41 (May 1985): 1,042–1,044.

Congenital dislocation of the hip is high in certain areas of France, Canada, and the United States. It may be due to manganese deficiency, which results from the practice of alkalinizing the soil, thereby impairing the absorption of manganese by plants. Further experimental work showed that a manganese-deficient diet leads to bone and joint malformation of the offspring. *South African Medical Journal* 63:12 (1983): 393.

## Epilepsy

In this study, blood manganese levels were measured in 197 young patients with convulsive disorders and 120 children without neurologic problems. The blood manganese levels were significantly lower in patients with convulsive disorders when compared with controls. The researchers conclude that low manganese levels may heighten a tendency to seizures. They also note that rats fed manganese-deficient diets have an increased susceptibility to convulsions. *Biochemical Medicine* 33 (March–April 1985): 246–255.

## The Immune System

Manganese stimulates microphage, phagocyte, granulocyte, and antibody activity. *American Journal of Clinical Nutrition* (Supplement) 35:2 (February 1982): 456.

Manganese deficiency reduces superoxide dismutase, a substance that prevents free radical damage. *Journal of Nutrition* 114 (1984): 1,438–1,446.

## Glucose Tolerance

The offspring of manganese-deficient laboratory rats were maintained on a manganese-deficient diet. They experienced significantly greater hyperglycemia and lower blood insulin levels than did rats fed a diet sufficient in manganese. The authors concluded that manganese deficiency during prenatal and postnatal periods may result in an impaired ability to synthesize insulin. *Journal of Nutrition* 114 (August 1984): 1,438–1,446.

Guinea pigs born to manganese-deficient mothers and fed manganese-deficient diets had abnormal glucose tolerance. *Journal of Nutrition* 94 (1968): 89–94.

The authors report on an 18-year-old male who had been controlling his diabetes with an alfalfa extract, which is high in manganese. When the hospital allowed this man to use his extract, it was found that his blood sugar could be reduced from 648 milligrams per milliliter to 68 milligrams per milliliter within 2 hours. This was repeated on 12 occasions, with the same response. The authors suggest that the manganese contained in the extract was responsible for the blood sugar-lowering effect. *The Lancet* (December 29, 1962): 1,318.

## Toxicity

Toxicity to manganese may occur with environmental exposure such as mining. Toxicity may appear as delusional thinking and hyperactivity. Subsequently, symptoms similar to Parkinson's disease appear. *Environmental Research* 34 (1984): 242–249.

## CHAPTER 28: CHROMIUM

### Glucose Tolerance

In a double-blind crossover study, 76 volunteers were given 200 micrograms of chromium per day. The researchers noted significant improvements in the glucose tolerance of a number of subjects. The authors point out that marginal dietary intake of chromium apparently is widespread in the United States and other developed countries, and that often well-balanced meals do not provide adequate chromium. *American Journal of Clinical Nutrition* 36 (December 1982): 1,184–1,193.

In this study, 5 hyperglycemic people were given 218 micrograms of chromium daily for 6 months. All of them had improved blood glucose control. They also had significant lowering of total serum-to-HDL cholesterol ratios, corresponding to halving their risk of coronary heart disease. *Nutrition Report International* 30 (October 1984): 911–918.

In this study, 6 noninsulin-dependent diabetics were given approximately 20 micrograms of chromium daily in the form of brewer's yeast. After 2 weeks of supplementation, their mean fasting serum glucose and insulin resistance were both closer to normal. The authors postulate that chromium replenished the cells' stores of chromium and increased the effects of insulin. *General Pharmacology* 15 (November–December 1984): 535–539.

Glucose-intolerant monkeys deficient in chromium were supplemented with chromium. Some improvement was seen after 3 weeks. After 22 weeks on chromium, 8 of 9 previously impaired animals had normal test results. This report also cites data demonstrating that chromium-deficient rats are less responsive to insulin than are rats given sufficient chromium. More than half of the 185 chromium-deficient rats showed a positive test for urine sugar, compared with only 9 of 87 chromium-supplemented controls. *Physiological Reviews* 49 (April 1969): 165–203.

In this study, 16 healthy elderly volunteers were divided into three groups and given 200 micrograms of chromium, 100 milligrams of nicotinic acid, or 200 micrograms of chromium and 100 milligrams of nicotinic acid daily for 28 days. Only the chromium-nicotinate complex caused a 15-percent decrease in the glucose area integrated total, and a 7-percent decrease in fasting glucose. It is possible that the inability to respond to chromium supplementation may result from suboptimal levels of dietary nicotinic acid. *Metabolism* 36:9 (September 1987): 896–899.

In this study, 10 elderly people were supplemented with chromium. Four out of the ten experienced a disappearance of all abnormal features of the glucose tolerance test.

The pattern of response in these individuals suggests the possibility that the nonresponders were suffering from such a severe chromium deficiency that a longer period of supplementation may have been required for them to show a response. *Metabolism* 17 (February 1968): 114–125.

Chromium picolinate was shown to significantly lower serum lipids including total cholesterol and LDL cholesterol, to raise HDL cholesterol, and to lower glucose in human subjects. It is an effective agent for the treatment of lipid disorders. *Western Journal of Medicine* 152 (1990): 41–45.

## Lean Body Mass and Decreased Body Fat

In this study, 42 football players were randomly given either 1.6 milligrams of chromium picolinate (200 micrograms of trivalent chromium) or a placebo for 42 days. In the group given chromium picolinate, lean body mass increased significantly after only 14 days and continued to increase until the end of the study. Total body weight decreased significantly by 2.63 pounds, and total body fat decreased from 15.8 percent to 12.2 percent—a loss of 22 percent of body fat. The results of this study confirm previous findings that chromium picolinate accelerates the development of lean body mass and concurrent loss of body fat. It may be a safe alternative to anabolic steroids. *International Journal of Biosocial and Medical Research* 11:2 (December 1989): 163–180.

## High Cholesterol

This report reviews several animal and human studies that show a correlation between chromium deficiency and diabetes as well as high cholesterol levels in the blood. *Southern Medical Journal* 70 (December 1977): 1,449–1,453.

In this study, subjects were given 24 to 48 micrograms of GTF (organic) chromium, in the form of brewer's yeast, daily for 8 weeks. The treatment resulted in decreased levels of total cholesterol and increased levels of HDL cholesterol. The authors found it striking that treatment with organic chromium raised HDL cholesterol in physically active, relatively young adults with normal blood lipid levels, as well as in subjects with high blood lipid levels. They also noted that previous investigations have shown that GTF chromium influenced blood glucose levels, insulin response, and lipid levels. *Journal of the American College of Nutrition* 1 (1982): 263–274.

In this study, 200 micrograms of chromium plus 100 milligrams of niacin lowered serum cholesterol levels in patients with hypercholesterolemia. Supplementation for 4 months resulted in a further decrease in serum cholesterol. These results are similar to those seen with the administration of 2,000 milligrams of niacin. *Journal of Family Practice* 27 (December 1988): 603–606.

## Psoriasis

This study examined the role of insulin resistance in psoriasis. Sores of psoriatic severity improved in response to chromium in patients with insulin resistance. Chromium supplementation may improve psoriasis and insulin resistance in these patients. *Journal of the American College of Nutrition* 12 (1993): 588/abstract 35.

## Deficiencies

A sizable portion of the American subjects studied had low or negligible amounts of chromium in their tissues compared with individuals in other countries. The total amounts indicated that Africans had 1.9 times, Near Easterners 4.4 times, and Far Easterners 5 times as much chromium as did Americans. In addition, the aortas of American subjects showed less chromium than did those of other Caucasian, Black, and Asian subjects from around the world. American Journal of Clinical Nutrition 21 (March 1968): 230–244.

Marginal dietary chromium intake is widespread in the United States and other developed countries. In a double-blind study of 76 people, chromium or a placebo was given for three months. Chromium was used as well as absorbed by the subjects, as indicated by a significant improvement in the glucose tolerance of a number of subjects. American Journal of Clinical Nutrition 36 (December 1982): 1,184–1,193.

In a study of 9 healthy male runners, the authors found that strenuous running led to significant losses of chromium, presumably because of its increased use in glucose metabolism. *Biological Trace Element Research* 6 (1984): 327–336.

## CHAPTER 29: SELENIUM

### Cancer

The authors review the anticancer properties of selenium in humans and experimental animals. Dietary selenium intake is inversely correlated with death from leukemia and cancers of the breast, ovary, lung, colon, rectum, and prostate. Selenium should be considered not only as a preventive, but also as a therapeutic agent in cancer treatment, and may act additively or synergistically with drug and X-ray treatments. *Journal of Agricultural Food Chemistry* 32 (May–June 1984): 436–442.

Many animal studies demonstrate a cancer-protective effect of selenium. Human epidemiological studies suggest that cancer risk is reduced in people living in high-selenium areas, in people with high-selenium food supplies, and in people with higher blood levels of selenium. *Seminars in Oncology* 10 (September 1983): 305–310.

Selenium supplementation in animals reduces the frequency of chemically induced cancers and inhibits the growth of transplanted tumors. In a study of over 10,000 people, the average selenium level of 111 subjects who subsequently developed cancer was lower than that of the 210 matched controls. Also, the risk of cancer was twice as high for people in the lowest quintile of selenium levels. *The Lancet* (July 16, 1983): 130–134.

In this study involving 240 patients with skin cancer and 103 controls, the mean selenium level of all skin cancer patients was significantly lower than that of controls. This study supports the hypothesis that higher blood selenium levels reduce the risk of developing some cancers. *Nutrition and Cancer* 6 (January–March 1984): 13–21.

A population of over 8,000 with low selenium levels was followed for 6 years. Cancer was subsequently diagnosed in 128 people who had significantly lower selenium levels than the controls. The authors suggest that selenium may act by reducing the mutagenicity of carcinogens, by affecting carcinogen metabolism, or by protecting against oxidative damage. *American Journal of Epidemiology* 120 (September 1984): 342–349.

The authors studied 12,000 people in Finland, 51 of whom died of cancer during the following 4 years. They found that selenium levels were significantly lower in cancer patients than in controls, and that the difference was greater in smokers than in nonsmokers. The risk of cancer mortality in people with the lowest selenium levels was nearly 6 times greater than that of the controls. For people with both low selenium levels and low vitamin E levels, the risk of death from cancer was more than 11 times that of people who had higher levels of both these nutrients. The data suggests that dietary selenium deficiency is associated with an increased risk of fatal cancer, that low vitamin E intake may enhance this effect, and that decreased vitamin A intake contributes to the risk of lung cancer among smoking men with low selenium intake. *British Medical Journal* 290 (February 9, 1985): 417–420.

This study showed that vitamin E enhances selenium's ability to inhibit the development of breast cancer in laboratory rats treated with a potent carcinogen. In general, the chemopreventive effect of selenium is manifested in the form of lower tumor incidence, a reduction in the size of tumors, and a longer latency period. *Cancer Research* 43 (November 1983): 5,335–5,341.

The combined effect of selenium and vitamin A on breast cancer development in rats was studied. This investigation provided evidence that vitamin A increases the protective effect of selenium. The authors suggest that the results warrant further study. *Cancer Research* 41 (April 1981): 1,413–1,416.

Several geographic studies have suggested that states or countries with higher selenium levels in the soil and in locally grown foods experience lower death rates from cancer. The author of this review article found that the results of such studies indicate a decreased mortality from cancer of the lung, colon, rectum, bladder, esophagus, pancreas, breast, ovary, and cervix. Lower selenium levels have been found in patients with various types of cancer, as well as lower levels of vitamins E and A and beta-carotene. The author emphasizes the need to consider several nutrients in diet and cancer studies, instead of focusing on just one nutrient per study. He also points out that current selenium trials are limited to 200 micrograms per day, which may not be the optimum amount needed to prevent cancer. *Federation Proceedings* 44 (June 1985): 2,584–2,589.

In a study of 1,458 healthy adults in 24 regions of China, low blood selenium levels were associated with higher deaths from cancer of the stomach, esophagus, liver, and other sites. The authors expect that selenium supplementation will reduce cancer incidence. *Biological Trace Element Research* 7 (January–February 1985): 21–29.

This letter to the editor reviews the research concerning selenium and other antioxidants in protecting the skin from the damages of ultraviolet radiation. In an animal study, selenomethionine was effective in protecting them against UV radiation-induced skin cancer. Selenium retarded the onset and number of lesions and reduced inflammation, blistering, and pigmentation. The author notes that he has given as much as 600 micrograms to patients without any toxic side effects. He recommends daily doses of 3 grams of vitamin C, 800 international units of vitamin E, and 200 micrograms of selenium to protect against excessive UV radiation. *Canadian Medical Association Journal* 147 (September 15, 1992): 839–840.

## Cardiovascular Disease

The authors studied over 8,000 people in Finland. During a follow-up period of 7 years, 367 of these people had heart attacks or died of heart disease. Their mean serum selenium levels were lower than those of the controls. Those with the lowest selenium levels had a 6- to 7-fold increase in the risk of death from heart disease. *The Lancet* (July 24, 1982): 175–179.

## Skin Conditions

In a study of patients with acne, those given 400 micrograms per day of selenium and 25 international units per day of vitamin E showed improvement in their condition. In patients not treated, there was a marked worsening of the acne. A few patients who were previously treated with zinc and tetracycline experienced complete healing of the acne when given the supplements. In addition, 3 patients with seborrheic dermatitis also improved with this treatment. *Acta Dermatologica Venerealogica* 64 (1984): 9–14.

## Rheumatoid Arthritis

The authors measured the selenium levels of 87 rheumatoid arthritis patients. Low selenium levels were found in all patients, with lowest levels in those with the most severe disease. Although selenium deficiency is probably not a primary etiological factor in rheumatoid arthritis, patients with low selenium levels may develop more severe disease.

Selenium supplementation might have some therapeutic benefit in rheumatoid arthritis. *Scandinavian Journal of Rheumatology* 14 (April–June 1985): 97–101.

In this study, 7 rheumatoid arthritis patients who no longer responded to conventional treatment were given 350 micrograms of selenium and 400 international units of vitamin E daily. Ten to fourteen days later, their normal treatment was resumed. In 4 patients, joint pain disappeared. In the remaining 3 patients, joint pain was diminished and mobility was markedly increased. *Biological Trace Element Research* 7 (May–June 1985): 195–198.

## Muscular Dystrophy

The author notes that it is well known that muscular dystrophy in cattle and sheep is a selenium-deficiency disease preventable by supplementation. In this study of 24 patients with muscular dystrophy, serum selenium levels were lower for patients than for controls. Patients who were more severely disabled had lower selenium levels than did patients with mild symptoms. One patient received selenium therapy and experienced considerable functional improvement. The authors suggest that muscular dystrophy may be a selenium-deficiency disease. A long-term study is being undertaken. *Acta Medica Scandinavica* 211 (1982): 493–499.

## The Elderly

In a double-blind study involving 30 elderly people, half received 1,720 micrograms of sodium selenate, 45 micrograms of organic selenium, and 400 milligrams of vitamin E. The other half received a placebo. After 2 months, the supplemented group showed obvious improvement in mental well-being when compared with controls. They showed significant improvement in fatigue, anorexia, depression, anxiety, emotional stability, hostility, mental alertness, motivation and initiative, self-care, and interest in the environment. There were no adverse effects after one year of treatment. *Biological Trace Element Research* 7 (April–May 1985): 161–168.

## Immunity

Selenium is needed for a fully functioning immune system. In studies with mice, the offspring of selenium-deficient mice have had impaired immune responses, and selenium supplements have enhanced the effects of vaccines. When a modest excess of selenium was given to dogs, it stimulated their immune systems. This effect was greatest when they were fed diets high in polyunsaturated fats. *American Journal of Clinical Nutrition* (Supplement) 35:2 (1982): 452–453.

## Absorption and Deficiencies

According to this study, selenium levels were significantly greater in humans with selenomethionine than with a selenite supplement. *American Journal of Clinical Nutrition* 42 (1985): 439–448.

In this study, 46 alcoholics were compared with 45 nonalcoholic individuals. Alcoholics had low blood selenium levels, especially if their livers were diseased. The authors conclude that inadequate selenium intake is likely in alcoholics. Impaired absorption, increased requirements, or altered metabolism of selenium may also be factors. Selenium deficiency, by reducing glutathione peroxidase activity, may contribute to liver damage in alcoholics. *American Journal of Clinical Nutrition* 42 (July 1985): 147–151.

In this study, 30 young women were given 150 micrograms of sodium selenate per day, 600 milligrams of vitamin C per day, or both. After 4 weeks, selenium levels were increased by 34 percent in the women taking selenium only, by 29 percent in those taking vitamin C only, and by

63 percent in those taking both. The authors conclude that vitamin C improves the bioavailability of dietary selenium. *Human Nutrition. Clinical Nutrition* 39C (May–June 1985): 221–226.

The authors found that TPN (total parenteral nutrition) patients have lower blood levels of selenium and vitamin E, and recommend supplementation with these nutrients in these individuals. *American Journal of Clinical Nutrition* 42 (1985): 432–438.

Blood selenium levels were measured in 16 patients with celiac disease and in 32 healthy controls. Selenium levels in plasma, leukocytes, and whole blood were significantly lower in celiac patients than in the controls. The authors hypothesize that gluten-free diets might be deficient in selenium, or that selenium may be poorly absorbed by celiac patients. Decreased selenium levels in these individuals may explain the increased incidence of cancers of the gastrointestinal tract and other parts of the body that has been reported in celiac patients. *British Medical Journal* 288 (June 23, 1984): 1,862–1,863.

The authors studied 23 patients with Down's syndrome and found significantly lower plasma selenium levels than in controls. They encourage further studies, including a trial of selenium supplementation. *Acta Paediatrica Scandinavica* 73 (1984): 275–277.

The authors studied 86 Texas oil refinery workers. Selenium levels were significantly lower in industrial workers than in controls. Their glutathione peroxidase levels were also lower. The authors conclude that lower selenium was not due to dietary inadequacy, but may have been due to exposure to environmental oxidants that may affect selenium status. *Nutrition Research* 3 (1983): 805–817.

There is a continuing but controversial interest in the use of hair as a diagnostic tool for the assessment of trace element status. The authors of this paper studied blood and hair selenium before, during, and after selenium supplementation. Selenium supplementation for 6 weeks caused no increase in plasma selenium levels, but did cause an increase in selenium levels in new hair growth. There was a significant decline in hair selenium levels during the final 6 weeks after the selenium supplement was withdrawn. There was no correlation between hair and blood selenium levels. *Nutrition Research* 4 (1984): 577–582.

## Toxicity

The authors report that the average daily selenium intake in an area that was high in selenium but free of toxicity was 750 micrograms. The authors indicate that the chronically toxic dose of dietary selenium is likely to be near 5 milligrams (5,000 micrograms) per day. The chronically toxic dose of sodium selenate is estimated to be lower, in the range of 1 milligram per day. *American Journal of Clinical Nutrition* 37 (May 1983): 872.

The authors review numerous data on the toxicity of selenium. Various studies have shown no adverse effects from the long-term consumption of 500 micrograms, 350 micrograms, or 600 micrograms daily. Selenium intake in China is reported to be 750 micrograms per day with no signs of toxicity. Toxicity for selenium, extrapolated from animal studies, may occur in humans ingesting 1,000 to 2,000 micrograms per day. The Food and Nutrition Board has stated that toxicity occurs in humans ingesting 2,400 to 3,000 micrograms daily. Based on these data, they point out the board's claim that the safe upper limit of 200 micrograms per day is a conservative one and has definite implications for chemoprevention studies based on supplementation. *Seminars in Oncology* 10:3 (1983): 311–319.

## CHAPTER 30: IODINE

### Overview

The author reviews the functions of iodine, its dietary sources, and geographical regions of high incidence of iodine deficiency. Corinne H. Robinson, *Normal and Therapeutic Nutrition*, 15th ed. (New York: Macmillan, 1977), 115–116.

## The Thyroid Gland

Iodine in the form of sodium iodide can be used to treat goiter and hyperthyroidism. A severe iodine deficiency can cause hypothyroidism. *The Merck Manual,* 14th ed. (Rahway, N.J.: Merck Sharp and Dohme Research Laboratories, 1982), 997–1,012.

## Hearing

Children in an area of China with endemic iodine deficiency had a lower hearing level than did children in an area without endemic iodine deficiency. After 3 years of iodine supplementation, thyroid function tests and hearing levels became normal. The authors suggest that hearing loss is one of the iodine deficiency disorders that are now being identified based on a broader understanding of iodine deficiency states. *The Lancet* (September 7, 1985): 518–520.

## Nuclear Accidents

A nuclear reactor accident could pose a hazard to the public because of the release of radioactive iodine, which could damage the thyroid and ultimately lead to thyroid cancer. In the event of such an accident, a single dose of 300 milligrams of potassium iodide would block the uptake of radioactive iodine by the thyroid, and may be advisable in high-risk individuals. *The Lancet* (February 1983): 451.

It is believed that predistribution of potassium iodide tablets to households near nuclear power plants may be worthwhile as a preventive measure in the event of a nuclear accident. *Public Health Reports* 98 (April 1983): 123–126.

## CHAPTER 31: POTASSIUM

## Overview

The author reviews the uses of potassium in the body, good dietary sources, and the causes and symptoms of deficiency. Corinne H. Robinson, *Normal and Therapeutic Nutrition,* 15th ed. (New York: Macmillan, 1977), 130–131.

## Cardiovascular Disease

### Blood Pressure

The authors studied the relationship between dietary nutrients and blood pressure in over 10,000 people. The 10 percent of the group with the highest blood pressure tended to have decreased intakes of calcium, potassium, vitamin A, and vitamin C. *Science* 224 (June 29, 1984): 1,392–1,398.

Only 2 percent of vegetarians have been found to have high blood pressure, as compared with 26 percent of nonvegetarians. Vegetarians with the highest potassium excretion, indicating a high intake, had the lowest blood pressure. *American Journal of Clinical Nutrition* 37 (May 1983): 755–762.

The authors of this article studied 12 subjects with mild hypertension. Some subjects responded to sodium restriction while others responded to potassium supplementation. The authors conclude that individuals respond differently to changes in sodium or potassium intake. *The Lancet* (April 7, 1984): 757–761.

## *Hypertensive Kidney Damage*

Salt-sensitive rats fed a high-salt diet developed hypertension and related symptoms. When potassium was added to their diet, blood pressure was unchanged, but there was less damage to the kidneys. The authors suggest that potassium exerts a protective effect and that blacks in the United States, who have a low potassium intake and a high rate of hypertensive kidney failure, might benefit from tripling their potassium intake. *Hypertension* (Supplement) 6 (March–April 1984): 1,170–1,176.

## *Stroke*

Hypertensive, stroke-prone rats were fed a stroke-inducing diet. After 6 weeks, the group supplemented with potassium had a systolic blood pressure of 187, versus 233 for the unsupplemented group. After 17 weeks, death (due mainly to strokes) was 2 percent in the supplemented group, versus 83 percent in the controls. Mortality was 7 times greater in the unsupplemented group than in the supplemented group, even when blood pressure was the same. The authors concluded that potassium intake at levels similar to those in prehistoric human diets (6 to 10 grams per day) may reduce stroke incidence even when blood pressure is not lowered. *Hypertension* (Supplement I) 7 (May–June 1985): I110–I114.

## Bioavailability and Retention

Since many potassium chloride supplements are distasteful, many physicians tell their patients to consume large amounts of potassium-rich foods, usually in the form of fruit. The authors measured the potassium levels in various fruits and concluded that the retention of potassium in these foods is poor. The authors conclude that potassium chloride supplements must continue to be the mainstays for potassium repletion. *The New England Journal of Medicine* 313 (August 29, 1985): 582–583.

Increasing potassium and decreasing sodium in diets could benefit people with hypertension, those who are overweight, and some diabetics. The authors suggest several approaches to achieving a more favorable sodium-to-potassium ratio in the diet: preserving potassium through steaming rather than boiling foods; adding modest amounts of potassium chloride salt substitute to cooking water; and adding less salt. *The Lancet* (February 12, 1983): 362–363.

## CHAPTER 32: BORON

A study examined the effects of boron on 12 women, ages 48 to 82. Daily supplementation of 3 milligrams of boron markedly reduced their urinary excretion of calcium and magnesium. It also markedly elevated the serum concentration of estradiol and testosterone, suggesting an endocrine mechanism. These findings suggest that supplementation of a low-boron diet induces changes in postmenopausal women consistent with the prevention of calcium loss and bone demineralization. Boron may be an important nutritional factor determining the incidence of osteoporosis. *FASEB Journal* 1 (1987): 394–397.

This review presents the concept that bone health doesn't depend only on estrogen and calcium, but on a wide range of other nutrients, including vitamins $B_6$, C, D, and K; folic acid; and magnesium, manganese, boron, zinc, copper, strontium, and silicon. The typical Western diet, high in sugar and refined foods, appears to be deficient in many of these nutrients. The requirement for certain nutrients may be increased by genetic factors or by metabolic changes that occur during menopause. Supplementation with a balanced combination of appropriate micronutrients may prove to be a useful adjunct to calcium and estrogen therapy. *Journal of the American Osteopathic Association* 4(2) (December 1988): 2–5.

Animal and human research suggests that boron enhances the utilization of vitamin $D_3$, and enhances and mimics some of the effects of estrogen therapy in postmenopausal women to positively affect mental alertness, psychomotor skills, and the cognitive processes of attention and memory. Experiments with humans show that people consuming about .25 milligram per day respond positively to boron supplementation, suggesting that boron intake should be higher than this. Based on both human and animal experimental data, humans may have a boron requirement between .5 and 1.0 milligram a day. *Journal of the American College of Nutrition* 15 (October 1996): 520 (abstract 27).

Analytical evidence reveals lower boron concentrations in femur heads, bones, and synovial fluid in people with arthritis than in those without this disorder. Moreover, bones of patients using boron supplements are much harder to cut than bones of unsupplemented people. Epidemiologic evidence reveals that in areas of the world where boron intakes are 1.0 milligram or less per day, the estimated incidence of arthritis ranges from 20 to 70 percent, versus the 0- to 10-percent incidence in areas where intakes are 3 to 10 milligrams per day. In a double-blind placebo-controlled trial, 50 percent of patients receiving 6 milligrams of boron a day experienced a significant improvement in their osteoarthritis symptoms, versus only a 10-percent improvement in those receiving the placebo. *Environmental Health Perspectives* 102 (November 1994): S83–S85.

## CHAPTER 33: COENZYME Q₁₀

### Overviews

This review of human and animal studies and reports documents the beneficial effects of CoQ for ischemic heart disease, congestive heart failure, toxin-induced cardiotoxicity, angina pectoris, arrhythmia, and hypertension. The authors found that the most intriguing property of CoQ is its potential to protect and preserve ischemic myocardium during surgery. *Medical Clinics of North America* 72 (January 1988): 243–257.

CoQ is capable of stabilizing cell membranes and preventing depletion of metabolites necessary for creating ATP. It may also help inhibit free radical formation. K. Folkers and Y. Yamamura, eds., *Biomedical and Clinical Aspects of Coenzyme Q*, vol. 3 (Amsterdam: Elsevier/North Holland Biomedical Press, 1981), 159–168.

This article reviews the biochemistry and use of coenzyme Q10. Double-blind studies have confirmed the efficacy of CoQ as an adjunctive treatment in heart failure. *Clinical Investigator* 71 (1993): S116–S123.

This study evaluated the effects of CoQ in the prevention of LDL oxidation. Doses of CoQ ranged from 100 to 300 milligrams. The results of the study demonstrated that CoQ is incorporated into plasma and all lipoproteins, increasing their resistance to oxidation. *Biochimica Et Biophysica ACTA* 1126 (1993): 247–254.

### Cardiovascular Disease

#### Angina

In a placebo-controlled trial of subjects with chronic stable angina, the group receiving CoQ was able to exercise significantly longer than the control group. K. Folkers and Y. Yamamura, eds., *Biomedical and Clinical Aspects of Coenzyme Q*, vol. 4 (Amsterdam: Elsevier Science Publ. BV, 1984), 291–301.

In a double-blind random crossover study of 12 patients with chronic stable angina, exercise time increased significantly in the CoQ-treated group. *American Journal of Cardiology* 56 (1985): 247–251.

In a double-blind crossover study of patients with chronic stable angina, CoQ was found to be as effective as drug therapy in reducing abnormal EKGs during exercise. K.

Folkers and Y. Yamamura, eds., *Biomedical and Clinical Aspects of Coenzyme Q*, vol. 5 (Amsterdam: Elsevier Science Publ. BV, 1985), 385–394.

## Congestive Heart Failure

Approximately 31 reports from Japan have described the beneficial effects of CoQ in small numbers of patients with various forms of congestive heart failure. G. Lenaz, ed., *Coenzyme Q Biochemistry, Bioenergetics, and Clinical Applications of Ubiquitone* (New York: Wiley-Interscience, 1985), 479–507.

In this study, 12 patients with congestive heart failure that was inadequately controlled with digitalis and diuretics were given CoQ daily. After one month, 67 percent showed clinical improvement in their symptoms of dyspnea (difficulty breathing) and fatigue. *Drug Experimental Clinical Research XI* 8 (1985): 581–593.

In a placebo-controlled double-blind crossover study of 19 patients with congestive heart failure, the group that received CoQ experienced better heart function. *Drug Experimental Clinical Research XI* 8 (1985): 577–579.

In a placebo-controlled double-blind crossover study of 12 patients with congestive heart failure, the group that received CoQ demonstrated a significant increase in stroke volume and ejection fraction (pumping action). *Proceedings of the National Academy of Science USA* 82 (1985): 4,240–4,244.

At the Seventh International Symposium on the biomedical and clinical aspects of CoQ in Copenhagen, Dr. Karl Folkers reviewed more than 35 years of research. On the basis of this research, he concluded that heart failure is caused by a dominant deficiency of CoQ, and that its clinical use is definitely positive to the health and well-being of the patient. *Clinical Investigator* 71 (1993): S51–54.

This study evaluated the use of CoQ at a dose of 50 milligrams per day in 1,715 patients with chronic congestive heart failure. Patients were stabilized on standard therapy for 3 months. In just 4 weeks, CoQ resulted in improvements in shortness of breath at rest, exertional dyspnea, palpitations, cyanosis, hepatomegaly, pulmonary rates, ankle edema, heart rate, and systolic and diastolic blood pressure. The authors conclude that CoQ treatment led to an improvement in the signs and symptoms and quality of life in these patients. *Clinical Investigator* 71 (1993): S129–S133.

This study evaluated the effect of CoQ supplementation on 2,500 patients with heart failure. Patients received 50 to 150 mg of CoQ, with the majority receiving 100 milligrams. After 3 months, there was improvement in: cyanosis, 81 percent; edema, 76.9 percent; pulmonary rates, 78.4 percent; palpitations, 75.7 percent; sweating, 82.4 percent; arrhythmia, 62 percent; insomnia, 60.2 percent; vertigo, 73 percent; and nocturia, 50.7 percent. *Clinical Investigator* 71 (1993): S145–S149.

This study evaluated 641 patients with heart failure in a double-blind trial. Patients received CoQ at a dose of 2 milligrams per kilogram per day (e.g., 140 milligrams of CoQ for a 154-pound man). Episodes of pulmonary edema or cardiac asthma were significantly reduced with CoQ supplementation. Results suggest that CoQ therapy, along with conventional therapy, reduces hospitalization for worsening of heart failure and the incidence of serious complications in patients with congestive heart failure. *Clinical Investigator* 71 (1993): S134–S136.

## Heart Surgery

This randomized study indicates that administering CoQ before surgery improves post-surgical cardiac output. *Thoracic Surgery* 33 (1982): 145–151.

When CoQ was given to patients prior to coronary bypass surgery, the CoQ group had less damage to the heart muscle. K. Folkers and Y. Yamamura, eds., *Biomedical and Clinical Aspects of Coenzyme Q*, vol. 4 (Amsterdam: Elsevier Science Publ. BV, 1984), 333–342.

The investigators reviewed the research on the use of CoQ for high-risk cardiac surgery patients who have a natural or clinically induced coenzyme $Q_{10}$ deficiency. The results support the use of oral CoQ in high-risk heart surgery patients. *Clinical Investigator* 71 (1993): S155–S161.

## Arrhythmia

In one of several studies using CoQ in patients with arrhythmia, the results suggest that 20 to 25 percent of patients experience improvement. *Tohoku Journal of Experimental Medicine* 141 (Supplement, 1983): 453–463.

Coenzyme $Q_{10}$ was found to be of therapeutic value in patients experiencing arrhythmia as a side effect of psychotropic drugs. Lenaz, G., ed., *Coenzyme Q* (New York: John Wiley & Sons, 1985), 479–505.

## Hypertension

In this small double-blind controlled study of subjects with essential hypertension, the group that received CoQ showed a decline in both systolic and diastolic blood pressure after 12 weeks. K. Folkers and Y. Yamamura, eds., *Biomedical and Clinical Aspects of Coenzyme Q*, vol. 5 (Amsterdam: Elsevier Science Publ. BV, 1986), 337–343.

This uncontrolled clinical trial suggests that CoQ may be effective in certain patients with essential hypertension. *Clinical Endocrinology* 25 (1977): 1,019–1,023.

The results of this uncontrolled clinical trial suggest that treatment with CoQ might be effective for essential hypertension. *Journal of Adult Disease* 6 (1976): 281–286.

In this study, 10 patients with hypertension were treated with 100 milligrams of CoQ for 10 weeks. At the end of the trial, CoQ had significantly decreased both systolic and diastolic blood pressure and total serum cholesterol levels, with a small increase in HDL cholesterol. CoQ's beneficial effects on cholesterol and hypertension is significant. *Current Therapeutic Research* 51 (1992): 668–672.

## Mitral Valve Prolapse

This study evaluated the use of CoQ in patients with mitral valve prolapse, chronic fatigue, or hypertension. CoQ supplementation reduced high blood pressure in 80 percent of the patients with hypertension, and improved diastolic function in all patients. A reduction in myocardial thickness in 53 percent of hypertensives and 36 percent of the combined prolapse and fatigue group also occurred. *Clinical Investigator* 71 (1993): S140–S144.

This study examined the use of CoQ in children, ages 6 to 16, with mitral valve prolapse. The normal Frank-Starling mechanism was recovered due to CoQ supplementation, which may improve disturbed bioenergetic function at a molecular level. Researchers used 3 to 3.4 milligrams per kilogram per day, with no adverse side effects noted. *Clinical Investigator* 71 (1993): S150–S154.

## Ischemia

Compared with controls, animal hearts pretreated with CoQ had significantly less depletion of ATP and reduced mitochondrial oxygen utilization following induced ischemia. Coenzyme $Q_{10}$ protects against ischemia. K. Folkers and Y. Yamamura, eds., *Biomedical and Clinical Aspects of Coenzyme Q*, vol. 2 (Amsterdam: Elsevier/North Holland Biomedical Press, 1980), 409–425.

## Cancer and AIDS

Cancer patients receiving CoQ with Adriamycin may experience less toxin-induced injury from Adriamycin. It is possible that pretreatment with CoQ might allow patients to receive higher and more effective doses of Adriamycin. *Journal of Molecular Medicine* 3 (1978): 289–298.

The researchers report a reduction in Adriamycin's toxic effect on the heart in cancer patients who received CoQ prior to chemotherapy treatment. K. Folkers and Y. Yamamura, Y., eds., *Biomedical and Clinical Aspects of Coenzyme Q*, vol. 3 (Amsterdam: Elsevier/North Holland Biomedical Press, 1981), 339–412.

Dr. Knud Lockwood, M.D., an oncologist from Denmark, described his successful treatment of 32 breast cancer patients who were treated with conventional therapy and were at high risk for recurrence. He used high-dose CoQ therapy (90 to 390 milligrams), and after 24 months, all were still alive when at least 6 deaths would have been expected. Six of the 32 patients showed partial tumor regression, and 2 had complete tumor regression. *Biochemical and Biophysical Research Communications* 199 (March 30, 1994): 1,504–1,508.

In this report, AIDS showed a striking clinical response to high-dose CoQ therapy. Also, 8 new case histories of cancer patients, plus 2 previously reported cases, showed survival periods of 5 to 15 years. *Biochemical and Biophysical Research Communications* 192(1) (April 15, 1993): 241–245.

## Chronic Fatigue and Immune Dysfunction

In this study, compared with healthy controls, a group of female patients, ages 28 to 43, who had had CFIDS for 2 to 5 years, had lower tissue levels of CoQ. Levels were further decreased after exercise. Supplementation with 100 milligrams of CoQ for 90 days resulted in 100 percent improvement in exercise tolerance; 85 percent improvement in postexercise fatigue; and 90 percent improvement in overall clinical symptoms. *Coenzyme Q10* presented at the American College of Nutrition Annual Meeting, 1996, San Francisco.

## Other Uses

A double-blind study was conducted with patients who had progressive muscular dystrophies and neurogenic atrophies, including Duchenne, Becker, limb-girdle dystrophies, myotonic dystrophy, and Welander disease. After a three-month trial using CoQ, improved physical well-being was observed. The results indicate that the subjects' impaired myocardial function and impaired skeletal muscle function may be associated, and that both may be improved with CoQ therapy. *Proceedings of the National Academy of Science* 32 (July 1985): 4,513–4,516.

CoQ markedly improved the course of treatment for periodontal disease in both double-blind and open trials. In one study, 100 percent of patients receiving CoQ improved, compared with 30 percent of the placebo group. *Communications in Chemistry, Pathology, and Pharmacology* 14 (1976): 715.

The benefits of CoQ supplementation for patients recovering from surgery for severe periodontal disease were dramatic. *Research Communication in Chemistry, Pathology, and Pharmacology* 12 (1975): 111.

In this study, 39 stable diabetics received CoQ. Fasting blood sugar was reduced by at least 80 percent in 12, and by at least 30 percent in another 12, while ketone levels fell in 13. *Journal of Vitaminology* 12 (1966): 293.

## Toxicity and Adverse Effects

Mice given CoQ orally, subcutaneously, intramuscularly, or intravenously showed no evidence of toxicity. *Applied Pharmacology* 6 (1972): 769–779.

Up to 600 milligrams per day of CoQ were given to rabbits. No toxic effects were observed. *Applied Pharmacology* 6 (1972): 781–786.

## CHAPTER 34: ESSENTIAL FATTY ACIDS

### Overview

This article reviews the therapeutic effects of diet and nutrients on dermatological disorders. Topics covered include fish oil, evening primrose oil, and Chinese herbal teas for atopic dermatitis; vitamins and wound healing; vitamins A and D for psoriasis; and antioxidants, vitamins, and skin cancer. *Journal of the American Academy of Dermatology* 29 (1993): 447–461.

### Omega-3 Fatty Acids (EPA, DHA, and Fish Oil)

#### Cardiovascular Disease

In this ground-breaking study, the researchers discovered that the diet of Greenland Eskimos, who have a low incidence of heart disease, is very high in a specific fatty acid called EPA, which is very low in the diets of individuals in North America. *The Lancet* II (1978): 117.

In a long-term investigation of middle-aged men in Holland, mortality from coronary heart disease was more than 50 percent lower among those who ate at least one ounce of fish per day, versus those who did not eat fish. *The New England Journal of Medicine* 312 (1985): 1,205.

This study was designed to determine whether fish oil or another constituent of fish affected heart disease. The researchers found that the fish oil diet decreased cholesterol up to 27 percent, and triglycerides to 64 percent, as compared with the control diet, which was a typical low-fat therapeutic diet. *The New England Journal of Medicine* 312 (1985): 1,210.

The author of this review article comments that it is not likely that lowering fat and cholesterol intake alone will eliminate the enormous disparity in heart disease between North America and countries such as Japan, with low rates of heart disease. There is considerable evidence to indicate that the consumption of fish oils containing omega-3 polyunsaturated fatty acids decreases both platelet aggregation and interactions between platelets and the vessel wall. It may be necessary to focus on recommendations that affect risk factors other than cholesterol, such as the consumption of fish 2 to 3 times weekly, or the consumption of EPA supplements. *Canadian Medical Association Journal* 139 (September 1, 1988): 377–381.

Omega-3 fatty acids decrease the tendency of platelets to clump or adhere to the vessel walls; they also dilate the blood vessels. Polyunsaturated fats, present in vegetable oils, encourage platelets to clump and adhere, and blood vessels to constrict. Including omega-3 fatty acids in a diet low in saturated fats and polyunsaturated fats appears to be a prudent and effective approach to preventing heart disease. *American Journal of Cardiology* 60 (October 30, 1987): 23G–32G.

In this study, healthy men and women were given either 3, 9, or 18 fish oil capsules per day. The results demonstrated that even low doses of fish oil given to subjects consuming a typical Western diet can have a beneficial effect on fats in the blood. *Nutrition Reports International* 38 (July 1988): 165–172.

In this study of men with high triglyceride levels, treatment with EPA and safflower oil reduced triglyceride levels by 44 percent. *American Journal of Clinical Nutrition* 48 (October 1988): 992–997.

In this double-blind study of patients with coronary artery disease, EPA was found to be an effective means of lowering fats in the blood, especially triglycerides. It also lowered blood pressure. (Presented at the American College of Cardiology, Atlanta, GA, March 13, 1986.)

The author of this overview of EPA and the multiple ways in which it protects against heart disease concludes that EPA may be even more effective than aspirin in this regard. *Annals of Internal Medicine* 107 (1987): 890–899.

This article reviews the many benefits of fish oil in relation to cardiovascular disease. The author suggests that a modest intake of fish oil will prove to be a safer, more efficacious alternative to mass prophylaxis with aspirin. *The Lancet* (May 14, 1988): 1,081–1,083.

In this controlled study of patients with exercise-induced angina, those given EPA for 4 weeks lowered their triglycerides and blood pressure. Half of the men did not experience chest pain during exercise, as compared with the placebo group. *American Journal of Medicine* 84 (January 1988): 45–52.

Men with hypertension taking 50 milliliters of EPA had a 35-percent reduction in triglycerides and a significant decrease in both systolic and diastolic blood pressure, compared with men taking vegetable oils. *The New England Journal of Medicine* 320 (April 20, 1989): 1,037–1,043.

The data suggests a dose-related effect of EPA on blood fats and blood pressure in subjects with mild hypertension. *Atherosclerosis* 62 (1986): 259–265.

In a study of 82 men who had successful angioplasty, only 17 percent of those who received supplements of EPA had recurrence of a serious amount of blockage, as compared with 46 percent of the control subjects. *The New England Journal of Medicine* 319 (September 22, 1988): 733–740.

The authors of this article suggest that fish oil can be used to prevent overgrowth of cells in vein grafts used for arterial bypass surgery. *Journal of Thoracic and Cardiovascular Research* 89 (1985): 351–357.

This is an analysis of 31 placebo-controlled trials evaluating the role of fish oil on blood pressure in 1,356 patients. There was a statistically significant dose-response effect observed in relation to the effects of EPA and DHA on blood pressure. The hypotensive effect of fish oil may be strongest in hypertensive subjects and those with clinical atherosclerotic disease or hypercholesterolemia. *Circulation* 88 (August 1993): 523–533.

The results of this analysis demonstrate that restenosis after coronary angioplasty is reduced by fish oil supplementation. The benefit is dose dependent, with doses ranging from 3,000 to 6,484 milligrams. *Archives of Internal Medicine* 153 (July 12, 1993): 1,595–1,601.

This is an extensive review on the role of fish oil in cardiovascular disease. Fish oils have been shown to: reduce triglycerides; reduce platelet reactivity; decrease blood pressure; reduce the use of nitroglycerin in patients with angina pectoris; reduce cardiac arrhythmias; and reduce LDL cholesterol. The increased risk of bleeding in patients taking fish oil is low and is less than with aspirin intake. *Drugs* 47 (1994): 405–424.

This article reviews the role of fibrinogen in cerebrovascular disease. Elevated fibrinogen levels result in generation of atherosclerosis. Fish oil supplementation has resulted in significant reductions in fibrinogen levels. In crossover trials, both serum triglycerides and fibrinogen levels were significantly reduced for up to 48 months in patients with hyperlipidemia who received EPA. *Heart Disease and Stroke* 2 (November–December 1993): 503–506.

This study examines the benefits of antioxidant supplementation added to fish oil supplementation in reducing LDL oxidation. The authors suggest vitamins E and C and probucol as antioxidants that may be of benefit. *Arteriosclerosis and Thrombosis* 13 (December 1993): 1,790–1,797.

In this study, 35 men on a controlled diet were given 15 fish oil capsules or a placebo. The fish oil capsules contained 1 milligram of vitamin E per gram of fat. Fish oil significantly lowered thromboxane levels by 38 percent, suggesting an antithrombotic effect. *Prostaglandins, Leukotrienes, and Essential Fatty Acids* 48 (1993): 305–308.

Three fish oil capsules daily in conjunction with low-dose aspirin was found to reduce the tendency to arterial thrombosis in patients who were being treated for atherosclerotic disease. Those receiving aspirin and fish oil experienced a reduced likelihood of developing symptoms of atherosclerotic disease, including cardiac arrest, heart attack, and stroke, compared with those taking only aspirin. In the Physician's Health Study, aspirin was associated with a slight but significantly increased risk of strokes. *Family Practice News* (December 1, 1992): 9.

Adipose-tissue biopsies and segments of coronary arteries were sampled from 40 consecutive autopsies. The group with the highest degree of coronary artery disease had lower concentrations of DHA in adipose tissue than did the group with the lowest degree. This study supports the hypothesis that a higher consumption of fish oil is associated with a reduced risk of coronary heart disease. *American Journal of Clinical Nutrition* 55 (1992): 1,117–1,119.

## Rheumatoid Arthritis and Other Inflammatory Conditions

In this study, 64 patients with rheumatoid arthritis taking NSAIDS were given 10 MaxEPA or placebo capsules daily for 12 months. There was a significant reduction in NSAIDS use in patients after 3 months of taking MaxEPA. The authors conclude that MaxEPA may be a useful therapy in patients with mild rheumatoid arthritis or those who cannot tolerate NSAIDS. *British Journal of Rheumatology* 32 (1993): 982–989.

This article reviews the role of fish oil in inflammatory conditions such as rheumatoid arthritis, Raynaud's phenomenon, systemic lupus erythematosus, psoriasis, psoriatic arthritis, gout, and osteoarthritis. The results of the study have shown modest clinical benefits. It may be a safer alternative than NSAIDS in some patients. *Seminars in Arthritis and Rheumatism* 21 (June 1992): 368–375.

In this study, 49 patients with RA completed a 24-week prospective double-blind randomized study of dietary supplementation with 27 milligrams per kilogram of EPA (18 milligrams per kilogram of DHA), 54 milligrams per kilogram of EPA (36 milligrams per kilogram of DHA), or olive oil capsules (6.8 grams of oleic acid). A total of 5 of 45 clinical measures were significantly changed from baseline in the olive oil group; 8 of 45 in the low-dose fish oil group; and 21 of 45 in the high-dose fish oil group. The authors conclude that clinical benefits of fish oil supplementation are more commonly observed at higher doses for time intervals that are longer than previously studied. The use of olive oil also requires further investigation. *Arthritis and Rheumatism* 33 (June 1990): 810–815.

In this study, 7 healthy subjects were given EPA supplements. The results suggest that diets enriched with fish oil-derived fatty acids may have anti-inflammatory effects. *The New England Journal of Medicine* 312 (1985): 1,217.

Supplementation of the diet with EPA reduces the synthesis of inflammatory prostaglandins, and so could offer a novel and nontoxic approach to treating inflammatory conditions. *Biochemical Pharmacology* 35: 5 (1986): 779–785.

Omega-3 fatty acids alter chronic inflammation and improve immunity. *Federal Proceedings* 46 (1987): 1,173.

In a controlled study, patients with rheumatoid arthritis who received EPA for 12 weeks had less morning stiffness and fewer tender joints. One to two months after stopping EPA, their condition deteriorated. *The Lancet* I (January 26, 1985): 184–187.

Fish oil results in the subjective alleviation of rheumatoid arthritis. *Annals of Internal Medicine* 106 (April 1987): 497.

Fish oil was shown to suppress lupus in mice. *Journal of Immunology* 134:3 (March 1985): 1, 914-1,919.

## Skin Conditions

In this study, 10 capsules of EPA were given to patients with atopic dermatitis for 12 weeks. Compared with controls, the EPA significantly reduced symptoms, particularly of itch and scale. Higher doses and longer treatment might have resulted in further improvement. *British Journal of Dermatology* 117 (1987): 463–469.

A double-blind randomized controlled study of psoriasis patients was conducted for 8 weeks. The group that received EPA had a significant lessening of symptoms, and tended to have less of their body surface affected. *The Lancet* (February 20, 1988): 378–380.

## Cancer

Eskimos eating diets high in EPA have a lower incidence of breast cancer than do Americans who ingest vegetable oils and animal fats that have almost no EPA. *Acta Medica Scandia* 192 (1972): 85.

In an animal study of advanced breast cancer, omega-3 fatty acid-rich diets prolonged survival and slowed tumor growth. This may have implications for the use of omega-3 diets at the time of diagnosis or surgical therapy for Stage II disease. *American Journal of Clinical Nutrition* 45 (1987): 859.

In a double-blind randomized crossover trial, 12 volunteers not at risk for colon cancer were given fish oil supplements or a corn oil placebo. A reduction in mucosal enzyme (ornithine decarboxylase) was seen with fish oil supplementation. Increased levels of this enzyme may be a risk factor for colon cancer in patients with familial polyps. *Gastroenterology* 105 (1993): 1,317–1,322.

## Dysmenorhea

In this study, 42 adolescent girls with dysmenorrhea (painful menstruation) were randomly assigned to 2 groups. Group 1 received 1,080 milligrams of EPA, 720 milligrams of DHA, and 1.5 milligrams of vitamin E. Group 2 received a placebo. At the end of 2 months, the supplemented group experienced a marked reduction in Cox Menstrual Symptom Scale, suggesting that omega-3 fatty acid supplementation has a beneficial effect on symptoms of dysmenorrhea in adolescents. *American Journal of Obstetrics and Gynecology* 174 (1996): 1,335–1,338.

## Kidney Disease

In an animal study, EPA supplements prevented the deterioration of kidney function in mice with kidney disease. *Prostaglandins, Leukotrienes, and Medicine* 22 (1986): 323–334.

Results from this study show that EPA produces potentially beneficial effects on blood fats, platelets, and blood pressure, and so may help protect against cardiovascular disease in high-risk dialysis patients. *Nephronology Research* (1986): 196–202.

## The Nervous System

Schizophrenia, manic-depressive-like illnesses, phobic and neurotic disorders, tinnitus, and fatigue appear to be helped by omega-3 fatty acids. *Biological Psychiatry* (September 1981): 1.

## The Retina

Results of an animal study suggest that omega-3 may be an essential nutrient and may have a specific function in the photoreceptor membranes of the retina. Prenatal and postnatal intake may influence retina development. *Journal of Clinical Investigation* 73 (January 1984): 272–276.

## Aerobic Exercise

In this study, 34 hyperlipidemic subjects were randomly assigned to one of 4 groups: fish oil and exercise; aerobic exercise; fish oil; or corn oil. The aerobic exercise improved the effects of fish oil on LDL cholesterol and apo-B, and improved fitness and body composition. *Medicine and Science in Sports and Exercise* 21 (1989): 498–505.

# Omega-6 Fatty Acids (GLA)

## Overview

This is an extensive review on the biochemistry of GLA and potential benefits in diseases such as diabetes, skin disorders (e.g., atopic eczema), reproduction, breast pain, PMS, inflammatory and autoimmune disorders, cardiovascular disease, and viral infections. A major source of GLA is evening primrose oil. The author argues that since high-dose fish oil may lower GLA levels, it should be given with GLA. *Progress in Lipid Research* 31 (1992): 163–194.

## Cardiovascular Disease

A mixture of EPA and GLA have synergistic activities. Blood platelet aggregation is inhibited more strongly with a mixture of these essential fatty acids than by either compound alone. *JPN Kokai Tokkyo Koho* (July 1986).

GLA as evening primrose oil has a cholesterol-lowering effect on rats. *Annals of Nutrition and Metabolism* 301 (1986): 289–299.

GLA weakened the cardiovascular responses to chronic stress in animals with a genetic predisposition to hypertension. These findings suggest that GLA may be useful in preventing hypertension in high-risk individuals. *Lipids* 20 (1985): 573–577.

Evening primrose oil offers the angina patient relief when given for a relatively short period of time. *Abstract Book, International Prostaglandin Conference,* Washington, D.C. (May 1979): 10.

## Rheumatoid Arthritis and Other Inflammatory Conditions

In this study, patients with rheumatoid arthritis and with gastrointestinal lesions from nonsteroidal anti-inflammatory drugs (NSAIDS) were supplemented daily with 6 grams of evening primrose oil (EPO) supplying 540 milligrams of GLA or a placebo in a double-blind controlled trial. EPO significantly reduced morning stiffness in 3 months. Pain and articular index were reduced in 6 months with the olive oil placebo. In both groups, 23 percent were able to reduce NSAIDS. The authors note other studies that have shown better effects with EPO with regard to reducing or eliminating NSAIDS. They suggest that olive oil should not be used as a placebo, and should be investigated for its own therapeutic effect. The authors feel they can recommend EPO for use in mild RA. *British Journal of Rheumatology* 30 (1991): 370–372.

This randomized double-blind controlled study compared daily supplementation of 1,400 milligrams of GLA from borage seed oil to a cotton seed oil placebo in patients with

RA. GLA resulted in a significant reduction of signs and symptoms. The placebo group had no change. This was a very high-dose GLA study with no adverse effects noted in any subjects. *Annals of Internal Medicine* 119 (November 1, 1993): 867–873.

Inflammation was suppressed in rats who were exposed to a potent inflammatory agent by the administration of evening primrose oil. Chronic proliferative adjuvant arthritis was also suppressed. *Progressive Lipid Research* 20 (1987): 885–888.

EPA and GLA were given to rats in which acute inflammation was induced. GLA significantly suppressed the cellular phase of inflammation. EPA suppressed the fluid phase. *Arthritis and Rheumatism Journal* 31 (December 1988): 1,543–1,551.

Observations of adults with atopic eczema and normal controls suggest that atopic eczema is associated with abnormal metabolism of essential fatty acids. Treatment with oral evening primrose oil partially corrected the abnormality. *British Journal of Dermatology* 11 (1984): 643–648.

In a controlled study on the effect of evening primrose oil on atopic eczema, the treatment group had a statistically significant improvement in the severity of symptoms and percentage of body surface affected. *British Journal of Dermatology* 117 (1987): 11–19.

## Cancer

Evening primrose oil has caused a highly significant inhibition of cancer growth without affecting normal cells. It is likely that GLA bypasses the block in the metabolic pathway of cancer cells that prevents them from producing an immunoactivating substance. The regression of cancer through such proposed normalization offers preliminary hope for a new effective and harmless approach to the treatment of cancer. *S.A. Medical Journal* 62 (October 2, 1982): 505.

Recent studies suggest that GLA may unblock the metabolic defect in cancer cells involving a substance that is responsible for the conversion of linoleic acid to gamma linoleic acid. This may explain some of its anticancer properties. *Medical Hypotheses* 12 (1983): 195–201.

In a study of breast cancer in rats, evening primrose oil inhibited the growth of the tumors. *Journal of Nutrition, Growth, and Cancer* 2 (1985): 41.

The cells of 2 types of human esophageal cancers were treated with GLA. After 7 days, the cells died. *S.A. Medical Journal* 62 (October 30, 1982): 681–683.

Malignant liver cells reverted back to normal when GLA was added to the cell culture. *S.A. Medical Journal* 62 (1982): 683.

## Premenstrual Syndrome

In a double-blind crossover study, patients received either evening primrose oil or a placebo for 2 menstrual cycles, and then a placebo for a further 2 cycles. Overall improvement in the treated group was 60 percent, compared with 40 percent for the placebo. The greatest results were for irritability and depression. *Journal of Reproductive Medicine* 28 (1983): 465–468.

In this study, 30 patients with severe PMS received evening primrose oil twice a day, or a placebo. After 4 menstrual cycles, the treated group showed decreased menstrual symptoms compared with the placebo group. *Journal of Reproductive Medicine* 39 (1985): 149–153.

## Diabetes

Seven noninsulin-dependent diabetics were given 4 grams of evening primrose oil, 2.4 grams of sardine oil, and 200 milligrams of vitamin E for 4 weeks. Fasting plasma glucose, hemoglobin A1C, total cholesterol, body weight, and percentage of body fat decreased significantly. These results suggest that these supplements are useful in improving abnormal lipid parameters in diabetic patients. *Prostaglandins, Leukotrienes and Essential Fatty Acids* 49 (1993): 569–571.

## Obesity

Researchers have observed that the more linoleic acid in the fat tissue, the less obese the person. This may be of particular significance in those with a family history of obesity. *2nd International Congress on Essential Fatty Acids, Prostaglandins, and Leukotrienes* (March 1985).

In this study, obese subjects received a daily supplement of evening primrose oil. After 6 to 8 weeks, half of those who were more than 10 percent overweight noted a reduction in appetite and had lost weight without dieting. The higher the dose of primrose oil, the greater the weight loss. *IRCS Journal of Medical Science* 7 (1979): 52.

## CHAPTER 35: FLAVONOIDS

### Overviews

These are 3 excellent reviews of all aspects of known plant flavonoid modulation of the immune system, cancer, and inflammatory cell function. They cover many topics, including T-lymphocytes, B-lymphocytes, natural killer cells, interferon, macrophages, monocytes, mast cells, basophils, neutrophils, eosinophils, and platelets. *Human Nutrition—A Comprehensive Treatise*, vol. 8, *Nutrition and Immunology*, ed. David M. Klurfeld (New York: Plenum Press, 1993), 239–266. J. B. Harborne, ed., *The Flavonoids: Advances in Research Since 1986.* (London: Chapman & Hall, 1993), 619–652. *Biochemical Pharmacology* 43 (1992): 1,167–1,179.

### Cancer and Viruses

Selected naturally occurring flavonoids (amentoflavone, scutellarein, and quercetin) had a concentration-dependent effect on inhibiting the reverse transcriptases of several viral and cancer cell lines. *Antiviral Research* 12 (1989): 99–110.

The flavonoid daidzein inhibited the replication of promyelocytic leukemia cells *in vitro* and *in vivo* in experimental models. *Anticancer Research* 13 (1993): 1,049–1,054.

Quercetin exhibits antitumor activity. In this study, it significantly inhibited the growth of squamous cell carcinoma of head and neck origin. Its inhibitory effect on malignant cells appears to be selective and dose dependent. *The American Journal of Surgery* 158 (October 1989): 351–355.

This study demonstrates the synergistic effect of vitamin C and two plant flavonoids on squamous cell carcinoma. Exposure of these cancer cells to ascorbic acid and either fisitin or quercetin resulted in 61-percent and 45-percent inhibition, respectively. Ascorbic acid may amplify the cancer growth inhibitory effect of flavonoids. *Anticancer Drugs* 4 (February 1993): 91–96.

The citrus flavonoids nobilitin and tangeretin markedly inhibited the growth of human squamous carcinoma cell lines. *Cancer Letters* 56 (1991): 147–152.

The flavonoid daidzein has been shown to have a potent differentiation-inducing effect on leukemia cells, both *in vitro* and *in vivo*. The medicinal plant *pueralia lobata* has high levels of daidzein, which may explain its therapeutic use since ancient times. *Anticancer Research* 13 (1993): 1,049–1,054.

A popular herbal medicine in Japan known as *Sho-saiko-to* has been used in the treatment of various chronic liver diseases. This study demonstrated that this herbal medicine inhibits the proliferation of a human hepatocellular carcinoma cell line and cholangiocarcinoma cell line. In fact, the combination of herbs in this medicine more strongly inhibited these cell lines than did any one of its major ingredients. *Cancer Research* 54 (January 15, 1994): 448–454.

Four flavonoids—baicalein, quercetin, quercitagentin, and myricetin—were found to be potent inhibitors of reverse transcriptases from Rauscher murine leukemia virus (RLV) and human immunodeficiency virus (HIV). Each of these flavonoids almost completely inhibited the activity of RLV. HIV reverse transcriptase was inhibited by these flavonoids 100 percent, 100 percent, 90 percent, and 70 percent, respectively. *European Journal of Biochemistry* 190 (1990): 469–476.

The ability of baicalin, a flavonoid purified from the Chinese medicinal herb *Scutellaria baicaleniss georgi*, to inhibit human T-cell leukemia virus type 1 (HTLV-1) was examined. Baicalin produced concentration-dependent inhibition of HTLV-1 replication in infected T- and B-cells. It also inhibited reverse transcriptase activity in the infected cells. These results suggest that baicalin may be a potential therapeutic agent against HTLV-1 associated T-cell disease. *The Journal of Infectious Diseases* 165 (1992): 433–437.

This study illustrates the variable spectrum of antiviral activity of several naturally occurring flavonoids against certain viruses. The viruses used in this study included herpes simplex virus type 1, polio virus type 1, parainfluenza virus type 3, and respiratory syncytial virus. For example, quercetin caused a concentration-dependent reduction in the infectivity of each virus and reduced intracellular replication. On the other hand, catechin inhibited only the infectivity of specific viruses. *Journal of Medical Virology* 15 (1985): 71–79.

Among 87 chemically defined tannins and related compounds, several were found to significantly inhibit both the cytopathic effect of HIV and the expression of HIV antigen in HTLV-I. *Antiviral Research* 18 (1992): 91–103.

## Phytoestrogens

This letter to the editor comments on potential explanations as to why Japanese women have less severe menopausal symptoms than Westerners. The excretion of flavonoids (i.e., genistein, daidzein) was as much as 100 to a 1,000 times higher than in American and Finnish women. Flavonoid excretion was associated with intakes of soy products such as tofu, miso, aburage, atuage, koridofu, soy beans, and boiled beans. This high level of flavonoid phytoestrogen intake may partly explain why hot flashes and other menopausal symptoms are reduced in Japanese women. *The Lancet* 339 (May 16, 1992): 1,233.

## Other Uses

In a controlled study, the authors found that 35 percent more vitamin C was absorbed when it was given with a citrus bioflavonoid extract than when it was given alone. They note that processing removes much of the bioflavonoids from frozen or reconstituted fruit juice. *American Journal of Clinical Nutrition* 48 (September 1988): 601–604.

Bioflavonoids scavenge free radicals. They also have an antibiotic-like action because of their influence on cell permeability. *Biochemical Pharmacology* 32:7 (1983): 1,141–1,148.

Experimental animals were given a drug to induce capillary fragility. Bioflavonoids were able to prevent this condition. *Farmaco Edizione Scientifica* 38:11 (1983): 67–72.

Bioflavonoids were effective in reducing cholesterol levels in the blood and liver in experimental animals. *Indian Journal of Experimental Biology* 19 (August 1981): 787–789.

Patients suffering from chronic venous insufficiency were treated with a combination of drugs containing bioflavonoids, which proved more effective in repairing tissue damage and alleviating symptoms. *Clinica Therapeutica* 108 (January 31, 1984): 91–98.

Bioflavonoids were shown to have pharmacological properties that may prove useful in the treatment of some connective tissue disorders, including rheumatoid arthritis. *Scandinavian Journal of Rheumatism* 12 (1983): 39–42.

Many bioflavonoids have anti-inflammatory effects that are considered to be superior to that of corticosteroids because of their low toxicity. Bioflavonoids are also useful for correcting capillary permeability and fragility. *Agents and Actions* 12:3 (1982): 298–302.

In this study, 13 out of 30 bioflavonoids tested inhibited the enzyme responsible for cataract formation. Animal studies have suggested that bioflavonoids may be useful in the prevention of cataracts in diabetics. *Biochemical Pharmacology* 31:23 (1982): 3,807–3,822.

In this study, 2 bioflavonoids were shown to inhibit cataract formation in humans. *Biochemical Pharmacology* 32:13 (1983): 1,995–1,998.

This review article highlights some potential therapeutic interventions for osteoporosis. Studies have demonstrated that the flavonoid ipriflavone increased the total amount of calcium retained in bones when orally administered to animals. In a Japanese study, a daily dose of 600 milligrams was found to be an optimal therapeutic regimen for the treatment of osteoporosis. Other regimens used dose levels of 1,200 milligrams per day. Ipriflavone appears to be a safe and rational alternative to estrogen replacement therapy in preventing bone loss. This review also highlights the use of vitamin D and its metabolites on both the prevention and treatment of osteoporosis. *The American Journal of Medicine* 95 (November 30, 1993, Supplement 5A): 69–74.

Angiogenesis is pathological during the development and progression of many diseases, including rheumatoid arthritis, psoriasis, retrolental fibroplasia, diabetic retinopathy, and hemangiomas; during the rejection of organ transplants; and in cancerous tumors and metastasis. The flavonoid genisteine is a powerful inhibitor of angiogenesis. *Proceedings of the National Academy of Sciences* 90 (April 1993): 2,690–2,694.

Pycnogenol, a naturally occurring plant flavonoid, significantly inhibited foam cell production by oxidized low-density lipoproteins (LDLs). *The International Conference on Pycnogenol Research*, Bordeaux, France (October 4–6, 1990).

In this study, 90 milligrams of pycnogenol were given daily to 110 persons with varicose veins. Of these subjects, 77 percent demonstrated improvement, and of those who complained of calf cramps, 93 percent had an improvement of symptoms. *Zeitschrift fur Allgemeinmedizin* 51 (June 30, 1975): 839.

Many other studies and reports on pycnogenol are contained in Richard A. Passwater, *The New Superantioxidant—Plus* (New Canaan, CT: Keats Publishing, 1992).

## CHAPTER 36: GARLIC

## Cardiovascular Disease

### *Atherosclerosis, Stroke, and Coronary Thrombosis*

In a review of the available data, the author suggests that garlic may be of value in preventing or treating atherosclerotic diseases. *Nutrition Research* 3 (1983): 119–128.

Garlic extract inhibited human platelet aggregation induced by common aggregating compounds such as ATP, epinephrine, collagen, thrombin, arachidonate, PAF, and the ionophore A-23187. *Thrombosis Research* 32 (1983): 155–169.

Garlic and onion oils inhibited *in vitro* platelet aggregation. *Biochemical Pharmacology* 29 (1980): 3,169–3,173.

Garlic is reputed to offer protection against stroke, coronary thrombosis, and atherosclerosis. These beneficial effects have been attributed to its ability to inhibit platelet aggregation. *American Chemistry Society* 106 (1984): 82–95.

Essential oil of garlic was given to 10 healthy individuals, 10 patients with old myocardial infarction, and 20 patients with acute myocardial infarction. The results indicate that garlic is of value in increasing the body's ability to overcome the clotting factor, fibrin. *Atherosclerosis* 28 (1977): 155.

This is a review article on the health benefits of garlic. Garlic has been shown to reduce cholesterol in human trials. It also reduces the susceptibility of LDL to oxidation. At the Fourth International Congress on Phytotherapy in Munich, Germany, September 1992, Dr. Jorg Grunwald concluded that the 3 main cardiovascular effects of garlic are: reduction of free radicals; reduction of oxidation of lipoproteins, particularly LDL; and inhibition of infiltration of lipids into the vascular wall. It is noted that Kwai garlic is made from Chinese garlic and is a licensed drug for the treatment of atherosclerosis in Germany. Kwai is noted to reduce LDL cholesterol, increase HDL cholesterol, and improve peripheral blood flow. *British Journal of Clinical Practice* 47 (March/April 1993): 64–65.

## Cholesterol

Lowering of cholesterol, triglycerides, LDL, and VLDL, with a rise in HDL, was observed in the majority of subjects who took odor-modified garlic extract. Garlic did not significantly affect the lipids in subjects whose initial levels were relatively low. Of special interest was the initial rise of lipids during the early part of the trial, suggesting possible mobilization of tissue lipids into the circulation during this phase. *Nutrition Research* 7 (1987): 139–149.

Essential oil of garlic significantly lowered serum cholesterol and triglycerides while raising the HDL in 20 healthy volunteers. Garlic was also given to 62 patients with coronary heart disease and elevated cholesterol; their serum cholesterol and triglycerides dropped and their HDL rose. Although blood lipids initially rise during garlic supplementation, and might cause alarm and possible discouragement, no adverse effects associated with this initial rise were noted. *American Journal of Clinical Nutrition* 34 (October 1981): 2,100–2,103.

In this study, 50 grams of freshly extracted juice of garlic or onion, or their essential oils, inhibited high cholesterol levels induced by feeding subjects 100 grams of butter. *Atherosclerosis* 21 (1975): 15–19.

Males ages 18 to 35 with cholesterol levels of 160 to 250 were given 10 grams of raw garlic daily for 2 months. Cholesterol levels decreased significantly in all subjects. *Indian Journal of Physiology and Pharmacology* 23:3 (July–September 1979): 211.

This study with human subjects confirms previous reports of lowered cholesterol and triglycerides with the use of various garlic preparations. Odor-modified garlic may be used in conjunction with dietary modification for control of hyperlipemia. *Nutrition Research* 7 (1987): 139–149.

Using a MEDLINE search, the studies revealed that patients treated with garlic consistently showed a greater decrease in total cholesterol levels when compared with the effects of a placebo. Analysis showed that half to a full clove of garlic (or the equivalent) resulted in a 9-percent reduction in serum cholesterol levels. *Annals of Internal Medicine* 119 (October 1, 1993): 599–605.

In this randomized double-blind trial, 10 volunteers took Kwai garlic or a placebo. After 2 weeks, blood samples revealed that lipoprotein susceptibility to oxidation was lowered by the garlic supplement by 34 percent. The authors note previous garlic studies demonstrating beneficial effects on serum lipids, platelet function, fibrinolysis, and blood pressure. *Lipids* 28 (1993): 465–477.

## Blood Pressure

A small study demonstrated the positive effects of garlic on hypertension. *The Lancet* II (1969): 962.

The author discusses garlic as a new hypertensive agent. *The Lancet* II (1969): 800.

In this study, 70 hypertensive patients were given the equivalent of 50 grams of raw garlic. Of these subjects, 33 had a marked lowering of blood pressure, and 14 had a moderate reduction. The overall reduction was over 60 percent. *Journal of Traditional Chinese Medicine* 6 (1986): 117.

## Infections and Immunity

Garlic has a long history of use for its medicinal antimicrobial and pesticidal properties. In this study, the growth of a variety of species of fungi was inhibited. *Mycologia* 67 (1975): 409.

A fresh extract of garlic was given orally to human volunteers. Within 30 minutes to an hour after administration, anticandidal and anticryptococcal activities were detected in the subjects' blood. *Antimicrobial Agents and Chemotherapy* 23:5 (May 1983): 700–702.

The effect of garlic juice on the growth and respiration of *staphylococcus*, *E. coli*, and *C. albicans* was studied. *Candida albicans* proved to be the most sensitive organism of the 3 examined. *Acta Microbiology Polonica* 5:22 (1973): 51–62.

A mouthwash containing 10 percent garlic produced a drastic reduction in the number of oral bacteria, suggesting a possible use of garlic or its extracts as an antiseptic in mouthwash or toothpaste. *Pharmazie* 38 (1983): 747–748.

Of 16 cases of cryptococcal meningitis given garlic therapy, 6 were cured and 5 improved, giving an effective rate of 68 to 75 percent. Preliminary studies show that garlic may kill fungi directly and improve the patients' immunologic function. The author points out that garlic is also cheap and plentiful, and causes no major side effects. *Chinese Medicine Journal* 93:2 (1980): 123–126.

## Cancer

Garlic extract and other immunotherapy agents were compared in this study, in which mice were injected with bladder cancer cells. Garlic was found to be more effective than 2 of the other agents. No tumor developed at all in mice that received 5 garlic injections directly into the tumor; indirect injections stimulated a moderate tumor reduction. The results suggest that garlic extract protects against cancer by acting directly on tumor cells and by stimulating macrophages and lymphocytes of the immune system. *The Journal of Urology* 136 (1986): 701–705.

In this study, mice were injected with bladder cancer cells and then treated with garlic extract or 3 other immunotherapeutic agents. Garlic was as effective or more effective than the other agents, which can cause side effects and complications. The results of this study are encouraging enough to suggest that clinical evaluation of garlic extract use in humans may be worthwhile. *The Journal of Urology* 137 (1987): 359–362.

Animal studies suggest that garlic and onions may have cancer-inhibiting properties. The authors studied diet and risk of stomach cancer in a high-risk Chinese population. An increased intake of allium vegetables (garlic and onions) was associated with a decreased risk of stomach cancer. *Journal of the National Cancer Institute* 81 (January 18, 1989): 162–164.

This study supports prior research that showed that garlic inhibits tumor formation in chemically induced cancers. In rats exposed to mammary carcinogen, raw garlic powder and garlic extract reduced DMBA-DNA adducts (biochemical markers) of breast cancer by an average of 40 percent. A commercial deodorized garlic powder reduced adducts by 64 percent, and a commercial high-sulfur garlic powder reduced adducts by 56 percent. *Carcinogenesis* 14 (1993): 1,627–1,631.

## Liver Disorders

In this laboratory study, aged garlic extract protected liver cells from potential damage caused by carbon tetrachloride. *Hiroshima Journal of Medical Science* 34:3 (September 1985): 303–309.

This animal study confirmed earlier data that aged garlic extract protects the liver from the damaging effects of carbon tetrachloride and another potent toxin. *Phytotherapy Research* 1 (1988): 1–4.

## Blood Glucose

The results of this animal study suggest that garlic reduces the production of lipids and influences the metabolism of glycogen in rat livers. The hypoglycemic effect of garlic seems to be associated with the increase of the insulin level. *Journal of Nutrition 110 (1980): 931–936.*

## CHAPTER 37: GLUTATHIONE AND N-ACETYLCYSTEINE (NAC)

### Overviews

Oral and intravenous N-acetylcysteine is an antidote for acetaminophen (Tylenol) toxicity. NAC shows promise in the treatment of chronic bronchitis and immune system disorders; as a cancer preventive agent; and in the treatment of diseases including acute pulmonary oxygen toxicity, septicemia, and endotoxin shock. NAC supports glutathione biosynthesis. *Toxicology Letters* 553 (1992): abstract W4-01. See also *Pharmacy Therapy* 60 (1993): 91–120.

Glutathione is important for the detoxification of free radicals, toxic oxygen radicals, thiol-disulfate exchange, and storage and transfer of cysteine. It is very important in organs that are exposed to toxins, such as the liver, kidney, lung, and intestine. *Pharmacological Therapy* 52 (1991): 287–305.

This comprehensive review article discusses the effects of glutathione and ascorbic acid in reducing oxidative stress. The administration of glutathione and vitamin C in patients experiencing high levels of oxidative stress from diseases such as aging, cancer, atherosclerosis, viral infections (including AIDS), stroke, myocardial infarction, and arthritis may be of clinical benefit. *Biochemical Pharmacology* 44 (1992): 1,905–1,915.

### Infection and Immunity

This article reviews the role of glutathione, NAC, and vitamin C supplementation in HIV infection and AIDS, with specific focus on the known fact that glutathione is frequently deficient in these individuals. Glutathione is the main intracellular defense against oxidative stress, and is decreased in the plasma, lung fluid, and T-lymphocytes in individuals with AIDS. NAC and other glutathione-replenishing substances can inhibit oxidative stress and HIV transcription or replication. *The Lancet* 339 (April 11, 1992): 909–912. See also *The Lancet* 339 (June 27, 1992): 1,603–1,604.

The intracellular concentration of glutathione was correlated with the absolute CD4 lymphocyte counts. The concentration of glutathione and mononuclear cells was significantly lower in patients with more advanced immunodeficiency. A single dose of NAC increased the concentration of cysteine in the plasma and mononuclear cells of HIV-infected patients. *AIDS* 6 (1992): 815–819.

An adequate supply of cysteine is important for maintaining the oxidant/antioxidant balance of the immune system. Since glutathione deficiency is prevalent in AIDS patients and important for lymphocyte function, NAC may be important in the treatment of HIV-infected patients. Anecdotal observations have reported that AIDS patients improve substantially on NAC. It is possible that NAC intervention in early-stage patients may help prevent progression of the disease. *Immunology Today* 13 (1992): 211–214.

This study reviewed the synergistic effects of NAC and vitamin C on HIV suppression. NAC caused approximately a 2-fold inhibition of HIV reverse transcriptase activity and had a synergistic effect when tested simultaneously with ascorbic acid. These results support the potent antiviral effects of ascorbic acid and suggest its synergistic effect with compounds such as NAC. *American Journal of Clinical Nutrition* 54 (1991): S1,231–S1,235.

NAC suppresses HIV expression in chronically infected monocytic cells. It has been shown that HIV seropositive patients treated with NAC for 4 months show a normalization in plasma cysteine and a reduction in tumor necrosis factor. The expected decline in CD4 helper cells is diminished. *Toxicology Letters* 54 (1992): SW4–L5.

## Cancer

This review article discusses glutathione deficiency in association with aging and increased cancer risk. It is believed that glutathione is important in the detoxification of a wide variety of carcinogens and free radicals, and in the maintenance of normal immune function. *Experimental Gerontology* 27 (1992): 615–626.

Several studies have demonstrated that sulfur-containing compounds such as glutathione appear to optimize the effectiveness of cisplatin, a potent anticancer drug, in the treatment of ovarian cancer. This combined treatment demonstrated a superiority over conventional cisplatin treatment as follows: 21 out of 21 stage I or stage II patients, and 9 out of 11 stage III patients had no evidence of ovarian cancer. All patients with early disease were alive after a median follow-up of 18 months. In the advanced stage group, 10 out of 11 patients were alive after a median follow-up of 22 months. Glutathione also appears to protect against kidney toxicity of cisplatin. *Cancer Treatment and Reviews* 18 (1991): 253–259.

This article reviews the importance of total parenteral nutrition with L-glutamine and glutathione in cancer patients. Glutathione is important because it helps to protect the gut mucosa from methotrexate, which may damage the gastrointestinal tract. *Physician Assistant Practice* 12 (Summer 1993): 14–16.

Glutathione has been shown to have cancer prevention activity in experimental models. This study evaluated the use of vitamin E, beta-carotene, glutathione, and vitamin C alone or in combination in preventing DMBA-induced cancer in the hamster buccal pouch. The authors conclude that the mixture of antioxidants produced a significant synergistic chemoprevention of oral cancer. *Nutrition and Cancer* 20 (1993): 145–151.

NAC prevented chemotherapy-induced hair loss when administered intravenously or applied topically to animals. *Cancer Investigation* 10 (1992): 271–276.

## Detoxification

NAC given within 12 hours of carbon tetrachloride exposure may decrease the severity of liver and kidney damage. Oral NAC is available and may be of benefit in carbon tetrachloride exposure. *American Family Physician* (October, 1992): 1,199–1,207.

## Sperm Motility

In this study, 11 infertile men with dyspermia received glutathione at 600 milligrams per day intramuscularly for 2 months. This treatment significantly boosted sperm motility patterns and reduced atypical sperm. *Archives of Andrology* 29 (1992): 65–68.

This placebo-controlled double-blind study evaluated the use of 600 milligrams daily of injected glutathione over a 2-month period. The patients had dyspermia associated with unilateral varicocele or a germ-free genital tract inflammation. Glutathione significantly improved sperm motility and sperm morphology *Human Reproduction* 10 (1993): 1,057–1,062.

## Cataracts and Aging

This extensive review article discusses the role of antioxidant nutrients in defending the lens of the eye from oxidative stress. Recent work suggests that supplementing the diet with vitamins C and E decreases the risk of cataract by 50 percent. Keeping high concentrations of glutathione in the lens may also protect against oxidative stress. Abraham Spector, *Oxidative Stress: Oxidants and Antioxidants* (New York: Columbia University, 1991), 529–558.

## Cardiovascular Disease

NAC ingested at doses of 1.2 grams per day for 6 weeks showed a significant decrease in lipoprotein(a) concentrations of approximately 7 percent. *Journal of Internal Medicine* 230 (1991): 519–526.

This study examines the importance of glutathione and glutathione-dependent enzymes in the cellular defense against oxidized low-density lipoproteins. *Journal of Lipid Research* 43 (1993): 479–490.

## Pulmonary Disease

Several studies have demonstrated that the inhalation of NAC (i.e., Mucomyst) is efficacious in controlling chronic bronchitis. *European Respiratory Reviews* 2 (1992): 5–8.

## Parkinson's Disease

There is a reduced level of glutathione in the brains of Parkinson's patients. This may result in oxidative stress that may lead to or be derived from mitochondrial damage. *Annals of Neurology* 32 (1992): S111–S115. See also *Annals of Neurology* 32 (1992): 804–812.

## Surgical Complications

Oxidative stress may participate in creating surgical complications of cardiopulmonary bypass procedures. Antioxidants (e.g., glutathione peroxidase, NAC, and superoxide dismutase) may afford protection in cardiovascular surgery. *Klinische Wochenschrift* 69 (1991): 1,066–1,072.

## CHAPTER 38: L-CARNITINE

### Overview

This excellent review article discusses the metabolism and function of L-carnitine in humans and its therapeutic applications. *Annual Review of Nutrition* 6 (1986): 41–46.

### Sports Nutrition

This article reviews the use of carnitine as an ergogenic aid. For example, in long-distance runners and sprinters, it has been found that L-carnitine supplementation at 2 grams per day over 6 months can increase muscle L-carnitine levels. There were reduced lactate and pyruvate levels in an L-carnitine-supplemented group when 2 grams were given one hour before progressive incremental cycle ergometry exercise to maximal heart rate, exhaustion, or dyspnea. In another study, 5 grams of L-carnitine given for 5 days resulted in a small but significant decrease in heart rate during cycle ergometry. *International Journal of Sports Nutrition* 2 (1992): 185–190.

Several studies have examined the role of L-carnitine in athletic performance. Findings have indicated that trained subjects have greater muscle L-carnitine levels than do their untrained counterparts, and that the performance time of submaximal exercise (80 percent

VO2max) is greatly increased by L-carnitine loading. This study examined the effect of L-carnitine loading (4 grams per day), given over a period of 2 weeks, on the aerobic and anaerobic performance of 6 long-distance runners. It was concluded that as a consequence of L-carnitine loading, VO2max is slightly but significantly raised. *European Journal of Applied Physiology* 54 (1985): 131–135.

In this double-blind crossover trial on 10 moderately trained young men, 2 grams of L-carnitine or a placebo were administered orally. Treatment with L-carnitine significantly increased both maximal oxygen uptake and power output. Carbon dioxide production, pulmonary ventilation, and plasma lactate were reduced. Under these experimental conditions, L-carnitine favored aerobic processes, resulting in a more efficient performance. *European Journal of Applied Physiology* 61 (1990): 486–490.

## Chronic Fatigue Syndrome

Patients with Chronic Fatigue Syndrome appear to be deficient in acyl-carnitine. This deficiency may result in an energy deficit and an intramitochondrial condition in skeletal muscle, possibly resulting in fatigue, myalgia, muscle weakness, and post-exertional malaise. Patients who recovered from general fatigue had their levels of acyl-carnitine increased to normal. *Clinical Infectious Diseases* 18 (1994): S62–S67.

## Cardiovascular Disease

L-propionyl carnitine has been shown to improve the heart's mechanical recovery and other parameters after ischemia-reperfusion. It may act as an energy substrate, directly as an antioxidant, and as a mild iron chelating agent. When compared with D-propionyl carnitine, the L-form has a wider variety of benefits. *Archives of Biochemistry and Biophysics* 296 (August 1, 1992): 394–401.

In humans, supplementation with L-carnitine at a dose of 300 milligrams, 3 times a day, for 12 weeks significantly improved the exercise tolerance of patients with angina. In patients with chronic congestive heart failure, 55 percent improved with supplementation. The results suggest that L-carnitine is a useful therapeutic agent in conjunction with other pharmacologic therapy. *Japanese Circulation Journal* 56 (January 1992): 86–94.

This crossover study evaluated the use of propionyl carnitine supplementation on typical stable effort angina at 500 milligrams, 3 times a day, for 30 days, compared with a placebo. Subjects were 18 males, ages 37 to 70. The authors conclude from the results that propionyl carnitine appears to have an anti-ischemic effect. *Cardiovascular Drugs and Therapy* 4 (1990): 481–486.

## Hemodialysis

Some dialysis patients have abnormalities in carnitine metabolism, resulting in skeletal myopathy, cardiomyopathy, arrhythmias, and plasma lipid abnormalities. Muscle cramps, cardiac arrhythmias, and hypotension may also be related to carnitine metabolism. Given that oral carnitine tablets are the least expensive preparation, the authors believe that the time is ready for routine administration of L-carnitine in hemodialysis. They recommend 660 to 990 milligrams daily or 2 to 3 grams just prior to hemodialysis. *Seminars in Dialysis* 5 (April–June 1992): 94–98.

## The Nervous System

### *Alzheimer's Disease*

In a randomized double-blind trial, patients received 2 grams of acetyl-L-carnitine or a placebo. The patients receiving acetyl-L-carnitine showed a consistently reduced rate of progression that was statistically significant for the Blessed Dementia Scale and for 3 neuropsychological tests. The 2-gram dose used in this study contained 1.6 grams of carnitine—about 5 to 10 times the average U.S. daily intake. *Neurology* 41 (November 1991): 1,726–1,732.

## Rett Syndrome

This is a case report of the successful treatment of a 17-year-old female with Rett syndrome. She was treated with L-carnitine at 50 milligrams per kilogram per day. The authors conclude that L-carnitine appeared to be effective in the treatment for advanced Rett syndrome, a progressive neurological disorder for which there is no effective treatment. *Southern Medical Journal* 86 (December 1993): 1,411–1,412.

## Antioxidant Powers

This article discusses new information that acetyl-L-carnitine may have direct antioxidant activity, as well as the ability to repair other antioxidants that have already been used to quench free radicals. *American Heart Journal* 123 (June 1992): 1,726–1,727.

## Weight Reduction

This review article on chromium reports the possible synergistic effect of chromium picolinate, L-carnitine, and a high-fiber supplement on weight reduction. *The Nutrition Report* 11 (June 1993): 41, 46.

## HIV Infection and AIDS

Patients with AIDS are at risk for developing carnitine deficiency for many reasons, including decreased appetite, dysphagia, prolonged or recurrent gastrointestinal infections, cancer, and drug use. The authors conclude that carnitine supplementation may be important to help supply fatty acids as energy to the muscle, and to maintain immunocompetence in HIV-infected individuals. *AIDS* 6 (1992): 203–205.

## CHAPTER 39: MELATONIN

### Insomnia

Doses of melatonin (0.1 to 10 milligrams) or a placebo were given to 20 volunteers to assess its effects. All melatonin doses significantly increased sleep duration, as well as self-reported sleepiness and fatigue, relative to the placebo. *Proceedings of the National Academy of Science* 91 (1994): 1,824–1,828.

Volunteers received melatonin (0.3 or 1.0 milligrams) or a placebo at 6, 8, or 9 p.m. Latencies to sleep onset, to stage 2 sleep, and to rapid eye movement (REM) sleep were measured. Either dose given at any of the 3 time points decreased sleep onset latency and latency to stage 2 sleep. Neither melatonin dose induced hangover effects. *Clinical Pharmacologic Therapy* 57 (1995): 552–558.

The combined circadian and hypnotic effects of melatonin suggest a synergistic action in the treatment of sleep disorders related to the inappropriate timing of sleep and wakefulness. Adjuvant melatonin may also improve sleep disruption caused by drugs known to alter normal melatonin production (e.g., beta-blockers and benzodiazepines). *Journal of Pineal Research* 15 (1993): 1–12.

## Jet Lag

In this study, 15 subjects took either 8 milligrams of melatonin or a placebo on the day of a return flight from North America to France, and continued dosage for 3 consecutive days. On day 8, self-rating significantly discriminated between melatonin and a placebo for global treatment efficacy, morning fatigue, and evening sleepiness. *Biology and Psychiatry* 32 (1992): 705–711.

This double-blind placebo-controlled study investigated the efficacy of and optimal time for taking melatonin in 52 international cabin crew members assigned to 3 groups. The early melatonin group used 5 milligrams, starting 3 days prior to arrival and ending 5 days after the return home. The late melatonin group used a placebo for 3 days, and then took 5 milligrams of melatonin for 5 days. The third group used a placebo only. The late melatonin group experienced the best recovery and improvements in mood, jet lag, and sleepiness. The late melatonin group also reported significantly less jet lag and sleep disturbance 6 days after arrival when compared with the placebo group, and had a significantly faster recovery of energy and alertness when compared with the early melatonin group. *Biology and Psychiatry* 33 (1993): 526–530.

## Aging

Transplantation of the pineal glands of younger mice to older mice extended the life span and enlarged the thymus glands of the older mice within 5 months. In a series of experiments, when old mice were given melatonin in their nighttime water, they experienced cataract-free eyes; improved digestion; increased strength, energy, and muscle tone; a thick, shiny coat of fur; and sexual interest and capacity until the end of their lives, as well as behavior of mice half their age. Their life span was increased to the human equivalent of adding 25 extra years. The aged mice not receiving the melatonin developed all the signs and symptoms of old age. Walter Pierpaoli and William Regelson, *Melatonin Miracle* (New York: Simon & Schuster, 1995).

## Antioxidant Powers

Melatonin scavenges and neutralizes the hydroxyl radical 5 times more effectively than does glutathione, and is twice as effective in deactivating the peroxyl radical as vitamin E. It stimulates glutathione peroxidase activity and inhibits nitric oxide synthase, thereby reducing the production of the highly toxic hydroxyl and nitric oxide free radicals. *Journal of Pineal Research* 18 (1995): 1–11.

## Hormone-Related Problems

Follicular fluid samples were obtained from the largest pre-ovulatory follicle of 120 women undergoing *in vitro* fertilization, and were examined for melatonin levels. The concentrations of melatonin and progesterone during the autumn and winter (dark) months were significantly higher than those of the spring and summer (light) months. By contrast, estradiol concentration were significantly lower during the dark months than during the light months. There was a positive correlation between follicular fluid melatonin and progesterone concentration, and a negative relationship between melatonin and estradiol. The results of this study suggest that melatonin may be involved in the regulation of steroidogenesis by the human ovaries. *Human Reproduction* 10 (1995): 50–55.

There is evidence that pineal melatonin is an anti-aging hormone, and that menopause is associated with a substantial decline in melatonin secretion and an increased rate of pineal calcification. Animal data indicates that pineal melatonin is involved in the regulation of calcium and phosphorus metabolism by stimulating the activity of the parathyroid glands, by inhibiting calcitonin release, and by inhibiting prostaglandin synthesis. The researchers propose that the fall of melatonin during the early stage of menopause may be an important contributory factor in the development of post-menopausal osteoporosis. Plasma melatonin levels measured in early menopause could be used as an indicator or marker for osteoporosis. Light therapy or administration of melatonin (2.5 milligrams), or of other agents that induce a sustained release of mela-tonin, could be useful agents in the prophylaxis and treatment of postmenopausal osteoporosis. *International Journal of Neuroscience* 62 (1992): 215–225.

## Cardiovascular Disease

Patients with coronary heart disease have increased nocturnal noradrenaline. Melatonin suppresses sympathetic activity, and its insufficiency may play a role in these elevated levels. It was determined in this study that patients with coronary heart disease have significantly lower levels of melatonin than healthy controls. Impaired nocturnal secretion of melatonin was shown to be associated with coronary heart disease. *The Lancet* 345 (1995): 1,408.

## Cancer

In this study, 10 milligrams per day of melatonin were given to 63 metastatic lung cancer patients. The survival at one year was significantly higher in patients treated with melatonin than in patients who were treated only with supportive care. *Oncology* 49 (1992): 336–339.

In this phase II study, 14 women with metastatic breast cancer who had disease progression despite tamoxifen therapy were given 20 miligrams per day of melatonin, along with tamoxifen therapy, for approximately 8 months. A partial response was achieved in 4 out of the 14 patients—a 28.5-percent response rate. Patients on melatonin experienced a relief of anxiety and a reduction of insulin-like growth factor (a growth factor for breast cancer). *British Journal of Cancer* 71 (1995): 854–856.

In this study, 14 patients with inoperable hepatocellular carcinoma (HCC) were given 50 milligrams per day of melatonin with interleukin-2 (IL-2). Over a 7-month period, tumor regression occurred in 5 out of the 14 patients (36 percent)—there was 1 complete response, and 4 partial responses. In addition, 6 patients had stable disease and 3 patients progressed. *European Journal of Cancer* 30A (1994): 167–170.

In this study, 22 patients with progressing metastatic renal cell carcinoma entered a phase II trial on the effect of a long-term regimen (12 months) with interferon and melatonin (10 milligrams per day). There were 7 remissions (33 percent): 3 complete, involving lung and soft tissue, and 4 partial, with a median duration at the time of 16 months. In addition, 9 patients achieved stable disease, and 5 progressed. Toxicity was mild, and side effects (fever, chills, arthralgias, myalgias) occurred rarely. *Cancer* 73 (1994): 3,015–3,019.

In this study, 14 patients with metastatic gastric cancer received IL-2 with 50 milligrams per day of melatonin. Tumor regression was obtained in 3 out of 14 patients (21 percent). There was 1 complete response and 2 partial responses, with a median duration of over 13 months. The disease stabilized in 6 out of 14 patients (43 percent), and progressed in the remaining 5 (36 percent). Survival was significantly longer in patients with response or stable disease than in those with progression disease. Toxicity was low in all cases. *Tumori* 79 (1993): 401–404.

## CHAPTER 40: DHEA

### Overview

This extensive article on DHEA reviews the published studies and personal communications of researchers. Topics covered include: studies on DHEA relieving gout, psoriasis, and congestive heart failure; animal studies demonstrating anticancer effects; protection against heart disease in men with higher DHEA levels; animal studies demonstrating reversal of diabetes, weight loss, alleviation of stress, and restoration of memory by encouragement of neurite growth; beneficial effects on elderly subjects receiving flu vaccines; and beneficial effects on sleep and joint soreness in humans. There is one report of liver damage in rats given very high doses of DHEA that far exceed the normal levels occurring in the animal even at a young age. *The Sciences* (September-October 1995): 26–31.

### Aging

In this study, 13 men and 17 women of ages 40 to 70 were given 50 milligrams per day of DHEA in a randomized placebo-controlled crossover trial. DHEA and DS serum levels were restored to those found in young adults within 2 weeks of DHEA replacement, and were sustained throughout the 3 months of the study. A 2-fold increase in serum levels of androgens was observed in women, with only a small rise in androstenedione in men. Levels of sex hormone-binding, globulin, estrone, or estradiol in either gender were unchanged. IGF-1 levels increased significantly in both groups, and were associated with a remarkable increase in perceived physical and psychological well-being for men (67%) and women (84%). These observations, together with the absence of side effects, constitute the first demonstration of novel effects of DHEA replacement in age-advanced men and women. *Journal of Clinical Endocrinology and Metabolism* 78 (June 1994): 1,360–1,367.

DHEA in appropriate replacement doses appears to have remedial effects with respect to its ability to induce anabolic growth factor, increase muscle strength and lean body mass, activate immune function, and enhance quality of life in aging men and women, with no significant adverse effects. Further studies are needed to confirm and extend our current results, particularly the gender differences. *Annals of the New York Academy of Sciences* 774 (1995): 128–142.

### Immune Function

Human volunteers above age 65 were given DHEAS and the influenza vaccine, resulting in a 4-fold increase in response to the vaccine, compared with the response of the group that did not receive DHEAS. However, when DHEAS was administered along with the tetanus vaccine, it did not improve immune response. *Annals of the New York Academy of Sciences* 774 (1995): 232–248.

In this study, 8 patients with hereditary angioneurotic edema (HAE), a clinical disorder with a deficiency of the C1 esterase inhibitor protein, were treated with DHEAS for 3 to 28 months. DHEAS treatment resulted in dramatic improvement of the subjects' clinical state and a moderate increase in the serum concentration of the C1 inhibitor. *Klinische Wochenschrift* 61 (1983): 715–717.

### Cardiovascular Disease

Studies on humans and animals have suggested that DHEAS has an antiatherogenic effect. DHEAS levels are significantly decreased in insulin-dependent diabetes mellitus patients, who are at high risk for atherosclerosis. It appears that these depressed DHEAS levels are a result of chronic insulin administration therapy. DHEAS, then, may provide a novel way to follow up and improve the outcome of patients with this form of diabetes. *Minerva Endocrinologia* 19 (1994): 113–119.

A double-blind placebo-controlled study was conducted that assessed the effects of DHEA administration on plasma plasminogen activator inhibitor type 1 (PAI-1) and tissue plasminogen activator antigen (tPA). In this study, 18 men received 50 milligrams of DHEA and 16 men received a placebo daily for 12 days. Androstenedione and estrone levels significantly increased, while PAI-1 and tPA levels significantly decreased. Reductions of PAI-1 and tPA are associated with a blood thinning effect by enhancing fibrinolytic (the breakdown of fibrinogen) potential. *American Journal of Medical Science* 311 (May 1996): 205–210.

## Diabetes

In this study, 50 milligrams per day of DHEA were given to 11 postmenopausal women in a placebo-controlled, randomized, blinded, crossover trial. DHEAS, DHEA, testosterone, and free testosterone increased up to twice the premenopausal levels in the group receiving the DHEA. Fasting triglycerides declined, and T-lymphocytes insulin binding and degradation increased. Since 50 milligrams per day give supraphysiologic androgen levels, 25 milligrams per day may be more appropriate. *Fertility and Sterility* 63 (1995): 1,027–1,031.

## Lupus

In this study, 10 female patients with systemic lupus erythematosus (SLE) were given 200 milligrams per day of DHEA for 3 to 6 months. Indices for overall SLE activity, including the SLE Disease Activity Index score and physician's overall assessment, were improved. DHEA was well tolerated. The only frequently noted side effect was mild dermatitis. *Arthritis and Rheumatism* 37 (1994): 1,305–1,310.

## GENERAL REFERENCES

I have drawn on several reference works for much of the background information presented in this book. Although they are geared primarily toward the professional, the average reader may also find them of interest.

Bland, Jeffrey. *The Justification for Vitamin Supplementation.* Bellevue, WA: Northwest Diagnostic Services, 1981.

Goodhart, Robert S., and Maurice E. Shils. *Modern Nutrition in Health and Disease,* 6th ed. Philadelphia: Lea and Febiger, 1980.

Marks, John. *A Guide to the Vitamins: Their Role in Health and Disease.* Lancaster, England: Medical and Technical Publishing Co., n.d.

The National Research Council. *Recommended Dietary Allowances,* 10th ed. Washington, D.C.: National Academy of Sciences, 1989.

Robinson, Corinne H. *Normal and Therapeutic Nutrition,* 15th ed. New York: Macmillan, 1977.

# INDEX